CONDUCTING SCHOOL-BASED ASSESSMENTS OF CHILD AND ADOLESCENT BEHAVIOR

The Guilford School Practitioner Series

EDITORS

STEPHEN N. ELLIOTT, PhD
University of Wisconsin–Madison

JOSEPH C. WITT, PhD
Louisiana State University, Baton Rouge

Recent Volumes

ADHD in the Schools: Assessment and Intervention Strategies
GEORGE J. DuPAUL and GARY STONER

School Interventions for Children of Alcoholics
BONNIE K. NASTASI and DENISE M. DeZOLT

Entry Strategies for School Consultation
EDWARD S. MARKS

Instructional Consultation Teams: Collaborating for Change
SYLVIA A. ROSENFIELD and TODD A. GRAVOIS

Social Problem Solving: Interventions in the Schools
MAURICE J. ELIAS and STEVEN E. TOBIAS

Academic Skills Problems: Direct Assessment
and Intervention, Second Edition
EDWARD S. SHAPIRO

Brief Intervention for School Problems:
Collaborating for Practical Solutions
JOHN J. MURPHY and BARRY L. DUNCAN

Advanced Applications of Curriculum-Based Measurement
MARK R. SHINN, *Editor*

Medications for School-Age Children: Effects on Learning and Behavior
RONALD T. BROWN and MICHAEL G. SAWYER

DSM-IV Diagnosis in the Schools
ALVIN E. HOUSE

Effective School Interventions
NATALIE RATHVON

Designing Preschool Interventions: A Practitioner's Guide
DAVID W. BARNETT, SUSAN H. BELL, and KAREN T. CAREY

Conducting School-Based Assessments of Child and Adolescent Behavior
EDWARD S. SHAPIRO and THOMAS R. KRATOCHWILL, *Editors*

Conducting School-Based Assessments of Child and Adolescent Behavior

♦♦♦

Edited by

Edward S. Shapiro
Thomas R. Kratochwill

♦

THE GUILFORD PRESS
New York   London

© 2000 The Guilford Press
A Division of Guilford Publications, Inc.
72 Spring Street, New York, NY 10012
www.guilford.com

Printed in the United States of America

This book is printed on acid-free paper.

Last digit is print number: 9   8   7   6   5   4

Library of Congress Cataloging-in-Publication Data

Conducting school-based assessments of child and adolescent behavior / Edward S.
   Shapiro, Thomas R. Kratochwill, editors.
       p.   cm.—(The Guilford school practitioner series)
   Includes bibliographical references and index.
   ISBN 1-57230-567-3 (hardcover: alk. paper)   ISBN 1-57230-822-2 (pbk.)
       1. Behavioral assessment of children—Handbooks, manuals, etc.   2. School
psychology—Handbooks, manuals, etc.   I. Shapiro, Edward S. (Edward Steven), 1951
II. Kratochwill, Thomas R.   III. Series.

LB1124   C66 2000
370.15′3—dc21   00-035421

*To Dan and Jay, who keep baseball in their hearts
and keep me young*

—E. S. S.

*To Tyler Thomas Kratochwill, a boater at heart and
my best buddy*

—T. R. K.

About the Editors

♦

Edward S. Shapiro received his doctorate in school psychology from the University of Pittsburgh in 1978. He currently is Professor of School Psychology and Chairperson of the Department of Education and Human Services at Lehigh University, Bethlehem, Pennsylvania. In 1987, Dr. Shapiro received the Lightner Witmer Award from the Division of School Psychology of the American Psychological Association, in recognition for early career contributions to school psychology. From 1990 to 1995, he was editor of *School Psychology Review,* official journal of the National Association of School Psychologists. The author or coauthor of several books, including *Academic Skills Problems: Direct Assessment and Intervention, Academic Skills Problems Workbook,* and *Behavior Change in the Classroom: Self-Management Interventions,* all published by The Guilford Press, Dr. Shapiro has numerous publications in the areas of curriculum-based assessment, behavioral assessment, behavioral interventions, and self-management strategies for classroom behavior change. Currently, he is codirecting a project focused on training doctoral school psychologists as pediatric school psychologists. This model attempts to train students to integrate children's health care, psychological, and educational needs within in school settings.

Thomas R. Kratochwill received his PhD in educational psychology from the University of Wisconsin–Madison in 1973 with a specialization in school psychology. He joined the faculty at the University of Arizona in 1973 in the Department of Educational Psychology, School Psychology Program, serving as coordinator of the Office of Child Research. In 1983 he returned to the University of Wisconsin–Madison to direct the School Psychology Program and Psychoeducational Clinic.

Dr. Kratochwill has been associate editor of *Behavior Therapy, Journal of Applied Behavior Analysis,* and *School Psychology Review.* He was selected as the founding editor of the APA Division 16 journal *Professional School Psychology*

(now *School Psychology Quarterly*) from 1984 to 1992. He is president of the Society for the Study of School Psychology and cochair of the Task Force on Empirically Supported Interventions in School Psychology.

An active researcher and contributor to the scientific psychological literature, Dr. Kratochwill has written or edited 23 books and made more than 100 presentations at professional meetings. Among his books, several are classic contributions, including *Single Subject Research: Strategies for Evaluating Change* (1978); *Selective Mutism: Implications for Research and Treatment* (1981); a series devoted to advances in research, theory, and practice in school psychology *(Advances in School Psychology*, Volumes I through VIII, 1981–present); a book (with Richard J. Morris) on treatment of children's fears and phobias (*Treating Children's Fears and Phobias: A Behavioral Approach*, 1983); and (also with Richard J. Morris) a book on child therapy (*The Practice of Child Therapy*, 1983, and now in a third edition). He has also written (with John R. Bergan) a text on mental health consultation (*Behavioral Consultation and Therapy*, 1990) and is coeditor (with Karen Callan Stoiber) of the *Handbook of Group Interventions for Children and Families* (1998).

Contributors

♦

Barbara Rybski Beaver, PhD, Department of Psychology, University of Wisconsin–Whitewater, Whitewater, Wisconsin

Mary H. Bull, MA, School Psychology Program, University of Massachusetts at Amherst, Amherst, Massachusetts

R. T. Busse, PhD, Department of Psychology, School Psychology Program, University of Wisconsin–Whitewater, Whitewater, Wisconsin

Elisa M. Castillo, MS, Department of Counseling Psychology, University of Wisconsin–Madison, Madison, Wisconsin

Robin S. Codding, BA, Department of Psychology, Syracuse University, Syracuse, New York

Christine L. Cole, PhD, Department of Education and Human Services, Lehigh University, Bethlehem, Pennsylvania

Erin K. Dunn, MS, Department of Psychology, Syracuse University, Syracuse, New York

Tanya L. Eckert, PhD, Department of Psychology, Syracuse University, Syracuse, New York

Katie M. Guiney, BA, Department of Psychology, Syracuse University, Syracuse, New York

John M. Hintze, PhD, School Psychology Program, University of Massachusetts at Amherst, Amherst, Massachusetts

Hannah Hoch, BA, Department of Psychology, The Graduate School and University Center of the City University of New York, New York, New York

Thomas R. Kratochwill, PhD, Department of Educational Psychology, University of Wisconsin–Madison, Madison, Wisconsin

F. Charles Mace, PhD, School of Psychology, University of Wales, Bangor, Gwynedd, United Kingdom

Tamara Marder, MS, Department of Education and Human Services, Lehigh University, Bethlehem, Pennsylvania

Lori McCann, MA, Department of Education and Human Services, Lehigh University, Bethlehem, Pennsylvania

Jennifer J. McComas, PhD, College of Education and Human Development, The University of Minnesota, Minneapolis, Minnesota

Stephanie H. McConaughy, PhD, Department of Psychiatry, University of Vermont, Burlington, Vermont

E. Constance McDaniel, MS, Department of Counselor Education and Educational Psychology, Mississippi State University, Mississippi State, Mississippi

Kenneth W. Merrell, PhD, Division of Psychological and Quantitative Foundations, The University of Iowa, Iowa City, Iowa

Stephen M. Quintana, PhD, Department of Counseling Psychology, University of Wisconsin–Madison, Madison, Wisconsin

Katrina N. Rhymer, MS, Department of Counselor Education and Educational Psychology, Mississippi State University, Mississippi State, Mississippi

Edward S. Shapiro, PhD, Department of Education and Human Services, College of Education, Lehigh University, Bethlehem, Pennsylvania

Christopher H. Skinner, PhD, School Psychology Programs, Department of Educational Psychology, The University of Tennessee, Knoxville, Tennessee

Gary Stoner, PhD, School Psychology Program, University of Massachusetts at Amherst, Amherst, Massachusetts

Manuel X. Zamarripa, MS, Department of Counseling Psychology, University of Wisconsin–Madison, Madison, Wisconsin

Preface

♦

The assessment of children and adolescents from a behavioral perspective has evolved into an accepted, state-of-the-art practice among school professionals. Although several volumes currently exist to assist practitioners and students in training in conducting this process, few texts synthesize the practice of conducting this assessment from a school perspective. New instruments, refinement of observational strategies, the use of computer technology, and newly developed concepts in assessments in schools have all emerged in the last several years. Additionally, care and concern to make assessments culturally sensitive have become critical in the practice of psychology in schools.

This text was developed with the school practitioner in mind. Using the conceptual framework described in our initial chapter, the reader is moved through the multiple methodologies that are used in conducting assessments of child and adolescent behavior. Although the emphasis throughout the book is on assessing school-based problems, the methods described easily translate across nonschool settings. Of particular importance in this text is the focus on the implementation of each method with many case studies, illustrations, and learning aids to better assist practitioners in conducting their evaluations.

A unique feature of this text is its link to a companion text, *Behavioral Assessment in Schools* (2nd ed.): *Research, Theory, and Clinical Foundations,* also edited by us. Each of the senior authors of this text have also written a related chapter in the companion text, describing more of the research and conceptual foundations that underlie the particular method that they are discussing. The idea behind these two companion texts is the recognition that covering research, theory, and practice in a single volume can be overwhelming. The current text offers the reader enough background to place the assessment process in context, but a reader seeking more background and conceptual

foundations for the method should examine the corresponding chapters in our companion text.

We would like to offer sincere appreciation to our colleagues who have contributed to this volume. Their responsiveness to our requested revisions was much appreciated and allowed us to bring this text to life. In addition, we give special thanks to Stephen N. Elliott, Series Editor, who first suggested that we consider editing a practitioner-oriented text such as this one. He has remained a consistent driving force behind our efforts. Finally, special thanks as always to our families, who have continued to support us in our efforts to contribute to our much loved profession.

EDWARD S. SHAPIRO, PhD
THOMAS R. KRATOCHWILL, PhD

Contents

♦

CONDUCTING SCHOOL-BASED ASSESSMENTS OF CHILD AND ADOLESCENT BEHAVIOR

CHAPTER 1

♦♦♦

Introduction:
Conducting a Multidimensional
Behavioral Assessment

♦

EDWARD S. SHAPIRO
THOMAS R. KRATOCHWILL

Behavioral assessment of children and youth has gone through a substantial amount of growth and change over the past three decades. Beginning with the emerging interest in and impact of interventions often called "behavior modification" in the late 1960s and early 1970s, psychologists began to recognize the growing gap between the technology of behavioral intervention and the technology of behavioral assessment. Indeed, as the success of behavioral interventions was demonstrated and the methodologies refined, practitioners and researchers began looking for and demanding a similar development in the processes used to conduct assessments of the individuals for whom intervention was implemented. Journals such as the *Journal of Applied Behavior Analysis* and *Behavior Modification,* born in the late 1960s and early 1970s, published volumes that described effective ways to improve student academic performance (e.g., Hewett, 1967; McKenzie, Clark, Wolf, Kothera, & Benson, 1968), reduce disruptive behavior (e.g., Barrish, Saunders, & Wolf, 1969; Thomas, Becker, & Armstrong, 1968), or improve attending behavior (Craig & Holland, 1970; Schutte & Hopkins, 1970). Many early books on the use of behavioral principles for the behavior change process emphasized the effectiveness of these techniques (e.g., Brown & Stover, 1971; O'Leary & O'Leary, 1972).

In the late 1970s, behaviorally oriented researchers noted that the conceptual foundations of the assessment process had never been clearly articu-

lated. Although the underlying conceptual frameworks of behavioral and psychodynamic intervention methods had been frequently discussed (Bond, 1974; Kanfer & Phillips, 1970; Lazarus, 1971), the translation of behavioral perspectives to the assessment process was just beginning.

Early attempts to draw distinctions between the existing assessment techniques and behavioral assessment methods were often targeted on the assessment of observable responses alone. Researchers attempted to establish direct, systematic observation as the sine qua non of behavioral assessment. In what was often cited as a reaction to the high-inference, very indirect methods of assessment commonly used (such as projective measures), behavioral assessors stressed the importance of direct and systematic observation of behavior as the criterion against which other methods of assessment should be compared. Individuals such as Bijou (Bijou, Peterson, & Ault, 1968; Bijou, Peterson, Harris, Allen, & Johnson, 1969), Werry and Quay (1969), and Ullman (1968) highlighted the importance of observational methodology alone as the defining method of behavioral assessment.

Behavioral assessment was closely linked to the theoretical developments within the broader field of behavior modification or behavior therapy. The term "behavior modification," popular in the 1970s and 1980s, was often used interchangeably with "behavior therapy," but in early work in the field, typically reflected a heavy operant influence. As the field of behavior therapy grew, broader theoretical models were included within the field and integrated into what we would characterize as a behavior assessment eclecticism. The models of behavior therapy included applied behavior analysis, neobehavioristic mediational stimulus–response (S-R) models, cognitive-behavior modification, and social learning theory. Each model differed in terms of what was defined as behavior (Kazdin, 1998), and assessment of these different variables varied in emphasis according to the theoretical model embraced. For example, individuals in the field of applied behavior analysis placed a premium on direct observation and relied on direct samples of behavior within the Cone (1978) formulation, described later in this chapter. In contrast, individuals in the field of cognitive-behavior therapy placed strong emphasis on self-report and methods designed to tap cognitions as part of the diagnostic, assessment, and treatment process. Thus, considerable variation in methods of assessment was associated with variations in theoretical focus. More detailed information on theoretical issues in the field of behavior therapy are presented in O'Donohue and Krasner (1995) and Wilson and Franks (1982). The point we wish to emphasize is that as the field developed, the eclectic characteristics of assessment began to be featured in diverse areas of practice.

In the late 1970s, Hartmann, Roper, and Bradford (1979), Cone (1978), and Nelson and Hayes (1979) were key figures among those offering conceptual frameworks for understanding the assessment process from a behavioral

perspective. Although they did not completely agree with each other on all points, their early writing noted the main assumptions underlying the behavioral assessment process.

One of the major outcomes of their writings was the broadening of behavioral assessment beyond direct, observable behavior. In particular, Cone (1978) described the behavioral assessment grid (BAG). The BAG consisted of a three-dimensional view of evaluation that incorporated modes, methods, and generalization. Within modes, Cone (1978), along with others (e.g., Ciminero & Drabman, 1977; Nelson & Hayes, 1979), recognized that the complexities of human behavior were too vast to be judged by observable behavior alone. For example, two individuals fearful of heights are observed while crossing a high suspension bridge. Upon their safe arrival on level ground, one individual states, "That wasn't as bad as I thought," while the other says, "Thank God I am back on level ground." Both individuals are observed to exhibit similar behaviors indicative of anxiety (i.e., sweating, clenched teeth, statements of impending doom). Yet if asked to predict which individual is likely to successfully reattempt to walk across the bridge, an assessor most likely would select the individual who had viewed the event as not as dreadful as he had expected. Clearly, the variable that predicts the outcome is less the observable behavior but, rather, the thought process (i.e., cognitions) that had been going on at the time the individual was being observed. In this sense, Cone (1978), among others, recognized the importance of assessing the cognitive modality as well as the observable. Likewise, the physiological modality could also be playing a part in the understanding of behavior. In sum, many investigators began to influence the behavioral assessment process to recognize the complex, interrelated, and multidimensional nature of behavior.

During the early and mid-1980s, there was a proliferation of writing on the methodology and concepts of behavioral assessment. No less than 9 such books were published during this time (Ciminero, Calhoun, & Adams, 1986; Cone & Hawkins, 1977; Haynes, 1978; Hersen & Bellack, 1981; Mash & Terdal, 1981, 1988; Nelson & Hayes, 1986; Shapiro, 1987; Shapiro & Kratochwill, 1988). Two professional journals (*Behavioral Assessment* and the *Journal of Behavioral Assessment*) also emerged. Clearly, the area of behavioral assessment was defining itself.

In schools the movement to adopt a behavioral assessment framework was also emerging, although it was somewhat more slowly than in clinical fields. This trend was evidenced by surveys published initially in 1983 by Goh and Fuller (1983), replicated in 1992 by Hutton, Dubes, and Muir (1992), and again in 1996 by Wilson and Reschley (1996). Results of these studies demonstrated that although school psychologists still clung tightly to their use of published norm-referenced, standardized tests and projective measures, an increasing acceptance and use of behavior rating scales and direct system-

atic observation, hallmarks of behavioral assessment, was evident (Anderson, Cancelli, & Kratochwill, 1984).

Over the past decade, the publication of efforts in behavioral assessment has diminished, reflecting a decreasing interest. For example, both behavioral assessment journals were subsumed within larger journals dedicated to both behavioral interventions and assessment. The number of books published on behavioral assessment was reduced to a small trickle (Bellack & Hersen, 1998; Breen & Fiedler, 1996; Mash & Terdal, 1997; Merrell, 1999; Prinz, 1991). Most noteably, the text by Mash and Terdal (1997), one of the defining and lasting texts in the field, changed its title by dropping the word "behavioral." The authors stated that they believed that the concepts of behavioral assessment that had been developed and had emerged in the 1970s and 1980s had become commonplace and accepted practices in the assessment of children and youth. The distinctions between behavioral and nonbehavioral assessment had thus blurred to such an extent as to be meaningless.

The historical development of behavioral assessment can be likened to the developmental phases in the process of growing up. Its infancy and early childhood were characterized by strong rejection of methods that incorporated nonobserved events. Although the presence of such private events were never doubted, their importance and relevance in the process of assessment were questioned. As might be insisted by a child in a preoperational stage of development, only one strategy was viewed as "correct," and evidence to the contrary was ignored.

During the childhood years, behavioral assessment began to mature and recognize that simple explanations of behavior based on observable events alone were not sufficient to understand and predict future behavior. During this period of formal operations, behavioral assessment attempted to define its identity by a method consistent with its philosophical roots in behaviorism, but at the same time incorporated other nonobservable events into the assessment paradigm. In particular, the developments in behavior therapy and child clinical psychology had to be integrated within a behavioral assessment context.

As behavioral assessment entered its adolescence, substantial questions about its identity were being raised. Clinicians began to recognize the importance of cognitive and emotional events to behavioral outcome, as well as the importance of environmental context in understanding behavior. Practitioners began again to define the identity of behavioral assessment as a blur between what had typically been viewed as traditional methods and interpretations of behavior (such as intrapsychic and family systems perspectives) and those more consistent with perspectives derived from behaviorism (such as functional relationships between antecedents, behavior, and consequences). In addition, research advances in developmental psychopathology, an increased emphasis on the interrelated influence of child and family cogni-

tions, and a conceptual and methodological convergence of ecosystems as explanatory models to understand behavioral pathology, have led to a recognition that behavioral assessment methods have to be multidimensional (Mash & Terdal, 1997).

Behavioral assessment has entered its young adulthood as a much more mature discipline. A concomitant link has been recognized between various subareas of behavioral psychology such as child and family behavior therapy, applied behavior analysis, behavioral pediatrics, and cognitive-behavioral therapy. The process of assessment is viewed as needing to accomplish a successful examination across these disciplines and their potential influences on behavioral outcomes. Mash and Terdal (1997) labeled this a behavioral–systems assessment (BSA), which effectively defines a "best practice" methodology for conducting assessments of children and youth. Contrasting traditional and behavioral assessment methods is no longer considered a meaningful comparison. At the same time, functional assessment and functional analysis, a methodology of behavioral assessment reliant primarily on direct observation and determining antecedent–behavior–consequence relationships, has reemerged as a very powerful and crucial part of the evaluation process for specific purposes and situations.

In this chapter, we begin by reviewing briefly the basic assumptions and methods that underlie behavioral assessment. This discussion is followed by a conceptualization of multidimensional behavioral assessment (MDBA), which we believe defines where the practice of child-based assessment is today, in both clinical and school settings, and where assessment is likely to head at the start of the 21st century. A review of the contents of this text and its organization are also provided.

ASSUMPTIONS UNDERLYING BEHAVIORAL ASSESSMENT

Early researchers defined behavioral assessment by contrasting the approach to that often called "traditional assessment." Basic assumptions of how personality was conceptualized, the causes of behavior, the role of behavior and history, and the consistency of behavior were considered (see Table 1.1; Hartmann, Roper, & Bradford, 1979). In these contrasts, behavioral assessment was viewed as a perspective that included the impact of environmental conditions, and the idiographic nature of comparisons rather than intrapsychic and/or psychodynamic interpretations, and considered history to be of low-level importance. Behavioral assessment viewed observable behavior as samples of a larger repertoire of possible behaviors rather than as signs of an underlying pathology that was manifesting itself through observable actions. Data in behavioral assessment was specifically aimed at target selection,

TABLE 1.1. Differences between Behavioral and Traditional Approaches to Assessment

	Behavioral	Traditional
I. Assumptions		
1. Conception of personality	Personality constructs mainly employed to summarize specific behavior patterns, if at all	Personality as a reflection of enduring underlying states or traits
2. Causes of behavior	Maintaining conditions sought in current environment	Intrapsychic or within the individual
II. Implications		
1. Role of behavior	Important as a sample of person's repertoire in specific situation	Behavior assumes importance only insofar as it indexes underlying causes
2. Role of history	Relatively important, except, for example, to provide a retrospective baseline	Crucial in that present conditions seen as a product of the past
3. Consistency of behavior	Behavior thought to be specific to the situation	Behavior expected to be consistent across time and settings
III. Uses of data	To describe target behaviors and maintaining conditions	To describe personality functioning and etiology
	To select the appropriate treatment	To diagnose and classify
	To evaluate and revise treatment	To make prognosis; to predict
IV. Other characteristics		
1. Level of inferences	Low	Medium to high
2. Comparisons	More emphasis on intra-individual or ideographic	More emphasis on inter-individual or nomothetic
3. Methods of assessment	More emphasis on direct methods (e.g., observations of behavior in natural environment)	More emphasis on indirect methods (e.g., interviews and self-report)
4. Timing of assessment	More ongoing; prior, during, and after treatment	Pre- and perhaps post-treatment, or strictly to diagnose
5. Scope of assessment	Specific measures and of more variables (e.g., of target behaviors in various situations, of side effects, context, strengths as well as deficiencies)	More global measures (e.g., of cure, or impowerment) but only of the individual

Note. From Hartmann, Roper, and Bradford (1979). Copyright 1979 by Plenum Press. Reprinted by permission.

treatment selection, and evaluation of interventions rather than being used for purposes of diagnosis or describing personality functioning.

Perhaps most notable among all the assumptions that distinguished behavioral from nonbehavioral assessment was the assumption of situational specificity. Within a behavioral assessment framework, all behavior was assumed to be situationally specific and only after empirical validation would one determine that a behavior was cross-situational. In contrast, nonbehavioral assessment assumes behavior to be cross-situational. In this case, one makes generalizations from observable behaviors that represent personality or trait characteristics likely to be evident across time and place.

The implications of this assumption and empirical findings for the interpretation of assessment results cannot be underestimated. For example, when a student referred for disruptive classroom behavior is removed to a small room for evaluation and his or her behavior is compliant, pleasant, and respectful, from a cross-situational perspective the evaluator may draw the conclusion that the student's behavior in that setting is indicative of general personality characteristics and traits. The evaluator may assume that the student's actions under the conditions of assessment are likely to occur in other settings. Such an assumption may be evaluated by observations of the student in differing settings, but such observations may not be performed. In contrast, from a situationally specific perspective an evaluator may assume that the student's behavior in the small room is indicative of events that surround the behavior, such as having been removed from the classroom (and thereby avoiding aversive events like work), working one-to-one with an adult, working in a restricted environment, and a host of other confounding variables. Only after the student is assessed across multiple settings and found to have similar behavior will the evaluator make a personality- or trait-based characterization of the student.

Behavioral assessment was also influenced by the empirical literature on what has been called "empirically based assessment" (Achenbach, 1998). Behavioral assessors noted that behavior is not consistent across situations, but some of the early formulations in the field of behavioral assessment were conceptual rather than empirical. As research using broad-band checklists and rating scales was conducted, researchers found that behavior varies across situations and by various informants (i.e., parent–teacher–child) (Achenbach, McConaughy, & Howell, 1987). Empirically based assessment, therefore, created an important knowledge base that behavioral assessors could point to as supporting the basic tenets that at one time operated only within the conceptual realm.

Although these comparisons served to offer distinctions that characterized and separated behavioral from nonbehavioral assessment approaches to evaluation, such distinctions have blurred over the last decade to the extent that what may have been viewed at one time as behavioral conceptualiza-

tions of assessment have now become accepted best practice in the evaluation of children and youth. It would be unusual for evaluators, regardless of their theoretical perspective, not to consider the influence of environment and setting in the development of behavior. It would be unusual to assume that observed behavior is not situationally specific. It would be unusual to assume that assessment is being used for diagnostic purposes only.

At the same time as the distinctions have blurred, there has also been a resurgence of the efforts of early behavioral assessors to recapture the importance of observable behavior and its relationship to surrounding stimuli. In particular, the strong interest in functional assessment (e.g., Schill, Kratochwill, & Gardner, 1996) and functional analysis (e.g., DuPaul & Ervin, 1996; Ervin, DuPaul, Kern, & Friman, 1998; Gresham, & Lambros, 1998; Volmer & Northrup, 1996) that has emerged, especially in school settings, has offered a clear place in the assessment process for the types of methods that were common in the earliest days of the development of behavioral assessment. Perhaps one of the best examples of the acceptance of this method and its importance in the evaluation of children is its explicit inclusion within the newly enacted law, the Individuals with Disabilities Education Act (IDEA) of 1997.

Although the assumptions underlying behavioral assessment appear to have been included in accepted practices for conducting child and youth assessments, distinctions are still quite evident in the overall methods that are linked to the assumptions. In particular, although methods such as interviews, self-report, informant report, and direct observation are the defining strategies of all psychological assessment, it is the interpretation of the outcomes of these methods that truly distinguish behavioral from nonbehavioral assessment (Kratochwill, Sheridan, Carlson, & Lasecki, 1999).

BEHAVIORAL ASSESSMENT: MODES, METHODS, AND GENERALIZATION DIMENSIONS

Cone's (1978) BAG (see Figure 1.1) offered a conceptual framework for behavioral assessment by considering the modalities targeted for assessment, the methods used to conduct the evaluation, and the dimensions across which generalization of behavior would be examined. This investigator identified three modalities of assessment that define the potential range of targets—motoric, cognitive, and physiological.

Modalities of Assessment

The motoric modality consists of the overt, observable responses that are the basis of behavioral assessment. These behaviors are those that can be direct-

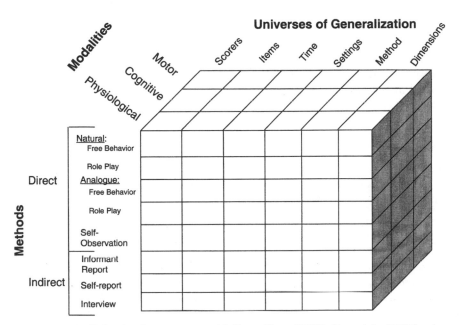

FIGURE 1.1. Behavioral assessment grid. From Cone (1978). Copyright 1978 by the Association for Advancement of Behavior Therapy. Reprinted by permission.

ly observed and are evident across raters. In schools, these are behaviors such as calling out, being out-of-seat, being on-task, engaging in social interaction, and similar responses.

A second modality of assessment considers those responses known as "private events." These responses are the thoughts, emotions, and other covert behaviors that cannot be observed directly. As noted previously, Cone (1978), Nelson (1983), and others recognized that the motoric modality alone was insufficient to adequately capture the complexity of behavior. Indeed, it became important to incorporate within the behavioral assessment framework those internal responses such as thoughts, perceptions, and feelings to complete the entire assessment picture. Access to this modality, however, is only indirect—through the verbal or written output of the individual being assessed. Clearly, because we cannot access and verify what a person tells us she was thinking or feeling, relying on this modality of assessment alone is insufficient to complete the picture of behavioral problems.

The third modality of assessment is the physiological. This mode of evaluation requires obtaining physiological measurement of internal events that may be related to behavior evident via other modalities. For instance, a youth who is asked to present a speech in front of his peers may report that he was relaxed and not very nervous, yet physiological indicators taken dur-

ing the speech (i.e., heart rate, blood pressure, respiration) may reveal an elevated set of indices consistent with a high level of anxiety. Likewise, another individual may report a high level of "nervousness" in a social situation, but physiological measurement may reveal no substantial change in anxiety-based indicators. Again, the necessity of assessment that crosses modalities is clear.

Methods of Assessment

The methods of behavioral assessment can be placed on a continuum ranging from direct to indirect, as illustrated in Figure 1.2. The key feature that distinguishes direct from indirect methods of assessment is the degree to which the method measures behavior under its naturally occurring conditions. If one is assessing behavior at the time it is actually occurring, the measure belongs on the direct side of the continuum. When the behavior is assessed at time and or place removed from its actual occurrence, the method becomes indirect.

On the direct side of the continuum, observing behavior in its natural setting as it is naturally occurring is the most direct form of behavioral assessment. For example, collecting data on a student's academic responses during a required math lesson, and observing a group of students interact on the playground (to note prosocial behavior) are forms of direct observation in the

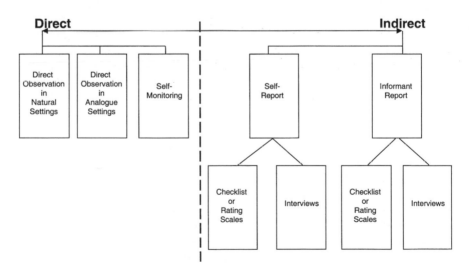

FIGURE 1.2. Continuum of behavioral assessment methods. From Shapiro and Browder (1990). Copyright 1990 by Plenum Press. Reprinted by permission.

natural setting. These methods usually require minimal inferences to interpret what is observed. Such a direct form of behavioral assessment offers opportunities to confirm or disconfirm the results of other forms of assessment.

Certain categories of behavior present problems in trying to observe while they are naturally occurring. For example, the opportunities to observe the use of social skills in interactions in a classroom are quite limited. Although one could assess such behavior using direct observation in the natural environment, the cost of placing an observer in that setting to observe the few or rare instances of such behavior would be prohibitive. For behaviors of this type it is possible to simulate the natural environment by creating analogue settings. When such an environment is created and the behavior is directly observed within that setting, one is still conducting direct behavioral assessment (i.e., the assessment occurs when the behavior actually occurs). However, because the setting is no longer natural and represents a situation of real events, one must make many inferences to interpret how the observable behavior reflects what may happen under more naturally occurring conditions.

A third form of direct assessment is self-monitoring. For this form of assessment, individuals collect data on themselves as the behavior occurs. Because the act of data collection and the actual occurrence of behavior are simultaneous, the method is viewed as direct. However, because the process of self-monitoring does not involve the observation of the particular behavior by another, one must make inferences that the reported self-monitored behavior indeed reflects accurately the behavior that occurred. Further, because the act of self-monitoring alone can potentially result in behavior change and its validity is influenced by numerous factors (see Chapter 5), self-monitoring is viewed as a less direct measurement method than others whereby behavior is directly observed by another individual.

Crossing the divide to indirect assessment, two methods are encountered. Self-report is considered indirect because data are gathered about behavior that has occurred at another time. Frequently, this form of data collection involves asking individuals to tell the evaluator about their own behavior (i.e., interviews) or asking students to complete checklists or rating scales that reflect the self-reporting of behavior. The behaviors being discussed have occurred at previous times and in settings other than where the interview or rating scale is completed.

The most indirect form of assessment is the use of informant reports. Under these conditions of assessment the evaluator is asking someone else about an individual's behavior at a time when the behavior is not actually occurring. Again, the disconnect from behavioral occurrence places this method on the indirect side of the equation. As with self-report measures, data are often gathered through interviews and the use of checklists and rating scales.

Dimensions of Generalization

In Cone's original conceptualization of behavioral assessment, the third element of the BAG was what he called the universes of generalization. Cone recognized that the value and validity of behavioral assessment was based on the degree to which measures used reflected outcomes that could be generalized across various aspects of the assessment. One could conceptualize the assessment process as reflecting a degree of consistency across scorers (to what degree do two independent judges report the same events), items (to what degree do different items on a measure reflect similar behaviors), time (to what degree do different measures find similar outcomes across time), setting (to what degree do different measures find similar outcomes across settings), methods (to what degree do different methods designed to measure the same behavior result in similar outcomes), and dimensions (to what degree do classes of behavior co-vary).

Cone (1986) later altered his conceptualization of this aspect of behavioral assessment by replacing the concept of dimensions of generalization with differing forms of accuracy in behavioral assessment. He identified occurrence accuracy as the degree to which measures were sensitive to the occurrences of behavior. For example, if one is using a measure of on- and off-task behavior to observe playground aggression, it is likely that the measure would have poor sensitivity to identifying the target behavior and thus have low levels of occurrence accuracy. Temporal accuracy is the degree to which an instrument is sensitive to the repeated occurrence of a behavior over time within the same setting. If a measure being used in behavioral assessment identifies an early occurrence during independent work in math class but fails to depict similar behavior later during the same independent work period in math, the measure would be viewed as lacking in temporal accuracy. In a similar way, the setting accuracy of a measure is determined by its degree of sensitivity to picking up occurrences of a behavior across different environments in which the behavior is present. Convergent accuracy is a reflection of the degree to which multiple measures, supposedly assessing similar behavior, converge on a similar conclusion. This is a particularly important point to consider inasmuch as changing methods alone may alter outcomes, irrespective of the actual occurrence of the behavior.

MULTIDIMENSIONAL BEHAVIORAL ASSESSMENT

As researchers have more carefully examined the variables and interrelationships among variables, it has become clear that the complex nature of the development of behavioral pathology in children and adolescents required that the assessment methodologies used are equally complex. It is impossible to

determine accurately the nature of a problem, the concomitant environmental events that are related to the maintenance of the problem, the immediate and delayed antecedents and consequences that surround the behavioral occurrences, the nature of reinforcers that affect the behavior, and other such variables, without conducting an assessment that examines the problem from different perspectives and uses different modalities of evaluation. The solutions to better understanding a problem and making effective predictions of intervention outcomes result from looking at the interrelatedness of these variables. Each of these perspectives and methods of assessment represents a particular dimension of behavior.

Conducting a Multidimensional Behavioral Assessment

It is especially important to recognize that data collected from one method are not inherently better than data collected from others. That is, data obtained through an indirect method from a parent (such as a rating scale) are not "less true" than data obtained by directly observing a student within a natural setting. Likewise, data collected through interviews with the student are not inherently more accurate than those collected through direct observation of analogue settings. The key to good assessment is to find conceptual links and relationships between methods and modalities of assessment. Each form of behavioral assessment contributes potentially unique elements to solving the assessment puzzle. Emphasis should be placed on treating the assessment process as problem solving. The perspective of a parent obtained through an interview may not be consistent with what that parent reports on a rating scale. The behavior of a student observed during a work session in reading may not be consistent with that reported by the teacher in a checklist. The self-monitored responses of a student may not match at all with those observed by an independent observer. For each individual, putting together and understanding the aspects of a problem, arriving at logical conclusions about its origins, and making effective recommendations for intervention requires the evaluator to have successfully integrated the various methods of assessment to complete a full picture of the student's functioning. Relying on any single method can result in a biased and potentially erroneous set of conclusions about the referral problem.

The assessment process typically begins with interviewing the referral source. In schools, that source is typically the teacher. From this indirect informant report, the evaluator can define the parameters necessary for direct observation (within the natural or analogue setting) and can begin to obtain the teacher's perspective of the child's difficulties. To supplement the interview, an evaluator generally uses other informant report methods such as checklists and/or rating scales. These measures offer confirmation (or discon-

firmation) of verbally reported items. An evaluator may also want to obtain the perspective of the individual who is the target of the assessment. Thus, interviews and other self-report measures are collected as well. Often this assessment includes the use of checklists and/or rating scales, again to help confirm or disconfirm verbal reports. Finally, a parental perspective is sought to obtain both developmental understanding of the problem and to assess the consistency of parental views against those of the student and/or the teacher.

Together, the data obtained from these perspectives and through the various methods provide a rich store of knowledge that can better define the problem, offer a sense of the environmental context within which the behavior occurs, and identify potential intervention strategies. It is this multidimensional analysis that the evaluator should seek.

ORGANIZATION OF THIS VOLUME

The material in this text is organized along a continuum of the methods of a Multidimensional Behavioral Assessment (MDBA) starting with the most direct methods and ending with the most indirect. Each chapter offers a practitioner-oriented review of the strategies that make up the method under discussion. The final chapter provides a broad discussion of the importance of cultural and linguistic diversity in conducting a thorough and nonbiased behavioral assessment.

In Chapter 2, Skinner, Rhymer, and McDaniel provide a solid grounding in the basic principles and procedures of direct observation. In particular, there is an excellent feel for the issues and concerns facing the psychologist in collecting classroom-based observation data. The chapter reviews the principles, but does assume that readers have a more than simple understanding of the methods, and offers practical advice on the data collection process.

Moving down the method path to analogue assessment, Hintze, Stoner, and Bull (Chapter 3) offer descriptions and examples of the methodology, highlighting especially the use of enactment measures. An excellent conceptual framework for discussing the techniques, which is strongly practitioner-driven, is provided.

In Chapter, 4 McComas, Hoch, and Mace describe functional analysis, a form of analogue assessment involving direct observation. This method has emerged as a critical skill needed within the repertoire of a psychologist conducting school-based assessment. Considered a form of functional assessment, functional analysis is a specific method designed to offer clear and extensive examination of the antecedent–response–consequence relationships that underlie the occurrence of behavior problems. The methodology of functional analysis has become a widely applied strategy, especially for children with severe behavior disorders such as self-injury, self-stimulation, and aggressive forms of attack such as biting, scratching, and hitting peers and

teachers. McComas et al. offer a good description of this methodology as applied to typical cases of severe behavior problems. Case studies are included, with illustrative examples that feature the forms and data collection methods underlying this approach.

In Chapter 5, Cole, Marder, and McCann complete the description of direct methods in their discussion of self-monitoring (SM). This chapter provides an easily followed description of the methods and processes of using self-monitoring. Although the chapter accurately points out the primary use of SM as an intervention rather than an assessment technique, it does offer numerous practitioner-friendly examples of the methodology. These can easily be applied in the school-based processes of assessment.

Eckert, Dunn, Codding, and Guiney (Chapter 6) give a practitioner-friendly description of common paper-and-pencil, self-report rating scale measures. They divide these measures between broad- and narrow-band configurations, a distinction also made by Shapiro and Kratochwill (1988) for informant measures. In addition, a problem-solving heuristic in conducting the assessment is provided, which moves the reader from the broad-band to the specific narrow-band measure linked to different syndromes. The important concept of comorbidity is discussed. This chapter illustrates key components of (MDBAs), that is, recognizing the range across which behavior occurs, how the specific syndromes match with broader conceptualizations of externalizing and internalizing disorders, and how one assesses using a multi-method approach.

The indirect method includes the use of interviews with the individuals who are the targets of the assessments. McConaughy provides a practical chapter (Chapter 7) on the techniques of interviewing children. Specific advice on style, method, and approaches relevant to obtaining excellent clinical information directly from children and adolescents are offered. She also offers a good description of a specific measure, the Semistructured Clinical Interview for Children and Adolescents (SCICA), and how it can be useful in the interviewing process. Finally, two strong case illustrations are provided to demonstrate the impact of interviewing within a multidimensional assessment. It is clear from the cases that interviewing alone cannot bring together the full sense of a child's difficulties, but combined with other strategies as discussed throughout the text, interviewing has a powerful role in the MDBA process.

The last and most indirect methods of behavioral assessment involve the collecting of data from informants. In Chapter 8, Merrell offers a practitioner-oriented overview of the major rating scale instruments used in schools for the assessment of behavior problems. The chapter focuses exclusively on teacher-completed measures and does not cover parent-completed companions to the measures (such as the Child Behavior Checklist or the Behavior Assessment System for Child–Parent). Measures are divided into two categories—general and specific. Within general measures, the major instru-

ments, such as the Teacher Rating Form, the Behavior Assessment System for Children—Teacher Rating Form, and the Revised Behavior Problem Checklist, are covered in enough detail that practitioners should be easily able to use and evaluate their effectiveness. Merrell breaks down the category of specific measures into two subsections—one on measures designed to assess attention-deficit/hyperactivity disorder (ADHD) and the other, more broadly, on social behavior problems. Again, the major instruments in use are covered. The chapter ends with practical recommendations for the effective use of these measures.

Busse and Beaver's chapter (Chapter 9) offers a practical description of the generic and specific skills needed for effective interviewing of informants in conducting behavioral assessments. They note that the skills inherent in any good interviewing process—that is, those derived from active listening and known effective counseling skills—are equally relevant and important in the behavioral assessment process. In addition, the chapter covers in detail the steps in conducting problem-identification interviews, especially those within a conjoint consultation framework. A case study offers an excellent illustration of completing such an interview.

The final chapter discusses the importance and value of culture and language in conducting the behavioral assessment process. Indeed, Chapter 10 provides something rarely seen in any assessment texts, especially those involving schools. Castillo, Quintana, and Zamarripa provide a context for conducting culturally competent assessments. Emphasizing the assessment of students with ethnic and linguistic minority (ELM) backgrounds, they provide a broad discussion of the theoretical and conceptual framework within which behavioral assessment must be placed in working with children and youth from culturally and linguistically diverse backgrounds. The authors further provide a relevant example to illustrate the issues in culturally competent assessment, along with many practical suggestions and methods for approaching this goal.

In total, this book offers a practitioner-oriented approach to the concepts and methods that make up a strong MDBA. Readers interested in delving deeper into the conceptual, theoretical, and research backgrounds of these techniques, as well as other issues related to behavioral assessment, should examine our companion volume (Shapiro & Kratochwill, 2000). Each of the senior authors of this book have companion chapters in the other book that take the reader further into the topic on which they have written.

SUMMARY

As noted at the beginning of this chapter, behavioral assessment of children and youth has evolved considerably over the past three decades. Moving

from infancy to young adulthood, the field has expanded its theoretical and conceptual base, now including diverse theoretical approaches within the broad field of behavior therapy—a field that has itself become remarkably diverse. It seems no longer relevant to contrast behavioral and traditional assessment according to method. Yet the orientation of behavioral assessors remains focused on a variety of characteristics that have maintained consistency throughout the development of behavioral assessment (Cone, 1978, 1986). Thus, although some of the traditional distinctions reviewed earlier can be invoked in describing behavioral assessment, many individuals who adhered to more traditional models have now embraced many of the tenets of behavioral assessment. They have come to accept these features from an empirical rather than a conceptual or theoretical basis. We also note that some of the more traditional aspects of behavioral assessment have become prominent not only in practice, but in the special education arena. Functional assessment, which emphasizes analyzing behavior in terms of antecedents and consequences, has become a prominent feature within education settings.

As behavioral assessment matures into adulthood, we will likely see a continuation of many existing dimensions of behavioral assessment. It is likely that the field will broaden and that others will embrace its basic tenets for empirical reasons. We look forward to its evolution as a methodology to improve the diagnostic, assessment, and treatment services for children and youth in educational settings.

REFERENCES

Achenbach, T. M. (1998). Diagnosis, assessment, taxonomy, and case formulations. In T. H. Ollendick & M. Hersen (Eds.), *Handbook of child psychopathology* (3rd ed., pp. 63–87). New York: Plenum Press.

Achenbach, T. M., McConaughy, S. H., & Howell, C. T. (1987). Child/adolescent behavioral and emotional problems: Implications of cross-informant correlations for situational specificity. *Psychological Bulletin, 101,* 213–232.

Anderson, T., Cancelli, A. A., & Kratochwill, T. R. (1984). Self-reported assessment of school psychologists. *Journal of School Psychology, 22,* 17–29.

Barrish, H. H., Sauders, M., & Wolf, M. M. (1969). Good behavior game: Effects of individual contingencies for group consequences on disruptive behavior in a classroom. *Journal of Applied Behavior Analysis, 2,* 119–124.

Bellack, A. S., & Hersen, M. (Eds.). (1998). *Behavioral assessment: A practical handbook* (4th ed.). Boston: Allyn & Bacon.

Bijou, S., Peterson, R. F., & Ault, M. H. (1968). A method to integrate descriptive and field studies at the level of data and empirical concepts. *Journal of Applied Behavior Analysis, 1,* 175–191.

Bijou, S., Peterson, R. F., Harris, F. R., Allen, K. E., & Johnson, M. S. (1969).

Methodology for experimental studies of young children in natural settings. *Psychological Record, 19,* 177–220.

Bond, J. A. (1974). Behavior therapy, learning theory, and scientific method. *Psychotherapy: Theory, Research, and Practice, 11,* 118–132.

Breen, M. J., & Fiedler, C. R. (Eds.). (1996). *Behavioral approach to assessment of youth with emotional/behavioral disorders: A handbook for school-based practitioners.* Austin, TX: Pro-Ed.

Brown, R. M., & Stover, D. G. (1971). *Behavior modification in child treatment: An experimental and clinical approach.* Chicago: Aldine-Atherton.

Ciminero, A. R., Calhoun, K. S., & Adams, H. (Eds.). (1986). *Handbook of behavioral assessment* (2nd ed.). New York: Wiley.

Ciminero, A. R., & Drabman, R. S. (1977). Current developments in the behavioral assessment of children. In B. Lahey & A. E. Kazdin (Eds.), *Advances in child clinical psychology* (Vol. 1, pp. 47–82). New York: Plenum Press.

Cone, J. D. (1978). The behavioral assessment grid (BAG): A conceptual framework and a taxonomy. *Behavior Therapy, 9,* 882–888.

Cone, J. D. (1986). Psychometric considerations and the multiple models of behavioral assessment. In M. Hersen & A. S. Bellack (Eds.), *Behavioral assessment: A practical handbook* (3rd ed., pp. 42–66). Elmsford, NY: Pergamon Press.

Cone, J. D., & Hawkins, R. P. (Eds.). (1977). *Behavioral assessment: New directions in clinical psychology.* New York: Brunner/Mazel.

Craig, H. B., & Holland, A. L. (1970). Reinforcement of visual attending in classrooms for deaf children. *Journal of Applied Behavior Analysis, 3,* 97–109.

DuPaul, G. J., & Ervin, R. A. (1996). Functional assessment of behaviors related to attention-deficit/hyperactivity disorder: Linking assessment to intervention design. *Behavior Therapy, 27,* 601–622.

Ervin, R. A., DuPaul, G. J., Kern, L., & Friman, P. C. (1998). Classroom-based functional and adjunctive assessments: Proactive approaches to intervention selection for adolescents with attention deficit hyperactivity disorder. *Journal of Applied Behavior Analysis, 31,* 65–78.

Goh, D. S., & Fuller, G. B. (1983). Current practices in the assessment of personality by school psychologists. *School Psychology Review, 12,* 240–243.

Gresham, F. M., & Lambros, K. M. (1998). Behavioral and functional assessment. In T. S. Watson & F. M. Gresham (Eds.), *Handbook of child behavior therapy* (pp. 3–22). New York: Plenum Press.

Hartmann, D. P., Roper, B L., & Bradford, D. C. (1979). Some relationships between behavioral and traditional assessment. *Journal of Behavioral Assessment, 1,* 3–21.

Haynes, S. N. (1978). *Principles of behavioral assessment.* New York: Gardner Press.

Hersen, M., & Bellack, A. S. (1981). *Behavioral assessment: A practical handbook* (2nd ed.). New York: Pergamon Press.

Hewett, F. M. (1967). Educational engineering with emotionally disturbed children. *Exceptional Children, 33,* 459–467.

Hutton, J. B., Dubes, R., & Muir, S. (1992). Assessment practices of school psychologists: Ten years later. *School Psychology Review, 21,* 271–284.

Kanfer, F. H., & Phillips, J. S. (1970). *Learning foundations of behavior therapy.* New York: Wiley.

Kazdin, A. E. (1998). *Research design in clinical psychology* (3rd ed.). Boston: Allyn & Bacon.

Kratochwill, T. R., Sheridan, S. M., Carlson, J., & Lasecki, K. L. (1999). Advances in behavioral assessment. In C. R. Reynolds & T. B. Gutkin (Eds.), *The handbook of school psychology* (3rd ed., pp. 350–382). New York: Wiley.

Lazarus, A. A. (1971). *Behavior therapy and beyond.* New York: McGraw-Hill.

Mash, E. J., & Terdal, L. G. (Eds.) (1981). *Behavioral assessment of childhood disorders.* New York: Guilford Press

Mash, E. J., & Terdal, L. G. (Eds.) (1988). *Behavioral assessment of childhood disorders* (2nd ed). New York: Guilford Press.

Mash, E. J., & Terdal, L. G. (Eds.) (1997). *Assessment of childhood disorders* (3rd ed.). New York: Guilford Press.

McKenzie, H. S., Clark, M., Wolf, M. M., Kothera, R., & Benson, C. (1968). Behavior modification of children with learning disabilities using grades as tokens and allowances as back-up reinforcers. *Exceptional Children, 34,* 745–752.

Merrell, K. W. (1999). *Behavioral, social, and emotional assessment of children and adolescents.* Mahwah, NJ: Erlbaum.

Nelson, R. O. (1983). Behavioral assessment: Past, present, and future. *Behavioral Assessment, 5,* 195–206.

Nelson, R. O., & Hayes, S. C. (1979). Some current dimensions of behavioral assessment. *Behavioral Assessment, 1,* 1–16.

Nelson, R. O., & Hayes, S. C. (Eds.) (1986). *Conceptual foundations of behavioral assessment.* New York: Guilford Press.

O'Donohue, W. T., & Krasner, L. (1995). Theories of behavior therapy and scientific progress. In W. T. O'Donohue & L. Krasner (Eds.), *Theories of behavior therapy: Exploring behavior change* (pp. 695–706). Washington, DC: American Psychological Association.

O'Leary, K., & O'Leary, S. G. (1972). *Classroom management: The successful use of behavior modification.* New York: Pergamon Press.

Prinz, R. J. (Ed.). (1991). *Advances in behavioral assessment of children and families: A research annual* (Vol. 5). London: Jessica Kingsley.

Schill, M. T., Kratochwill, T. R., & Gardner, W. I. (1996). Conducting a functional analysis of behavior. In M. J. Breen & C. R. Fielder (Eds.), *Behavioral approach to assessment of youth with emotional/behavioral disorders: A handbook for school-based practitioners* (pp. 83–179). Austin, TX: Pro-Ed.

Schutte, R. C., & Hopkins, B. L. (1970). The effects of teacher attention on following instructions in a kindergarten class. *Journal of Applied Behavior Analysis, 3,* 117–122.

Shapiro, E. S. (1987). *Behavioral assessment in school psychology.* Hillsdale, NJ: Erlbaum.

Shapiro, E. S., & Browder, J. L. (1990). Behavioral assessment: Applications for persons with mental retardation. In J. L. Matson (Ed.), *Handbook of behavior modification with the mentally retarded* (pp. 93–120). New York: Plenum Press.

Shapiro, E. S. & Kratochwill, T. R. (Eds.). (1988). *Behavioral assessment in schools: Conceptual foundations and practical applications.* New York: Guilford Press.

Shapiro, E. S., & Kratochwill, T. R. (Eds.). (2000). *Behavioral assessment in schools (2nd ed.): Theory, research, and clinical foundations.* New York: Guilford Press.

Thomas, D. R., Becker, W. C., & Armstrong, M. (1968). Production and elimination

of disruptive classroom behavior by systematically varying teacher's behavior. *Journal of Applied Behavior Analysis, 1,* 35–45.

Ullman, L. P. (1968). A sample of operant studies. *Journal of Special Education, 2,* 319–321.

Vollmer, T. R., & Northup, J. (1996). Some implications of functional analysis for school psychology. *School Psychology Quarterly, 11,* 76–92.

Werry, J. S., & Quay, H. C. (1969). Observing the classroom behavior of elementary school children. *Exceptional Children, 35,* 461–467.

Wilson, G. T., & Franks, C. M. (Eds.). (1982). *Contemporary behavior therapy: Conceptual and empirical foundations.* New York: Guilford Press.

Wilson, M. S., & Reschly, D. J. (1996). Assessment in school psychology training and practice. *School Psychology Review, 25,* 9–23.

CHAPTER 2

♦♦♦

Naturalistic Direct Observation in Educational Settings

♦

CHRISTOPHER H. SKINNER
KATRINA N. RHYMER
E. CONSTANCE McDANIEL

School psychologists use assessment data to make a variety of decisions regarding special education eligibility, placement recommendations, screening, referral, and evaluation of students' progress and performance under different conditions (Salvia & Ysseldyke, 1985). Because interpreting direct observation in natural environments requires low levels of inference, school psychologists should find these assessment procedures useful when making such decisions. Leaders in the field of school psychology have begun to focus more attention on the prevention and remediation of problems as opposed to the mere identification and verification of problems (Reschly & Ysseldyke, 1995). Based on behavioral theory, it is often the case that the conditions maintaining assessed behaviors are also directly observable. School psychologists, therefore, can collect data on these causal conditions. In many instances it is possible for school personnel to directly manipulate these causal, maintaining conditions (Bergan & Kratochwill, 1990). Direct observation of target behaviors and causal conditions in natural environments is a procedure school psychologists can use that allows educational personnel to construct applied interventions clearly indicated by the assessment data. This direct link between assessment procedures and applied interventions is one of the most important strengths of behavioral theory, because it allows practitioners to collect assessment data that directly lead to intervention procedures (Shapiro, 1996).

TARGET BEHAVIORS FOR DIRECT OBSERVATION

Direct observation merely requires one to observe behaviors and record behaviors and/or events. This assessment technique is best thought of as a flexible process that allows for collection of a variety of data across behaviors and ecologies. Because this process is flexible, a variety of decisions must be made before implementing direct observation procedures. Such decisions can have a profound impact on the assessment results and, consequently, on the decisions made based on those assessment data.

Target behaviors can vary across many dimensions. To a large degree, these dimensions will impose limitations on the assessment and recording procedures that are used. Attempting to collect direct observation data without considering the various characteristics of behavior may yield invalid or unreliable data.

Behaviors That Do Not Lend Themselves to Direct Observation

As noted, behaviors can vary across several dimensions. One dimension is the location of the behavior relative to the person being observed. To avoid making qualitative or functional distinctions between behaviors, Skinner (1945) began to refer to behaviors as being either public or private. Private or covert behaviors, (e.g., behaviors that occur within the skin) include emotional and cognitive behaviors. For example, a student's fear of school may be an important emotional behavior that school psychologists would want to measure and treat. However, because fear cannot be directly observed, school psychologists may use other assessment procedures (e.g., clinical interviews, checklists, and rating scales) to measure such internal behaviors.

The most common goal of assessing internal behaviors is to improve students' academic and/or cognitive skills. School psychologists often have confidence in standardized and nonstandardized assessment procedures designed to measure these behaviors, but because cognition cannot be directly observed, these assessment procedures also require some degree of inference (Skinner & Schook, 1995). For example, when a student produces an accurate answer to a mathematics problem, one often assumes that the student made appropriate cognitive responses to arrive at that answer.

Although some behaviors are difficult to observe because they are within the skin, other behaviors are difficult to observe because of the environmental or proximal context in which they occur. School psychologists may want to treat a child who is wetting the bed, but it is unlikely that they can directly observe the bedwetting behavior. It can also be difficult to directly observe inappropriate behaviors that occur in school settings. For example, it would be difficult for a school psychologist, especially a male school psychologist, to directly observe a female student smoking in the lavatory.

Other behaviors are difficult to observe directly because of the time when they occur. Some behaviors of interest occur infrequently, for short durations, and at unpredictable times. For example, consider a student who experiences infrequent seizures. Although a number of variables can influence seizure activity, it is often not possible to identify conditions under which seizures are likely to occur (Perry-Warner, 1996). Because they may occur infrequently, it would not be practical to have someone observing the student for weeks at a time, waiting to record seizure behavior and the conditions under which the behavior occurred.

Typical school- or classroom-based rules or procedures also affect behaviors that can physically be observed. For example, most schools have rules and punishments that are delivered contingent upon breaking those rules. One way to avoid being punished is to not break the rules. However, students quickly learn that another way to avoid being punished is to avoid being caught breaking the rules (Sulzer-Azaroff & Mayer, 1986). Moreover, when their behaviors are physically observable, many students quickly learn not to engage in inappropriate behavior when they are being observed (Henington & Skinner, 1998). For example, students tend not to copy from a peer's paper during an exam when the teacher or another educational professional is directly observing their behavior.

Assessment Procedures for Behaviors That Do Not Lend Themselves to Direct Observation

When target behaviors of interest do not lend themselves to direct observation, school psychologists have alternatives. One alternative is to use different assessment procedures such as analogue assessment, self-monitoring, self-report, and informant report (see Chapters 5, 6, 7, and 8). A second alternative is to directly observe and record correlates of the target behavior. A variety of the direct observation procedures described in this chapter can be used in these situations. When measuring correlates of target behaviors, cautious interpretation is required. For example, a variety of technological devices can be used to measure physiological behaviors, such as blood pressure and heart rate, which often correlate with students' reported fear and behavior problems associated with that fear. One cannot assume, however, that measures of internal behavior will always correlate with the behaviors of interest (Cone, 1978).

A more common example of measuring a corollary behavior using direct observation procedures is the collection of on-task data. "On-task" is typically operationally defined as a student having his head and/or eyes oriented toward assigned material, an appropriate speaker, or another presentation medium (e.g., blackboard, overhead projector, or TV screen). Such an orienting behavior is rarely the primary target behavior (Lentz, 1988;

Winette & Winkler, 1972). When this correlate is assessed, educational professionals often infer that the students with their heads oriented toward instructional or academic stimuli are responding to that stimuli. However, students oriented toward a teacher lecturing could be daydreaming. Students oriented toward assigned written material are not necessarily reading, and students who appear to be writing during assigned independent mathematics seat work may be drawing cartoons or scribbling.

Thus, in using direct observation to measure correlates of target behaviors, the inferences that must be made can lead to faulty conclusions or decision making. In these cases, if possible, other data should be collected that can either support or fail to support these inferences (Cone, 1979). For example, during a lecture a teacher may ask a student to answer a question regarding material just presented. If the student answers the question accurately, this would support the inference that when the student was oriented toward the teacher (i.e., on-task), she was indeed performing the unobservable behavior of interest (e.g., paying attention).

Another alternative to use when behaviors are not directly observable is to measure the permanent products of target behaviors. Wet bed sheets provide a highly reliable index for the behavior of bedwetting that can be directly observed and recorded. Requiring students to "show their work" in completing mathematics problems is another procedure that allows observers to confirm a hypothesis regarding cognitive behaviors.

MEASURABLE DIMENSIONS OF BEHAVIOR

Behaviors exist across both temporal and physical dimensions. Regardless of whether they are observing and recording target behaviors directly or correlates of target behaviors, before deciding how to record behaviors, observers must identify the characteristics of these target behaviors that are of interest. In behavioral theory, the context and environmental condition surrounding a target behavior can affect that behavior and the observation procedures. This section describes the characteristics of behaviors, including topography, intensity, duration, and environmental context.

Physical Characteristics of Behavior: Topography and Intensity

Topography refers to the shape of a behavior, or what the behavior looks like. Many topographical behavior problems are addressed by school psychologists. For example, hitting, biting, and leaving one's assigned seat typically refer to topographical characteristics of behavior. However, not all problems are related to topography. At times the issue is the intensity of the behavior. For example, a student's talking quietly with another student during free time

may not be a problem behavior. However, if the intensity of the behavior is increased (e.g., the student is screaming at another student), then the aspect of the behavior that is of concern is the intensity of the behavior, not the topography.

Because the topography or shape of a behavior can be observed, it is often easy to measure with the use of simple occurrence versus nonoccurrence recording procedures. However, special instruments are required to obtain precise measurement of behavioral intensity. For example, Greene, Bailey, and Barber (1981) conducted a study in which they decreased the intensity of noise on a school bus. Although no one would expect students riding a bus not to talk, students on this bus were getting so loud that the bus driver could not attend to his driving. Furthermore, a pattern had emerged in which intense levels of noise often preceded students' leaving their seats and engaging in aggressive behavior. An interdependent group contingency was implemented whereby the bus driver reinforced the group if they kept their overall noise level below a certain intensity. In this study the intensity of the noise was measured with a mechanical instrument mounted in the bus driver's seating area. Results showed that the procedure was effective in reducing noise levels, out-of-seat behavior, and aggression.

The Greene et al. (1981) study provides an example of intensity being measured precisely with the use of mechanical measuring devices. In contrast, observer judgments are often used to measure behavioral intensity. For example, inappropriate verbal behavior may involve students speaking too loudly (screaming and disrupting the class) or too softly (not speaking loudly enough to be heard). The major problem with making such judgments of intensity is that it is difficult for observers to remain consistent throughout the observation process. An observer may record the presence or absence of inappropriately loud verbal behavior in a classroom with much ambient noise. Initially, the observer may record some verbal behaviors as inappropriately loud. However, as the observer remains in the classroom, he or she can become habituated to the noise and as an observation session progresses may become less likely to record the same level of noise as intense. This phenomenon, called "observer drift" is discussed later in the chapter.

Temporal Characteristics of Behavior

Educational personnel are often concerned with temporal characteristics of behavior. The latency between a request and a student's beginning to respond is often a concern. Educators may complain of students who eventually comply with requests (e.g., a teacher tells a student to stop bothering a classmate and return to his own desk), but constantly take too long to begin to comply (e.g., the student eventually returns, but first smacks his peer on the arm and then slowly walks back to his seat while making faces and pestering

other students). Sometimes educators refer to this as passive–aggressive behavior.

Other behaviors are problems because of the rate at which they occur. Talking to a peer during independent seat work, leaving one's seat without permission, and calling out during recitation are inappropriate behaviors. However, educators expect such behaviors to occur occasionally and often do not express serious concern unless these behaviors occur at extremely high rates.

Temporal characteristics of academic behaviors are also important. For example, a child who can perform his mathematics problems with 100% accuracy, but is extremely slow, is likely to have difficulty in completing assignments and developing his mathematics skills (Binder, 1996). Thus, the time required to complete a task is the concern, not the topography or accuracy of the student's work. Some students can begin assigned work but have difficulty persisting in their tasks. For these students the issue is, again, temporal, and the observer may want to record data on the amount of time a student is continuously engaged in the assigned tasks.

CONTEXTUAL VARIABLES

All behavior has physical and temporal properties. However, the general context in which the behavior occurs and/or the assumed motivation, intention, or function of the behavior are often considered important and can often suggest interventions that may remedy the presenting problems. In collecting these data, observations sometimes require judgments about the valence of the behavior, the intent or purpose of the behavior, and/or the function of the behavior.

Valence of Behavior

Researchers have discussed behaviors in terms of valence (Cone, 1978). Negative valence behaviors are inappropriate behaviors, and positive valence behaviors are appropriate. Teachers often want to reduce inappropriate behaviors such as inappropriate language and touching. However, the appropriateness or inappropriateness of a behavior is situation-specific. For example, in a school setting, showing a peer how to do an assignment may be appropriate during scheduled peer tutoring, whereas the same behavior is considered inappropriate in testing situations.

It is sometimes difficult to make judgments of these types of behaviors. Therefore, in collecting data on behaviors that require such judgments, it is essential that the observer determine which behaviors are considered appropriate or inappropriate. Thus, obtaining information pertaining to school

and classroom rules and regulations and typical patterns of functions (e.g., is hand raising typically required? are students allowed to leave their seat without permission to sharpen their pencils?) is often necessary before collecting this kind of data. Data of this type are often collected via teacher interview.

Intent of Behavior

Judgments are also required when behaviors are defined in terms of intent. An excellent example of this is aggression. Aggression is often defined as behavior that is intended to harm a person or object. Aggression has also been broken down according to the purpose or function of the behavior. For example, the intended function of instrumental aggression could be to obtain an object (e.g., a toy a peer is playing with) or territory (e.g., the seat in the front of the class). However, the intended function of hostile aggression is to hurt another child. On the surface these definitions of aggression appear quite clear. However, the definitions are based on the intent of the behavior, and this intent is not directly observable.

Thus, any direct observation data collected on aggression is based on the observer's judgment with respect to the child's intentions. Typically, intent must be inferred from the general environmental context where the behavior occurs and the antecedent and consequent events that immediately surround the behavior. For example, one may label a behavior as instrumental aggression if immediately following the target behavior the child gains possession and begins to play with a toy that another child was using. However, if the child gains nothing, then one may infer that the intent of the behavior was to harm the other child and may thus label the behavior as hostile. Although determining the intent of a behavior is important, observers must exercise extreme care when reporting this type of data. Specifically, they should record and report the antecedent and consequent conditions that are directly observable and verifiable. Then they should make it clear that these data are being used to support their inferences.

Functions of Behavior

Although direct observation of intent is not possible, this does not mean that the reason a student is engaging in a particular behavior is not important. Behaviors are maintained by environmental conditions and past learning history. It is the identification of these conditions that allow for the construction of interventions designed to prevent and remedy problems. Thus, assessment procedures that allow for the identification of environmental conditions that cause or maintain behaviors of interest may be even more important than procedures designed to measure specific target behaviors (Carr, 1993).

Operant behavioral psychology assumes that behaviors are maintained

by contingencies of reinforcement, including both positive and negative reinforcing contingencies. Reinforcement contingencies specify a relationship between behaviors and consequences that increase the probability of those behaviors occurring under similar conditions. Although antecedent events are
not typically viewed as variables that cause certain behaviors, recording data
on antecedent events can often help indicate what consequences are reinforcing the behaviors. For example, when negative reinforcement is operating,
students may engage in target behaviors at higher rates under some antecedent conditions (e.g., high rates of inappropriate behavior during independent seat work in mathematics but not during reading or history) because
these behaviors allow them to escape or avoid specific academic stimuli or
demands (e.g., to avoid independent mathematics seat work).

One of the advantages of direct observation procedures is that observers can record antecedent and consequent events that surround target
behaviors. However, the contingent if-then relationship (if this behavior occurs under these antecedent conditions, then this consequence will follow) is
not directly observable; what can be observed and recorded is a sequence of
events. For example, during independent seat work in reading a child may
throw his books on the floor (target behavior). The teacher may then react by
yelling at the child and sending him to the principal's office (consequence).
Plausible reinforcers for this scenario include teacher attention or principal
attention (these are positive reinforcing events). By being sent to the principal's office, the student escapes schoolwork. Thus, the immediate demand to
do the schoolwork (reading) is removed, which may negatively reinforce the
inappropriate behavior. Finally, although these events followed the target behavior, none of them may actually be reinforcing the behavior. The actual reinforcement may be a delayed unobservable event, such as the student's peers
socially praising this behavior 6 hours later when school is out.

Therefore, when using direct observation to record target behaviors and
plausible antecedents, one must infer that the events that followed the target
behavior are causing or reinforcing the target behavior. For these reasons,
procedures that require observers to record behaviors, and the antecedent
and consequent conditions surrounding these behaviors, have been termed
descriptive functional analysis procedures (see McComas, Hoch, & Mace,
Chapter 4, this volume). Descriptive analysis procedures can lead to the identification of conditions that are reinforcing behaviors in the natural environment (Lalli, Browder, Mace, & Brown, 1993; Lewis & Sugai, 1996). However,
to clearly demonstrate the relationship between behaviors and their consequences, assessment procedures with more experimental control are needed
to rule out other causes of target behaviors. In natural environments, single-
subject research designs (e.g., withdrawal, reversal, multiple-baseline, and alternating treatments designs) are often used to establish functional relationships. Furthermore, experimenters have used analogue conditions and alter-

nating treatments designs to determine which conditions are reinforcing specific behaviors (see Mace and Lalli, 1991, for excellent examples of both descriptive and functional assessment procedures).

RECORDING PROCEDURES

The products of direct observation procedures are the recordings of the observer(s). Although the observation process is simple, there are many options for recording behaviors. Which option is most appropriate depends on the reason for collecting data (e.g., to verify a problem, to evaluate an intervention) and the characteristics of the behaviors being observed. In this section, narrative and empirical direct observation procedures are described and analyzed.

Narrative Recording Procedures

Narrative recording procedures require observers to record (typically in written narrative form) what they see occurring in the classroom. Data collected from narrative recordings can be used to (1) confirm problems, (2) operationally define target behaviors, (3) develop empirical recording systems, (4) develop future direct observation procedures (e.g., determine where to sit so that target behaviors can be observed), and (5) identify antecedent and consequent events that may be functionally related to target behaviors.

Narrative recordings generally yield topographical and sequential data. With respect to topography, observers can record narrative descriptions of student behaviors as they occur. Having the opportunity to observe student target behaviors and write narrative descriptions of these behaviors is often useful in attempting to define target behaviors that are highly idiosyncratic and variable. For example, a student may be referred for hand flapping or temper tantrums. However, these behaviors often vary with respect to their shape or topography, duration, and rate across students. Therefore, seeing these behaviors and making narrative recordings of their characteristics often helps observers in developing operational definitions of target behaviors and structuring empirical recording procedures.

Because narrative recording takes time and events in a classroom often proceed at a rapid rate, it is difficult to record narrative data continuously. A remedy may be to record narrative data at specified intervals. When this procedure is used, an observer may look up and observe a student's behavior at specified intervals (e.g., every 10 seconds) and record what the student is doing at that time. This procedure allows time for observers to record behaviors and may provide some idea of the amount of time students spend engaged in specific behaviors (Shapiro & Skinner, 1990). However, this procedure is not

very useful for determining environmental consequences that may be causally related to specific behaviors, as observers may miss opportunities to observe these events while they are writing narrative descriptions of the target behaviors.

Narrative recording can also be used in conducting antecedent–behavior–consequence (A-B-C) analysis data. When narrative A-B-C data are collected, the occurrence of a target behavior(s) serves as a cue for the observer to record narrative descriptions of (1) antecedent events and conditions that precede the target behavior, (2) the target behavior itself, and (3) events that follow the target behavior that may be functionally related to that target behavior.

A-B-C analysis can be used to help identify plausible functions of specific behaviors. At times there are clear antecedent events that precede target behaviors, that are functionally related to the target behaviors (e.g., a peer throws something at a child and the child leaves his area and becomes aggressive). In other instances, nothing dramatic occurs immediately before the target behavior (e.g., a student who appears to be working quietly during independent seat work suddenly throws a temper tantrum). In the latter case, an observer has little to record with respect to antecedent events that immediately precede the behavior. However, an observer should provide a detailed description of the general antecedent conditions, sometimes referred to as ecological conditions, as these conditions may be functionally related to the target behavior. Ecological conditions that should be recorded include the time the behavior occurred, the assigned tasks or activities that were occurring (e.g., independent seat work, group recitation), contingencies that were in place during that time (e.g., classroom rules and regulations for general behavior and specific rules related to the specific situation), the academic content area that was being covered (e.g., reading, mathematics), whether the teacher was instructing the entire group or a small group, whether students were engaged in independent seat work or other learning activities, and approximately how long the students were engaged in the current activities.

Recording general conditions may allow observers to identify the function of target behaviors. For example, students may engage in inappropriate behavior to avoid doing their assigned tasks. A student who finds mathematics very aversive (perhaps very difficult) may (1) act out, (2) put his or her head down and sleep, or (3) scribble in any answer. These behaviors are dissimilar with respect to topography. However, all of the behaviors may serve the same function, allowing the student to escape doing the independent seat work mathematics assignment. Therefore, describing the general environmental conditions that are in place before a behavior occurs may help observers to identify the function of a behavior and suggest interventions based on that identified function (Sprague, Sugai, & Walker, 1998).

Identifying and recording events that follow and reinforce target behav-

iors can also be more complex than it appears. Although reinforcement procedures tend to be strong when the events occur immediately following a behavior, delayed reinforcers can also maintain a behavior (Neef, Mace, & Shade, 1993). Observers may record events that immediately follow target behaviors (teacher yells, principal lectures), only to find that these events may not be serving as reinforcers. Rather, as previously indicated, unobservable events that occur later and perhaps in different environments may be reinforcing the behavior (e.g., peers praise these behaviors after school on the playground).

Another difficulty with recording consequences is related to observer judgments. Observers tend to think of punishers and reinforcers as stimuli that they believe to be satisfying or aversive. This can lead to problems, as secondary reinforcers and punishers are often idiosyncratic and shaped by an individual's learning history (Skinner, 1974). For many students, being reprimanded by a teacher serves as a punishing event; but for other students, the same event serves as a reinforcer. Therefore, it is important for observers to record all events that immediately follow a behavior.

The consistency of reinforcement can also lead to errors in forming hypotheses about reinforcing consequences. To maintain a behavior, reinforcing events do not have to follow every instance of that behavior. In fact, basic research on schedules of reinforcement indicates that intermittent reinforcement can maintain behavior(s) for longer periods of time (Ferster & Skinner, 1957). Thus, observers must be careful to avoid dismissing an event as a plausible reinforcer because it occurred only once or twice after a target behavior that occurred many times.

Narrative recording can be useful for identifying target behaviors and possible antecedent and consequence variables related to those target behaviors. However, because data are not recorded in a systematic fashion, narrative recording procedures can yield imprecise data that are difficult to verify. The next section describes empirical recording procedures that can yield both precise and verifiable data.

Empirical Recording Procedures

Although narrative recording is often useful, empirical recording procedures allow one to measure behavior more precisely. Such precision allows for comparisons of the behavior strength, as opposed to just the presence or absence of behavior, across conditions. For example, empirical data may show that a child engaged in an inappropriate behavior 30 times during reading class but only 3 times during mathematics class. This precision not only allows one to compare strength of behavior across naturally occurring conditions, but also allows for comparisons of the strength of behavior across baseline and intervention conditions. Therefore, with empirical data it is possible to evaluate

the effects of interventions, including immediacy of change, change in trends, and variability of data across baseline and intervention conditions (Barlow & Hersen, 1984; Johnston & Pennypacker, 1980).

Operational Definitions

A characteristic of all methods for recording empirical data is that target behaviors must be operationally defined. The definitions are based on the shape or topography of the behavior, not its intent or function (Heward, 1987). For example, aggressive behavior is defined as hitting or kicking another student. However, including intention in this definition, (e.g., hitting or kicking with the intention of hurting another student) requires observers to make judgments about unobservable events, which can lead to inconsistent and unverifiable data recording.

Another concern is the boundaries of the behavior. For example, suppose a student is disrupting class and annoying peers by throwing objects. If a peer were to ask this student for a dime and the target student flipped the dime to the other student, observers may record this event as an instance of throwing because it fits the topographical description of the behavior. Recording behaviors based solely on observable and verifiable events may result in some behaviors being recorded that are not actual target behaviors, owing to the context or assumed intent. In other instances behaviors may be excluded that are actually of concern. However, if observers consistently record behavior based solely on operational definitions, then these omissions or inclusions are likely to be equally distributed across conditions.

Several procedures can be used to help develop operational definitions. First, it is often useful to interview teachers and have them describe the behavior. Initially, teachers may provide broad, vague definitions of the behaviors (e.g., student has a bad attitude). When the goal is to operationally define the behaviors, questions are asked that require the teacher to narrow the definition of the behaviors to include observable events (e.g., What does she do that makes you say she has a bad attitude? What do these behaviors look like? How would I recognize these behaviors?). In other instances, descriptions of behaviors may not be sufficient and observers may have to directly observe the behavior in order to form an operational definition. As previously mentioned, these observations are extremely useful for idiosyncratic student behaviors (e.g., hand flapping, temper tantrums).

In developing operational definitions, it is often useful to provide examples of behaviors that fit and do not fit the operational definitions (Saudargas & Fellers, 1986). For example, prior to taking data on students' off-task behavior, observers should decide whether sharpening a pencil should be considered off-task.

Once behaviors are operationally defined, data recording systems can

be constructed. Although the operational definition of behaviors has been considered separately from data recording procedures, problems associated with recording behaviors can often be addressed through altering recording procedures and/or operational definitions. In the next sections, different methods of empirically recording behaviors are described. Furthermore, variables that may impact the validity and reliability of direct observation data are analyzed across each system. This analysis should allow readers to develop appropriate direct observation recording procedures for specific situations and behaviors.

Event Recording

Once a behavior is operationally defined, an observer can record each occurrence of that behavior. When these occurrences are summed, frequency data are collected. Frequency counts are sometimes useful to confirm the presence or absence of a behavior. However, in most instances recording either the time spent observing or the number of opportunities the student had to engage in the target behavior during the observation period can enhance the validity of event data.

PERCENTAGE OF OCCURRENCE DATA

The occurrence or nonoccurrence of some behaviors is dependent on other events that occur at inconsistent levels in school environments. For example, a teacher may want to increase a student's level of compliance with following directions. Compliance may be defined as the student's beginning to follow the teacher's direction within 5 seconds after the direction is issued. During one 40-minute observation session, the teacher may give the student 6 directions. During another 40-minute observation session, the teacher may give the student 18 directions. In the first session, the child may comply all 6 times. However, in the second session the student may comply 9 of the 18 times. If the observer merely recorded instances of compliance, the student's compliance levels would appear higher in the second session (9 instances) than the first (6 instances).

When the opportunity to perform a behavior varies across observation sessions, observers should also collect frequency data on the opportunities. The data can then be expressed as a ratio that can be converted to percentage data. In the previous example, reporting that the student complied with 6 out of 6 commands (100% compliance) in one session, versus 9 of 18 commands (50% compliance) in the other session, provides more information and enhances the validity of the data. Furthermore, converting data to percentages allows one to make empirical comparisons of behavior levels across sessions where opportunities to engage in target behaviors vary naturally.

RATE DATA

When frequency counts are divided by time observed, the data can be reported in terms of behavior rates. Rate data have many advantages over frequency data. First, rate data typically have much more social or educational significance. For example, if one were observing physical aggression in a child, frequency data may allow one to report two instances of aggressive behavior. If the purpose of the observation is merely to confirm that the student is sometimes aggressive, these data may be useful. However, when these data are converted to rates, the meaning can be altered dramatically. For example, two instances of aggression over a 10-minute observation period suggests a more serious problem than two instances over 360 minutes.

A second major advantage of collecting rate data is that it allows for comparisons of behavior strength across time or conditions. This is particularly useful when observation intervals are not equal. For example, an observer may record data during independent seat work in mathematics and reading. During these sessions, the student may have 25 minutes of independent seat work during mathematics but only 15 minutes during reading. By converting these rate data to number of instances of target behavior per minute (i.e., number of occurrences recorded/number of seconds observed × 60) an observer can compare the student's rate of behavior across observation sessions that are not equivalent in length.

LIMITATIONS ASSOCIATED WITH EVENT RECORDING

There are some limitations associated with event recording that are related to the topography, duration, and rates of target behaviors. With respect to topography and duration, behaviors are described across a continuum with continuous behaviors at one end of the continuum and discrete behaviors at the other end. A discrete behavior has a clear beginning and end. Event recording tends to lend itself to reporting discrete behaviors. For example, one could record the number of times a student calls out in class, because each instance of this behavior has a clear beginning and end.

Other behaviors—for example, physical aggression (e.g., hitting or kicking, throwing objects at another student)—are less discrete and tend to occur in bursts. Therefore, if a student hits another child five times, stops for 3 seconds and then hits the child three times, the observer may have difficulty determining how many instances of aggression to record. What may be more important than the number of actual acts of hitting (e.g., eight hits) is the number of instances of aggression. If this is the case, it can be useful to alter the operational definition of the behavior to include the point at which aggressive outbursts have stopped. In the previous example, an instance of aggression can be defined as acts of hitting, kicking, or throwing that begin following the first occurrence of any of these behaviors and end only when

none of the behaviors have occurred for 30 seconds. Thus, in the preceding above example, the observer would record one aggressive outburst and would not have to attempt to count the number of hits or kicks.

Although employing temporal variables to operationally define the end of a behavior may work in some cases, in other instances this strategy will not improve the validity or usefulness of the data. For example, suppose the target behavior is out-of-seat behavior and the operational definition of an instance of this behavior included the instance ending when the child returns to his assigned seat for 5 seconds. On one day the observer may observe the child leave his seat at the beginning of a 40-minute session and never return. Thus, the observer would record one instance of this continuous out-of-seat behavior. However, the next day the child may leave his seat 10 times for very brief periods (e.g., 10 seconds) and then return to his seat each time. In this case, if event recording procedures are used, 10 occurrences of out-of-seat behavior would be recorded for the second session. Thus, rate data would show one instance of out-of-seat behavior in 40 minutes versus 10 instances of out-of-seat behavior in 40 minutes. The rate data make it appear that the target behavior was at a high level during the second session when the child was in his seat for 39 of 40 minutes (scored as 10 instances), as opposed to the second session when the child was in his seat for only the first 1 of 40 minutes (scored as 1 instance). In this case, invalid data collection is caused by using the wrong recording procedure. Duration recording, as opposed to event recording, should have been used to measure this continuous behavior.

Duration Recording

Duration recording requires observers to record the amount of time a behavior occurs from beginning to end. In many instances, it is the duration of target behaviors that is of concern. For example, a goal may be to increase the time a student spends engaged in silent reading. Inappropriate behaviors are often a concern because of their duration, rather than the frequency or rate of the behaviors. For example, a teacher may become concerned over how long a child's tantrums last as opposed to how frequently they occur (Shapiro & Skinner, 1990). In such cases, an observer would need a clear definition of the target behavior, including when the behavior begins and ends, and a timing device (e.g., stopwatch) to record the duration of the target behavior.

Observers can collect duration data continuously. For this purpose, they need some type of timing device (e.g., a stopwatch, a computer with appropriate software running). For example, an observer may start a stopwatch when a student engages in a target behavior and then stop it when the student ceases to be so engaged.

This process appears to be very simple. However, there are several limi-

tations associated with collecting continuous duration data. Perhaps the greatest limitation is having to work the timing device. Although it is a simple process to start and stop a stopwatch, it is difficult to track whether the watch is running or not. For example, suppose an observer is collecting continuous data for on-task behavior defined as head and eyes oriented toward the speaker. Even children who are on-task most of the time will not stay oriented toward the speaker the entire time. Rather, they will make quick glances around the room, out the window, toward the door, and so on. These quick glances make it very difficult to accurately time the target behavior using continuous data recording. Furthermore, because the observer is required to observe certain behaviors and operate a timing device simultaneously, it is often extremely difficult to collect data on other behaviors or events (e.g., antecedents and consequences) that may be influencing the target behavior(s).

TIME SAMPLING PROCEDURES

Time sampling procedures are extremely useful for estimating the duration of behaviors that are more continuous rather than discrete, and for discrete behaviors that occur at high rates. When time sampling is employed, observation sessions are broken down into smaller units of time or intervals and the occurrences of the target behavior during those intervals are recorded. The recording intervals allow the observer to collect data on high-rate behaviors that are difficult to count (e.g., number of kicks) or to collect data on the duration of behaviors that are continuous (e.g., on-task behavior). Furthermore, because behaviors are not recorded in a continuous manner, time sampling procedures often allow observers to record multiple behaviors (e.g., on-task, aggression, out-of-seat) and other events (e.g., antecedent and consequent conditions) during the same observation session.

There are three methods of recording time sampling data: (1) momentary time sampling, (2) whole-interval time sampling, and (3) partial-interval time sampling. All three procedures require a recording device with the interval marked and a system to cue the observer when the interval occurs. Although a watch can be used to cue the intervals, it is often easier to employ an audiotape and tape player to cue recording, as this system does not require the observer to visually monitor the student behavior(s) and classroom events simultaneously with a watch or clock.

Making an interval recording tape is fairly simple. All that is required is a tape recorder, an audiotape, and a watch. After the observer decides on the length of intervals and the length of the session, the cues at each interval are recorded. Although any type of audible stimulus can be used to mark intervals (e.g., computers can be programmed to beep at specific intervals), it may be best to mark intervals by reading interval numbers onto a tape. By doing so, the observers can also construct data recording sheets with intervals num-

bered, and this allows the observer to keep track of the exact interval where the specific behavior(s) should be recorded.

During momentary time sampling, the observer records the presence of a target behavior only if it occurs during a specified instant or moment. Thus, if the target is out-of-seat behavior, at the specified interval the observer would record the target behavior. Because the only concern is whether the behavior is occurring at that instant, momentary time sampling can be used to record high-rate behaviors and behaviors that are continuous. Furthermore, because the behaviors are observed for only a moment, it is possible to collect data on several behaviors at once.

For example, suppose the behaviors of interest include time spent talking to a peer, on-task behaviors, and out-of-seat behavior during independent seat work. It would be extremely difficult for one observer to collect continuous data on all three of these behaviors using a stopwatch or a computer. However, using momentary time sampling, the observer, can (1) look up every 5 seconds (at the cue), (2) observe the student at that moment, and then (3) record the presence of each observed behavior during that moment. During the interval between observations (5 seconds), the observer would have time to record the behaviors without being concerned that other behaviors would be missed.

Recording the presence or absence of behaviors can be very simple. For example, if only one behavior is targeted, the observer can merely record the presence of the behavior on a sheet with a number for each interval (1, 2, 3, 4, 5, 6, etc). If the target behavior is not observed during an interval, then no mark is placed on the interval number. If the behavior is observed, then the observer can put a slash on the number. As previously mentioned, it is not always possible to observe during an entire session. Therefore, in some instances an observer may not be able to determine the presence or absence of a target behavior at the moment the interval cue is delivered (e.g., peer walked between observer and student). To prevent these intervals from being scored as non-occurrences, observers should use a different mark or code (e.g., circle the interval number) to indicate that no observation was made during that interval.

In partial-interval time sampling, behaviors are recorded if they occur at any time during an interval. If a 20-minute recording session is broken down into 5-second intervals, one would observe continuously and record the interval if the target behavior occurs at any time during each 5-second interval. As with momentary time sampling, this method of data recording works well with continuous behavior because there is no need to record the beginning and end of the target behavior. If a behavior begins in one interval and continues to the next interval, then the behavior is recorded as occurring in both intervals. Partial-interval time sampling works well with high-rate behaviors because observers are not required to record every instance of the

behavior. Rather, they record the behavior as occurring in that interval if it occurs just one time during the interval. A final advantage of partial-interval time sampling is that once the behavior occurs during an interval, the behavior does not have to be continuously monitored for the rest of the interval. Thus, partial-interval time sampling may be extremely useful when teachers are asked to record low-rate behaviors over long intervals (e.g., a tantrum every hour).

When whole-interval time sampling is used, the behavior is recorded only if it is observed for the entire interval. Thus, if an observer is recording on-task behavior using whole-interval time sampling, the student would have to remain on-task during the entire interval in order for the observer to score the interval. Because the behavior must exist throughout the entire interval to be scored, this procedure may be most useful when brief intervals are used to record common continuous behaviors (e.g., on-task behavior recorded, using 5-second intervals).

REPORTING AND INTERPRETING TIME SAMPLING PROCEDURES

Time sampling data yield duration estimates (Lentz, 1988). These estimates are affected by the time sampling method employed (i.e., momentary, whole-interval, or partial-interval), the length or number of intervals employed, and the interaction of these variables.

Time sampling data are often summarized in terms of number of intervals during which the behavior was observed and the number of intervals for which data were collected. Regardless of the time sampling method, if a student is recorded as on-task for 7 of 10 intervals observed, these data are reported and summarized as the student's being on-task during 70% of the intervals observed. Based on this sample, one can estimate that during the observation session the student was on-task 70% of the time.

Research has shown that the errors involved in duration estimates are likely to be effected by the time sampling procedure being used. Whole-interval recording tends to underestimate behavior duration, and partial-interval recording tends to overestimate behavior duration (Lentz, 1982; Powell, Martindale, Kulp, Martindale, & Bauman, 1977). These over- and underestimates may be affected by the length of the intervals. For example, partial-interval recording with extremely long intervals may increase overestimation, whereas whole-interval recording with long intervals may increase the number of underestimations. Although momentary time sampling neither consistently over- or underestimates behavior duration, sampling theory suggests that errors are more likely to occur if samples are taken less frequently (Lentz, 1982, Powell et al., 1977). Therefore, in reporting time sampling data it is essential that the type of time sampling procedure (e.g., whole-interval), the length of intervals (e.g., 5-second intervals), and the session length (20-

minute session) be reported along with the summary data (e.g., on-task in 70% of the intervals observed).

Comparison Child Data

In addition to taking direct observation data on target student behavior, observers should also consider collecting direct observation data on comparison children (Saudargas & Fellers, 1986; Shapiro, 1996). Data from comparison children can be used to verify problems and help establish empirical goals. For example, data may show that a comparison student's behavior is similar to the target student's behavior (e.g., comparison student was on-task in 75% of the observed intervals, and the target student was on-task in 72% of the observed intervals). Such comparison data suggest that the target behavior may not be the presenting problem or may be inappropriately defined. Thus, comparing data across comparison and target students can alert professionals to problems with their identified target behavior and/or recording procedures and prevent them from developing and implementing interventions that address an inappropriately targeted behavior.

There are several procedures for collecting comparison child data when interval recording is employed (Alessi, 1988; Shapiro, 1996). Observers can collect data on one or several comparison students. Furthermore, data can be collected on several students simultaneously or observers can use discontinuous data collection procedures whereby they collect data on comparison and target students at different intervals.

SIMULTANEOUS RECORDING

When momentary time sampling data are being collected on one behavior, it may be possible for observers to collect simultaneous data on several students, including the target student. Observers can then record the presence and absence of the target student's behavior and the proportion of comparison students who were also engaged in those behaviors. For example, an observer may be able to record a target student's behavior and five comparison students' on-task behavior simultaneously. For each interval the observer can record the number of comparison students on-task—for example, four, which would indicate that four of the five comparison students were on-task during this interval.

Simultaneous observation is possible when a group of students are located in close proximity (e.g., their assigned seats are adjacent). However, as they move around their educational environments, it may not be possible to observe all of these students simultaneously during each interval. When this occurs, observers should record ratio data for those intervals (e.g., three-fourths of students were on-task). In reporting the data for the observation

session, comparison data are aggregated across intervals (e.g., comparison student data showed that comparison students were on-task in 77 of 100 intervals observed).

It may be difficult to reliably record data simultaneously across students when observers are recording many different behaviors using complex recording systems. Because both whole- and partial-interval recording procedures often require continuous observation, simultaneous recording across students should not be used to collect comparison student data. In these situations, discontinuous data collection procedures allow observers to collect comparison student data.

DISCONTINUOUS RECORDING

When using discontinuous recording, observers establish intervals when they will cease collecting data on target student behavior so that they can collect comparison student data. If one student is chosen as a comparison student, it is important that the student be average or acceptable, not exceptional, in terms of target behavior. Thus, teacher reports play an important role in selecting a comparison student. Unfortunately, teachers may inadvertently select a comparison student who displays similar problems or is atypical in that he or she never engages in the behavior(s) being recorded (Alessi, 1988; Shapiro, 1996). To some degree, collecting data on several comparison students may address this problem by providing a more diverse sample of comparison student data.

When only one student can be observed during each interval, collecting comparison child data across comparison students can be accomplished by rotating comparison students across intervals. In conjunction with the teacher, observers select several comparison students. At each interval designated for collecting comparison student data, observers observe only one comparison student, but rotate their observations across comparison students as they move through data recording sessions. For example, comparison student data may be collected every 5th interval. During the 5th interval observers can record comparison student A's behavior. During the 10th interval, observers can record comparison student B's behavior. During the 15th interval, observers can record comparison student C's behavior. During the 20th interval, observers repeat this rotation by collecting data on comparison student A.

There are several limitations in using discontinuous data collection procedures. Observers may have to increase observation session length or the number of observation sessions in order to obtain an adequate sample of both target and comparison student behavior. Furthermore, while observing comparison students, observers may miss an opportunity to observe and record events that are functionally related to target behaviors. For example,

if a target behavior is being reinforced by infrequent peer attention, observers may miss the opportunity to observe and record this reinforcing event because they were observing and recording comparison children's behavior.

Summary of Procedures for Collecting Comparison Student Data

There are several procedures for collecting comparison student data. Each procedure has strengths and weaknesses that must be considered. Simultaneous data collection procedures may allow observers to obtain larger and more diverse samples of comparison student data in brief periods of time. In addition, simultaneous recording allows observers to continuously record data related to target behaviors. Discontinuous systems can be used with complex direct observation systems (e.g., multiple behaviors and events) and when observation procedures require whole- or partial-interval recording. However, to adequately sample both target and comparison student behaviors, these systems may require longer or more observation sessions, and observers may occasionally lose the opportunity to observe and record important antecedent and consequent events.

Recording Sequential Events Surrounding Target Behaviors

Collecting empirical data on target behaviors is extremely useful for (1) confirming behavior problems, (2) establishing precise baseline or pre-intervention behavior levels, trends, and patterns, and (3) evaluating the effects of interventions. In attempting to construct interventions, it is often useful to collect empirical data on antecedents and consequences surrounding target behaviors. For example, teacher attention may reinforce a variety of inappropriate behaviors. Observers can collect data on these teacher behaviors. However, merely collecting data on teacher attention does not indicate the sequential relationship between target behaviors and the hypothesized consequent events or antecedent events. Interval recording systems are useful for collecting this type of data because they can provide a temporal sequence of events. Furthermore, constructing operational definitions that include an interactive component (i.e., teacher and student behavior) can also be useful for indicating interventions.

Collecting frequency data on target behaviors and assumed antecedent or consequent events that may be functionally related to that target behavior does not yield data on events that precede or follow target behaviors. However, when event recording, is combined with interval recording, it is possible to obtain a record of a sequence of events. This sequence of events can help determine whether the hypothesized consequent events occurred immediately after the target behavior and whether antecedent events that may be relat-

ed to the target behavior occurred immediately prior to the target behavior. For example, assume that the target behavior is self-injurious behavior and one plausible reinforcer in the natural environment is teacher attention. Frequency count data may reveal that the child engaged in 10 instances of self-injurious behavior over a 20-interval observation session. The data may also suggest that the teacher approached the child 20 times during this session. However, the data do not reveal the temporal relationship of the target behavior and the hypothetical reinforcer (teacher attention).

Figures 2.1 and 2.2 provide examples of the same observation session showing where events were recorded within intervals. In both examples, continuous event recording is used, but data are recorded during 20-second intervals. Notice how the data in Figure 2.1 show that most of the teacher attention occurs early and the student's self-injurious behavior occurs after a long period of time (e.g., several intervals). Figure 2.2 provides data that show a strong temporal relationship between teacher attention and self-injurious behavior. Notice how teacher attention often occurs after intervals of the student's self-injurious behavior. The data suggest that the function of the self-injurious behavior may be to obtain teacher attention.

Another strategy for collecting data on target behaviors, antecedents, and consequences is to employ complex definitions of behavior that include interactions. One example of this strategy was developed by Saudargas (1992) and is used in the direct observation system, the State–Event Classroom Observation System (SECOS). The SECOS has an operational definition for a target child initiating a social interaction with another child either verbally or physically (i.e., "approach child"). If the child approaches another child *and* a social interaction between the children ensues, then the observer records a slash or line to indicate that the child made the approach and then circles this line to indicate the subsequent social interaction. If the approach

	1	2	3	4	5	6	7	8	9	10	11	12	13	14	15	16	17	18	19	20
Teacher Approach	//	//	///	/	///															
Self-Injurious Behavior									//	//	////	////	////	///	/					

FIGURE 2.1. Frequency data recorded across intervals.

	1	2	3	4	5	6	7	8	9	10	11	12	13	14	15	16	17	18	19	20
Teacher Approach		//					/	/					/	/				/	//	/
Self-Injurious Behavior	/					///	//					////	///					///	//	/

FIGURE 2.2. Frequency data recorded across intervals.

is ignored and no social interaction follows, then the line indicating the approach is not circled. Thus, this operational definition is interactive as it includes both peer behavior and target student behavior.

This type of interactive recording may lead to hypotheses regarding the function of specific behavior. For example, direct observation data may reveal that a student is off-task and out of his seat at high rates. Furthermore, the data may also show high rates of the student approaching other children while out of his seat and that a social interaction typically occurs following the approach. This may suggest that these social interactions may be reinforcing off-task, out-of-seat, and initiating-social-interaction behavior. In contrast, the direct observation data may also show that the same behaviors (off-task, out-of-seat, and approach child) are often ignored by peers, but are followed by teacher attention. This pattern of data may suggest that the behaviors are being reinforced by teacher attention, rather than peer attention.

QUALITY OF DIRECT OBSERVATION DATA

The quality of standardized assessment data is often evaluated by the psychometric properties of the assessment instruments including the reliability, validity, and normative sample. Some researchers have argued that behavioral assessment procedures can not and should not be subject to the same standards (e.g., Cone, 1988; Hayes, Nelson, & Jarrett, 1986), and others have argued that many of these standards should be applied to behavioral assessment procedures (e.g., Barrios & Hartmann, 1986; Strosahl & Linehan, 1986). Although it is beyond the scope of this chapter to cover this theoretical debate, there are procedures developed by researchers for empirically evaluating the quality of direct observation data.

Behavioral theory differs from more traditional theories of human behavior in that behaviors are not assumed to be stable (Hartmann, Roper, & Bradford, 1979). Thus, traditional procedures, such as test–retest reliability, that are designed to evaluate the amount of error or inaccuracy associated with assessment instruments would not be appropriate for use with behavioral assessment. In fact, variation in behavior levels across environments can be useful in that observers may be able to identify antecedent and consequent events that account for this variation. Once such events are identified, interventions can often be constructed based on these variables that may account for the instability (e.g., unusually high or low levels) in the behavior.

Although consistent behavior from students or clients is not assumed, it is essential that observers be consistent and reliable when recording their observations. The primary procedure used for evaluating observer-recorded behavior is interobserver agreement. In most instances, interobserver agreement data are gathered by having two observers independently record the

same behaviors or events at the same time (Johnston & Pennypacker, 1980). Thus, in order to collect interobserver agreement data it is necessary to have two trained observers, using the same empirical recording systems, collecting data at the same time.

Calculating Interobserver Agreement

House, House, and Campbell (1981) review 17 procedures for calculating interobserver agreement. It is beyond the scope of this chapter to review each procedure. However, one of the simplest and most often used statistical procedures for calculating interobserver agreement across two observers is percent agreement. The basic formula for calculating percent interobserver agreement is:

$$\frac{\text{Agreements on Occurrence}}{\text{Agreements on Occurrence} + \text{Disagreements on Occurrence}} \times 100$$

Suppose observers are recording the number of times a student engages in an inappropriate behavior during a 40-minute mathematics class. Both the primary observer and a secondary observer can collect data using event recording during the same class period. The primary observer may record 12 instances of the inappropriate behavior, and the secondary observer may record 9 instances of the behavior. Interobserver agreement for occurrence can then be calculated by dividing 9 by 12 and multiplying by 100. Thus, percent interobserver agreement would be 75%.

Just as statistical analysis procedures are often guided by convention or general rules of thumb, (e.g., p < .05), there are some guidelines associated with interobserver agreement data. Generally, 80% interobserver agreement is considered acceptable for research purposes. Furthermore, researchers generally collect interobserver agreement across a minimum of 20% of the observation sessions. Finally, because observers may alter their recording procedures over time, interobserver agreement data should be collected across the sessions rather than during consecutive sessions.

In the previous example, 75% interobserver agreement is fairly strong and approaches the minimum level that researchers prefer. However, this agreement percentage may not accurately reflect level of agreement. In fact, observers may have never actually agreed, as the primary observer could have recorded 12 instances of inappropriate behavior and the secondary observer could have recorded 8 other (no overlap or agreement) instances of inappropriate behavior.

When observation sessions are broken down to intervals and data are recorded within these intervals, a more rigorous and precise measure of percent interobserver agreement can be calculated. Figure 2.3 displays the data

from the previous example, which was recorded using 2-minute partial-interval time sampling. Recall that if the behavior is observed to occur at all during these intervals, the interval is scored.

When both a primary and a secondary observer record behavior for each interval, there are four possible outcomes: (1) They may agree on occurrence (see Figure 2.3, intervals 4, 5, 12, 13, 18, 19, and 20), (2) they may disagree, with the primary observer recording occurrence and the secondary observer recording nonoccurrence, (see Figure 2.3, intervals 1, 2, 9, 10, and 16), (3) they may disagree, with the primary observer recording nonoccurrence and the secondary observer recording occurrence (see Figure 2.3, intervals 14 and 15), and (4) they may agree on nonoccurrence (see Figure 2.3, intervals 3, 6, 7, 8, 11, and 17).

The data presented in Figure 2.3 have been summarized, and the intervals in which each of these agreement/disagreement conditions occurred is presented below the interval data. With each of the four possible outcomes

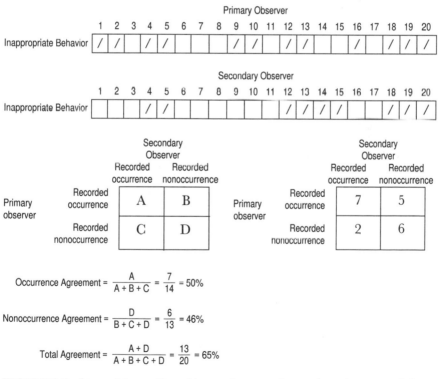

FIGURE 2.3. Interval data collected by a primary and secondary observer and three procedures for calculating interobserver agreement for interval recording.

totaled, it is possible to calculate three different percent interobserver agreement scores. In many instances these three formulas will yield different interobserver agreement percentage scores. These interobserver agreement percentages can be systematically influenced by the occurrence and nonoccurrence rates of recorded behaviors. In some instances, target behaviors occur infrequently and occurrence is rarely recorded. Thus, observers often agree on nonoccurrence. This can cause a high percentage of agreement in both total interobserver agreement and nonoccurrence interobserver agreement even when observers rarely agree on occurrence of the target behavior. In these cases, a more conservative estimate of interobserver agreement would be percent agreement for occurrence, because intervals in which both observers scored nonoccurrence are excluded. In other instances, behaviors occur frequently and occurrence is recorded for most intervals. In these cases, percent agreement for nonoccurrence provides a more conservative estimate of interobserver agreement.

Because target behavior levels can systematically affect percent interobserver agreement scores, in reporting interobserver agreement data it is essential to indicate which formula was used to calculate interobserver agreement. Typically, interobserver agreement is reported with a mean score (e.g., average interobserver agreement across sessions was 87%) and the range of session interobserver agreement scores (e.g., session interobserver agreement ranged from 72% to 95%).

Improving Interobserver Agreement

Several procedures can be used to improve interobserver agreement. One reason for the lack of interobserver agreement may be poor operational definitions. If operational definitions include unobservable events that require observers to make judgments, then it is often more difficult to obtain interobserver agreement.

Altering the recording system may increase observer accuracy and consistency. Lack of interobserver agreement can be caused by extremely complex systems that require observers to record many different behaviors consecutively. Reducing the number of behaviors recorded can enhance interobserver agreement. Altering the recording system to reduce continuous evaluation requirements may result in more accurate and consistent recording. For example, it is often easier to record data accurately using momentary time sampling as opposed to continuous whole-interval time sampling. Finally, increasing the amount of time observers spend training, using consistent training procedures across multiple observers or training multiple observers simultaneously, training observers in natural environments, and providing corrective feedback during training sessions can increase consistency of observer's recordings.

Although interobserver agreement is generally calculated by sessions, a phenomenon known as "observer drift" suggests that these data should also be collected over time. Observer drift occurs when observers do not consistently record behaviors. In fact, the process of collecting direct observation data can cause this drift. Kazdin (1977) suggests some procedures that may help reduce observer drift. First, continuous training is recommended. A useful method for assessing and correcting drift is to use videotapes. Tapes can be made of the target student in the natural setting, or training tapes can be designed to provide opportunities to practice recording direct observation data using a specific recording system. An observer can record data using these videotapes early on and then record data from the same videotapes after they have collected some direct observation data. By comparing their recording data on the same tapes, observers may be able to identify where drift is occurring and use this feedback to correct or prevent drift. Another procedure is to initially train three observers so that they are obtaining high levels of interobserver agreement. Because both the primary and secondary observer record data on a regular basis, they may be more susceptible to drift. However the third observer could then collect data very infrequently throughout the study. Because this observer has not been collecting data as often as the primary and secondary observers, this third observer may be less likely to alter her data collection procedures. Thus, comparing the third observer's data with the primary and secondary observer's data may allow one to identify, prevent, and remedy problems related to observer drift.

THE DATA COLLECTION PROCESS

Although school psychologists can enter the classroom and collect direct observation data using the procedures that have been described, more reliable and valid data may be obtained in a more resource-efficient manner when someone else collects the data. In this section we address procedural concerns related to school psychologists entering the classroom to collect direct observation data. Situations in which it may be preferable to have teachers and peers collect data are also described.

School Psychologist or Other External Observer

Even after data collection procedures are established, several process issues should be addressed before a school psychologist enters a classroom to collect data. Much of the information required to make these decisions can be collected during preobservation teacher interviews. A concern with having a school psychologist or other person who is not a typical part of the classroom milieu collect data is that his or her presence in the classroom is likely to be

conspicuous and cause reactivity. Such reactivity can threaten the validity of direct observation data. Several variables have been shown to cause reactivity, including the rationale for the observation, the personal attributes of the observer, and the conspicuousness of the observer (Johnston & Bolstad, 1973).

Although school psychologists cannot measure or predict the degree of reactivity that may occur, they can take steps to reduce the probability of its occurrence, even before entering a classroom to collect data. Students are likely to notice the presence of the observer in the classroom and will often ask the teacher about this person (e.g., Who is that person and what is he (she) doing in the room?). By no means should the teacher inform the children that the "psychologist" is there to observe the target child's (e.g., "Johnny's") behavior, as the students are likely to react very differently to that child and such information may stigmatize the target child. However, the teacher should not lie to the students. One option is for the teacher to tell the students that the person is there to observe the classroom (Saudargas & Fellers, 1986). Another option is for the teacher to tell the students nothing and instruct them to ignore the person. In any case, some reactivity is likely to occur, and there is no procedure to (1) predict how much reactivity will occur, (2) measure any reactivity that does occur, or (3) predict or measure the nature of that reactivity (e.g., increase or decrease in target behavior levels).

Students may attempt to interact with the observer. Observers should not respond to student questions or otherwise interact with them, as initial interactions may increase the probability of the student(s) attempting to engage the observer in future interactions. To avoid seeming rude, it may be best for the observer to appear to be extremely busy (fiddling with a taperecorder or shuffling papers). This strategy can be particularly useful during transition times when students may be more likely to attempt to interact with the observer as they are less likely to be engaged in competing behaviors (e.g., working on assignments). It is very difficult to enter a classroom full of students inconspicuously. Therefore, if possible, it may be best for the observer to arrange to enter the class before the students arrive.

The observer also must make decisions regarding when he or she is going to collect direct observation data. Obviously, if the target behavior tends to occur during independent seat work in mathematics, then the school psychologist will want to schedule observations during that time. However, the psychologist may also want to collect direct observation data when the target behavior is not a problem, as these data may allow the observer to identify antecedent and consequent events or general ecological conditions that differ and may be causally related to target behaviors.

Another concern is where the school psychologist will sit while collecting data. Ideally, the psychologist sits in an area where he or she is less conspicuous. Sitting in the back of the room away from the students' general area of

orientation should decrease conspicuousness of the observer and may therefore reduce reactivity. However, the observer must also position him- or herself so that target behaviors, and the environmental events that may affect those behaviors, can be observed. This may require the observer to make slight adjustments in his or her location in the room. Therefore, it is best for the observer to sit in a small, light chair with some open area around the chair so the observer can quickly and unobtrusively adjust his or her view.

Before entering the classroom, the school psychologist may perform a variety of other assessment procedures (e.g., a teacher interview, academic skills assessments). During teacher interviews, arrangements can be made for the direct observation (e.g., what to observe, when to enter the classroom, what the teacher will tell the students about the observer's presence, where the observer will position him- or herself in the room, etc.). Clearly the entire process can cause reactivity in the teacher (i.e., the teacher behaves differently because the observer is in the room collecting data). Because it is difficult to avoid such reactivity, the observer should instruct the teacher to behave in the usual manner and to avoid interacting with the observer while he or she is in the room.

A related, and perhaps more serious, concern is the impact preobservation assessment procedures may have on the target student(s)' behavior. If the student knows that the observer is there to observe him or her, then that student is likely to behave differently. Even if the target child is not directly informed that the observer is there to observe him or her, should the observer have recently conducted preobservation interviews or other assessment procedures with the target child, the child is likely to suspect that the school psychologist is there to observe him or her. Therefore, when attempting to determine whether to conduct such preobservation assessment procedures with the target child, the school psychologist must weigh the potential benefits of the preobservational data against the possibility of direct observation procedures producing invalid data as a result of reactivity. Another option is to have different people conduct the observations and the preobservation assessments that require direct contact with the child.

School psychologists should also monitor their own orientation and behavior while collecting direct observation data. If a school psychologist stares directly at the target child the entire time he or she is in the room, the behavior of the target child is likely to be affected. Thus, one should periodically reorient the head and body while observing the child so that the target child and other children are not aware of who is being observed.

It would be irresponsible to describe all the procedures and concerns related to collecting direct observation data without including a general note of caution. It is important that observers be prepared for the unexpected. For example, observations may be planned perfectly, only to be spoiled by the child being absent on the day observations are scheduled. Another problem

is that while an observer is in the classroom collecting data with the use of interval recording, the tape player may malfunction. Although not all problems can be prevented, it is best to bring a backup tape recorder with fresh batteries, an extra set of headphones or an extra earpiece, and a backup copy of the interval tape.

Internal Observers: Teacher or Peers

It is often difficult for a school psychologist or other observers to collect direct observation data on behaviors that occur at low rates and unpredictable times. In these instances, it is often more resource efficient for the teacher to collect this data. When teachers are collecting direct observation data, it is important for procedures to be constructed in a manner that requires little teacher time and does not cause frequent disruptions to all the teacher's other duties. Therefore, teacher recording is most appropriate when recording systems are simple and data are recorded infrequently on few behaviors. For example, if a behavior occurs at a low rate (e.g., aggression may only occur once or twice a week), a teacher may easily record these behaviors at the end of each school day.

When behaviors occur at high rates and require the teacher to record them immediately after they occur, several simple portable recording devices and procedures can be used. For example, a teacher may move a coin, from several in one pocket, to another pocket, or record behaviors using a simple golf score counter every time the child uses inappropriate language. Finally, teachers can use a form of momentary time sampling to collect direct observation data. For example, a teacher may set a cooking timer or a wristwatch to buzz after a set interval. When the buzz occurs, the teacher looks up and records momentary time sampling data. The audible cues associated with these systems may cause reactivity and disruptive classroom activity and, therefore, should probably not be used for marking brief intervals.

In some instances, a classmate may also observe and record peers' behavior (Fowler, 1986). A variety of interventions have been used that require peers to monitor and record classmates' academic behaviors (e.g., Greenwood, Delquadri, & Carta, 1988; Stern, Fowler, & Kohler, 1988). Furthermore, researchers have shown that same-age peers, younger peers, and students with disabilities can all be trained to accurately observe, evaluate, and record classmates' academic behaviors (Carden-Smith & Fowler, 1984; McCurdy & Shapiro, 1992). Because the process of observing, evaluating, and recording peers' behavior has been shown to enhance the observers' academic skills (Skinner, Shapiro, Turco, Cole, & Brown, 1992), engaging students to observe and evaluate peers' academic behaviors and responding may be an efficient procedure for collecting data that also enhances observer achievement.

Some inappropriate behaviors occur infrequently and are very obvious or intense. These behaviors are easier to monitor, but because they are often punished, students are not likely to perform such behaviors when a teacher is observing them. Therefore, peers may have more opportunities to observe these behaviors. Although there are many advantages to training students to observe, record, and report peers' incidental inappropriate behavior, Hening-ton and Skinner (1998) provide a detailed analysis of the possible negative side effects associated with such a system. First, students tend to focus much of their attention on their peers' incidental inappropriate behaviors. In fact, without any formal training, most students learn at a very young age to tattle (i.e., observe and report peers' inappropriate behaviors). Although this focus on monitoring peers' inappropriate behaviors may enhance students' skills at performing observations, it also tends to draw their attention away from peers' prosocial behaviors. A related issue is peer rejection. Children with high rates of inappropriate behavior may be more likely to be rejected by their peers (Coie, Dodge, & Kupersmidt, 1990). Having peers observe and record classmates' inappropriate behaviors may increase the probability of target students being rejected. Finally, students who misbehave may threaten peers who observe their behavior, in order to prevent them from reporting their observations to their teacher. Given the negative side effects associated with having peers observe, record, and report classmates' inappropriate be-haviors, peer monitoring should be used only when target behaviors are so-cially neutral or appropriate.

CONCLUSIONS

Direct observation in natural settings can provide highly reliable and valid data that can be used to make a variety of important educational decisions. This chapter provides readers with enough information to develop their own direct observation systems. However, the process of constructing these sys-tems is extremely complex, and observers often need to practice using the systems before they can record data in a reliable manner. Therefore, school psychologists should consider learning specific direct observation systems. Preconstructed systems for direct observation have been developed by Alessi and Kaye (1983), Saudargas (1992), and Shapiro (1996) among many others. Each of these systems was developed to measure student behavior in educa-tional ecologies (see Shapiro, 1996, for a brief review and analysis of each code). Martin (1993) has developed a computerized system for collecting these types of data. Learning to record data reliably using any system re-quires an investment in training time. However, school psychologists who ac-quire and master direct observation skills using one system will likely be able to generalize these skills to other systems and/or adapt the systems they learn

to meet their own needs. Given the many and varied uses of direct observation data and the low levels of inference required for interpreting these data, it appears that the time and resources spent in learning direct observation systems and/or procedures can be beneficial (Hintze & Shapiro, 1995).

REFERENCES

Alessi, G. (1988). Direct observation methods for emotional/behavior problems. In E. S. Shapiro & T. R. Kratochwill (Eds.), *Behavioral assessment in schools: Conceptual foundations and practical applications* (pp. 14–75). New York: Guilford Press.

Alessi, G., & Kaye, J. H. (1983). *Behavior assessment for school psychologists*. Kent, OH: National Association of School Psychologists.

Barlow, D. H., & Hersen, M. (1984). *Single case experimental designs: Strategies for studying human behavior*. New York: Pergamon Press.

Barrios, B., & Hartmann, D. P. (1986). The contributions of traditional assessment: Concepts, issues, and methodologies. In R. O. Nelson & S. C. Hayes (Eds.), *Conceptual foundations of behavioral assessment* (pp. 81–110). New York: Guilford Press.

Bergan, J. R., & Kratochwill, T. R. (1990). *Behavioral consultation in applied settings*. New York: Plenum Press.

Binder, C. (1996). Behavioral fluency: Evolution of a new paradigm. *The Behavior Analyst, 19,* 163–197.

Carden-Smith, L. K., & Fowler, S. A. (1984). Positive peer pressure: The effects of peer monitoring on children's disruptive behavior. *Journal of Applied Behavior Analysis, 17,* 213–227.

Carr, E. G. (1993). Behavior analysis is not ultimately about behavior. *The Behavior Analyst, 16,* 47–49.

Coie, J. D., Dodge, K. A., & Kupersmidt, J. B. (1990). Peer group behavior and social status. In S. R. Asher & J. D. Coie (Eds) *Peer rejection in childhood* (pp. 17–59). New York: Cambridge University Press.

Cone, J. D. (1978). The Behavioral Assessment Grid (BAG): A conceptual framework and a taxonomy *Behavior Therapy, 9,* 882–888.

Cone, J. D. (1979). Confounded comparisons in triple response mode assessment research. *Behavioral Assessment, 1,* 85–95.

Cone, J. D. (1988). Psychometric considerations and the multiple models of behavioral assessment. In A. Bellack & M. Hersen (Eds.), *Behavioral assessment: A practical handbook* (pp. 42–66). New York: Pergamon Press.

Ferster, C. B., & Skinner, B. F. (1957). *Schedules of reinforcement*. New York: Appleton-Century-Crofts.

Fowler, S. A. (1986). Peer-monitoring and self-monitoring: Alternatives to traditional teacher management. *Exceptional Children, 52,* 573–581.

Greene, B. F., Bailey, J. S., & Barber, F. (1981). An analysis and reduction of disruptive behavior on school buses. *Journal of Applied Behavior Analysis, 14,* 177–192.

Greenwood, C. R., Delquadri, J. C., & Carta, J. J. (1988). *Class-Wide Peer Tutoring (CWPT): Programs for spelling, math, and reading (training manual)*. Delray Beach, FL: Educational Achievement Systems.

Hartmann, D. P., Roper, B. L., & Bradford, C. C. (1979). Some relationships between behavioral and traditional assessment. *Journal of Behavioral Assessment, 1*, 3–21.

Hayes, S. C., Nelson, R. O., & Jarrett, R. B. (1986). Evaluating the quality of behavioral assessment. In R. O. Nelson & S. C. Hayes (Eds.), *Conceptual foundations of behavioral assessment* (pp. 463–503). New York: Guilford Press.

Henington, C., & Skinner, C. H. (1998). Peer monitoring. In K. Toppins & S. Ely (Eds.), *Peer assisted learning* (pp. 237–253). Hillsdale, NJ: Erlbaum.

Heward, W. L. (1987). Selecting and defining target behaviors. In J. O. Cooper, T. E. Heron, & W. L. Heward (Eds.), *Applied behavior analysis* (pp. 36–58). Columbus OH: Merrill.

Hintze, J. M., & Shapiro, E. S. (1995). Best practices in systematic observation of classroom behavior. In A. Thomas & J. Grimes (Eds.), *Best practices in school psychology–III* (pp. 651–660). Washington DC: National Association of School Psychologists.

House, A. E., House, B. J., & Campbell, M. B. (1981). Measures of interobserver agreement: Calculation formulas and distribution effects. *Journal of Behavioral Assessment, 3*, 37–58.

Johnson, S. M., & Bolstad, O. D. (1973). Methodological issues in naturalistic observation: Some problems and solutions. In L. A. Hamerlynck, L. E. Handy, & E. J. Mash (Eds.), *Behavior change: Methodology, concepts, and practices* (pp. 7–68). Champaign, IL: Research Press.

Johnston, H., & Pennypacker, H. (1980). *Strategies for human behavior research*. Hillsdale, NJ: Erlbaum.

Kazdin, A. E. (1977). Artifact, bias, and complexity of assessment: The ABC's of reliability. *Journal of Applied Behavior Analysis, 10*, 141–150.

Lalli, J. S., Browder, D. M., Mace, F. C., & Brown, K. (1993). Teacher use of descriptive analysis data to implement interventions to decrease students' maladaptive behavior. *Journal of Applied Behavior Analysis, 26*, 277–238.

Lentz, F. E. (1982). *An empirical examination of the utility of partial interval and momentary time sampling as measurements of behavior.* Unpublished doctoral dissertation, University of Tennessee, Knoxville.

Lentz, F. E. (1988). On-task behavior, academic performance, and classroom disruptions: Untangling the target selection problem in classroom interventions. *School Psychology Review, 17*, 243–257.

Lewis, T. J., & Sugai, G. (1996). Functional assessment of problem behavior: A pilot investigation of the comparative effects of teacher and peer social attention on students in general education settings. *School Psychology Quarterly, 11*, 1–19.

Mace, F. C., & Lalli, J. S. (1991). Linking descriptive and experimental analyses in the treatment of bizarre speech. *Journal of Applied Behavior Analysis, 24*, 553–562.

Martin, S. (1993). ! *Observe*. Denton, TX: Psychsoft. [Computer software].

McCurdy, B. L., & Shapiro, E. S. (1992). A comparison of teacher-, peer-, and self-monitoring with curriculum-based measurement in reading among students with learning disabilities. *Journal of Special Education, 26*, 162–180.

Neef, N. A., Mace, F. C., & Shade, D. (1993). Impulsivity in students with serious emotional disturbance: The interactive effects of reinforcer rate, delay, and quality. *Journal of Applied Behavior Analysis, 26*, 37–52.

Perry-Warner, E. (1996). Seizure disorders. In P. J. McLaughlin & P. Wehman (Eds.), *Mental retardation and developmental disabilities* (pp. 173–186). Austin TX: PRO-ED.

Powell, J., Martindale, B., Kulp, S., Martindale, A., & Bauman, R. (1977). Taking a closer look: Time sampling and measurement error. *Journal of Applied Behavior Analysis, 10,* 325–332.

Reschly, D. J., & Ysseldyke, J. E. (1995). School psychology paradigm shifts. In A. Thomas & J. Grimes (Eds.), *Best practices in school psychology–III* (pp. 17–31). Washington DC: National Association of School Psychologists.

Salvia, J., & Ysseldyke, J. E. (1985). *Assessment in special and remedial education* (3rd ed.). Boston: Houghton-Mifflin.

Saudargas, R. A. (1992). *State Event Classroom Observation System* (SECOS). Knoxville: University of Tennessee, Department of Psychology.

Saudargas, R. A., & Fellers, G. (1986). *State–Event Classroom Observation System: Research Edition* (SECOS-R). Knoxville: University of Tennessee, Department of Psychology.

Shapiro, E. S. (1987). *Behavioral assessment in school psychology.* Hillsdale, NJ: Lawrence Erlbaum.

Shapiro, E. S. (1996). *Academic skills problems: Direct assessment and intervention* (2nd ed.). New York: Guilford Press.

Shapiro, E. S., & Skinner, C. H. (1990). Best practices in observational/ecological assessment. In A. Thomas & J. Grimes (Eds.), *Best practices in school psychology–II* (pp. 507–518). Washington DC: National Association of School Psychologists.

Skinner, B. F. (1945). The operational analysis of psychological terms. *Psychological Review, 52,* 270–277.

Skinner, B. F. (1974). *About behaviorism.* New York: Knopf.

Skinner, C. H., & Schook, H. (1995). Assessing mathematics skills. In A. Thomas & J. Grimes (Eds.), *Best practices in school psychology–III* (pp. 731–741). Washington DC: National Association of School Psychologists.

Skinner, C. H., Shapiro, E. S., Turco, T. L., Cole, C. L., & Brown, D. K. (1992). A comparison of self- and peer-delivered immediate corrective feedback on multiplication performance. *Journal of School Psychology, 30,* 101–116.

Sprague, S., Sugai, G., & Walker, H. (1998). Antisocial behavior in schools. In T. S. Watson & F. M. Gresham (Eds.), *Handbook of child behavior therapy* (pp. 451–474). New York: Plenum Press.

Stern, G. W., Fowler, S. A., & Kohler, F. W. (1988). A comparison of two intervention roles: Peer monitor and point earner. *Journal of Applied Behavior Analysis, 21,* 103–109.

Strosahl, K., & Linehan, M. (1986). Basic issues in behavioral assessment. In A. Ciminero, K. Calhoun, & H. Adams (Eds.), *Handbook of behavioral assessment* (2nd ed., pp. 12–46). New York: Wiley Interscience.

Sulzer-Azaroff, B., & Mayer, G. R. (1986). *Achieving educational excellence using behavioral strategies.* New York: Holt, Rinehart, & Winston.

Winette, R. A., & Winkler, R. C. (1972). Current behavior modification in the classroom: Be quiet, be docile. *Journal of Applied Behavior Analysis, 5,* 499–504.

CHAPTER 3

♦♦♦

Analogue Assessment: Emotional/Behavioral Problems

♦

JOHN M. HINTZE
GARY STONER
MARY H. BULL

Mr. Miller, a school psychologist, has been asked by a sixth-grade teacher in his school to provide suggestions for a young girl who refuses to stand up and give a speech in front of the class. Dr. Matthews has been asked by the parents of a kindergarten student for some assistance in managing the noncompliant behavior of their son at home. A special education teacher, Ms. Provost, is interested in assessing the effects of a social skills curriculum she has been using with four students in her classroom. Dr. Brady has been asked to assess the friendship patterns of students in a third-grade classroom.

These are just a few examples of the myriad of assessment situations school psychologists and other school-based professionals encounter daily. However, for those who work in school settings, situations like these pose some of the greater challenges in assessment. Behavioral difficulties that are highly situation specific (e.g., lack of social or peer interaction skills), are hard to access in the natural environment (e.g., noncompliant behavior), or occur at a low frequency (e.g., trouble with public speaking) prove extremely difficult to systematically observe directly. In such situations, analogue measures provide a mechanism by which assessors can simplify and reduce complex behavioral constructs and observe isolated features of more global behavioral repertoires in a more manageable assessment arrangement (Kratochwill, Sheridan, Carlson, & Lasecki, 1999; Shapiro & Kratochwill, 1988).

The purposes of this chapter are to define what is meant by analogue assessment measures and to present the general characteristics of a number of analogue assessment measures used in assessing emotional, behavioral, and social relationship areas of functioning. As a supplement to our chapter that describes the theoretical and research-related background of analogue techniques (Hintze, Stoner, & Bull, 2000), the current chapter focuses on the various enactment and role-play analogues that school-based practitioners may find helpful in assessing complex behavioral patterns of school-age children and youth. Although by definition paper-and-pencil and audio/videotape measures can be considered analogue assessment techniques, attention is focused mainly on those situational analogues that employ enactments and role play, with limited discussion of self- and informant-report measures. For an expanded discussion of various paper-and-pencil and audio/videotape analogues, see Hintze et al. (2000), Eckert, Dunn, Guiney, and Codding (2000), Eckert, Dunn, Codding, and Guiney (Chapter 6, this volume), and Merrell (1999 and Chapter 8, this volume).

WHAT EXACTLY ARE ANALOGUE MEASURES?

Specifically, analogue assessment measures are indirect measurement procedures that reflect how an individual *might* behave in a real-life situation. In comparison to direct measures of behavior (e.g., observation of behavior in natural environments as it naturally occurs), analogue measures purposefully constrain some aspect of either the behavior of interest or the environment in which the behavior is observed. As such, analogue measures typically assess behavior in simulated or hypothetical situations that are set up to mimic the real-life situation in which the behavior of interest usually takes place. The assumption, therefore, is that there is some degree of similarity in how an individual behaves in the simulated setting or arrangement and how the individual behaves naturally (Prout & Ferber, 1988). The observation of the behavior in the analogue setting then serves as a predictor of how an individual is likely to behave in the natural environment.

However, because analogue assessment procedures are less direct than naturalistic observation, it is important that distinctions be made between how an invividual is observed to act in the analogue setting and how the individual behaves outside the analogue. That is, the relationship between behavior in the analogue and behavior in the natural setting is far from perfect. There is no guarantee that a person who is observed under contrived or simulated conditions will act or behave similarly under natural arrangements. For this reason, practitioners must be careful in drawing conclusions based on analogue assessment data. The level of the inferences made will vary as a

function of the extent to which the analogue assessment procedures deviate from the natural setting.

Although analogue assessment procedures have been conceptualized in a number of ways (Gettinger, 1988; McFall, 1977), school-based applications of the procedures are probably most easily categorized according to the method by which participants are asked to respond. Nay (1977), for example, identified four basic measures typically used in analogue assessment: (1) enactment or role-play procedures, (2) paper-and-pencil techniques, and (3) audiotape or (4) videotape procedures.

Enactment and role-play procedures, perhaps most common, require the subject to respond to contrived situations that are artificially arranged, away from the natural environment. More specifically, *enactments* are to those analogue arrangements whereby situations typical to the natural environment are recreated, with the behavior of the individuals systematically observed as it occurs. For example, a school psychologist may recreate a cooperative learning situation outside the classroom and simply observe the interaction patterns among a number of students as they naturally occur. In contrast, in *role plays* it is the behavior of the individual that is contrived or scripted. For example, a school psychologist may assess the social skills of a child by having the child behave as if he or she were meeting a new student for the first time. Unlike enactments, in which the behavior of an individual is free to vary, role plays require the subject to respond in a clearly defined fashion.

Paper-and-pencil analogues, also quite common, require the subject to respond to a stimulus situation presented in a written format. Once the material is read, the subject is asked to respond with either a written, oral, or physical response. For example, in the assessment of peer preference, students may be asked to identify peers whom they would like to accompany them on a "Journey to the Center of the Earth," or peers who should play certain characters in a class play (e.g., role of the "mathematician," the "athlete," etc.). Finally, as they imply, audio- and videotape analogues require that the subject listen to and/or view auditorially or visually presented arrangements and respond either orally, physically, or both.

ANALOGUE ASSESSMENT MEASURES FOR EMOTIONAL CONCERNS

Anxieties, Fears, Phobias, and Depression

Internalizing disorders are widely recognized as being among the most common emotional problems affecting school-age children and youth (Albano,

Chorpita, & Barlow, 1996; Bell-Dolan & Brazeal, 1993; Kashani & Or-vaschel, 1988). In practice, enactments and role plays typically involve simulating a depressive or anxiety-provoking stimulus. Once a child is placed in such a situation, specific behaviors that are representative of the anxious, fearful, or depressive responses are observed and recorded and/or the subject is asked to self-report his or her level of anxiety, depression, or fear, using some type of rating scale (King & Ollendick, 1989).

One of the most common analogue outcome measures used in enactment and role plays is the Behavioral Avoidance Test (BAT; Hamilton & King, 1991; Lang & Lazovik, 1963; Van Hasselt, Hersen, Bellack, Rosenblum, & Lamparski, 1979). In its most typical usage, the BAT follows one of two variations in structure. In the first variation, a situational enactment is created whereby the subject is brought into close proximity or contact with the depressive or anxiety-producing stimulus. Once the subject is placed in the situational enactment, systematic direct observational data are recorded on preestablished criteria. For example, the amount of time spent within the enactment may be recorded (i.e., duration), frequency of engaging in the feared behavior can be noted (e.g., petting a dog), or proximity to the fear- or anxiety-producing stimulus may be measured. It is important that the practitioner decide beforehand what behaviors will be observed and recorded. Guidelines for what to observe and record should be based on the most salient features of the subject's anxious or fearful behavior, or those behaviors that will be the targets for intervention. Unfortunately, there is no specific "test" per se available that specifies administration and scoring procedures. Rather, the practitioner is guided by sound systematic direct observation procedures (cf. Hintze & Shapiro, 1995) for determining target behaviors and recording strategies. In addition to systematic direct observation, self-report measures can also be used, whereby the subject reports on his or her own self-perceived level of discomfort. This procedure is usually conducted with some kind of rating scale, using a Likert-type response format.

In a second enactment and/or role-play variation, the subject is requested to perform each step of a graded hierarchy of observable behaviors that brings the subject closer and closer to the depressive or anxiety-producing stimulus. In addition to systematic direct observation and self-reporting of levels of discomfort, compliance with each step of the hierarchy can serve as an outcome measure. Steps within the hierarchy are best formulated by the practitioner using the process of task analysis (Sulzer-Azaroff & Mayer, 1991). In doing so, the practitioner breaks down a complex skill or behavior into its component parts by carefully observing the desired behavior and specifying the process or procedure that is presumed to be involved in performing the behavior. Each component is stated in order of its occurrence and should set the occasion or prompt the next component or behavior in the

chain. As each step in the process is identified, the subject is requested to perform that step, and the resultant behavior is recorded.

Examples

In an example of a BAT role-play analogue, Esveldt-Dawson, Wisner, Unis, Matson, and Kazdin (1982) treated a 12-year-old girl for anxieties and fears related to school and unfamiliar males. Response to treatment outcomes were assessed with the use of a series of situational analogues (treatment consisted of instructions, performance feedback, participant modeling, and social reinforcement). Five of the role-play analogues involved interactions with unfamiliar males: (1) asking an unfamiliar man for a donation to a children's hospital, (2) asking a salesman about trying on a new pair of shoes, (3) meeting a new male therapist, (4) welcoming a peer's father to the treatment session, and (5) sitting next to an usher at a wedding reception dinner. The five school-related role-play analogues consisted of (1) picking up a graded semester report with a poor mark, (2) being excluded by peers during an art project, (3) speaking in front of a class, (4) being accused of cheating by the teacher, and (5) being sent to the principal for being late.

Each role play lasted approximately 15 minutes. In each role-play analogue, direct observations were made of several target behaviors that included both avoidance (e.g., stiffness of body movements, nervous mannerisms, and a self-rating of anxiety) and prosocial behaviors (e.g., eye contact, quality and amount of appropriate affect, appropriate body movements, and overall social skills). Results showed a rapid reduction in the frequency and rate of avoidance behaviors and a concomitant increase in prosocial behaviors during all role plays. Follow-up role play and anecdotal reports suggested that treatment effects were maintained and generalized to everyday situations.

Butler, Miezitis, Friedman, and Cole (1980) used situational enactments and role plays in the assessment and treatment of 14 fifth- and sixth-grade children who exhibited elevated levels of depression. A series of ten, 1-hour role-play sessions were developed for use in a small group arrangement (approximately six to eight children). Each session followed a specific format: (1) warm-up, (2) review of previous session, (3) specification of a problem, (4) preparation for role play, (5), enactment, (6) discussion and successive enactments, (7) specification of a second problem, (8) summarizing discussion, and (9) homework assignment focusing on newly learned skill. Each session focused on a problem relevant to the depressive children—for example, acceptance and rejection by peers, success and failure, guilt and self-blame, and loneliness. The objectives of each role play were to (1) sensitize the children to personal thoughts and feelings, and to those of others, (2) teach skills that would facilitate social interaction, and (3) teach problem-solving approach strategies for similar situations. Outcomes were assessed with a vari-

ety of self-report instruments, including measures of self-esteem, depression, and locus of control. Results suggested significant reduction in depressive symptoms for children who experienced situational enactments and role plays, as compared with those who experienced cognitive restructuring and control conditions.

Bellak, Kay, and Murrill (1989) report on the development of a unique self-report measure called the Dysphorimeter. It is sometimes difficult for an individual to communicate verbally the exact level and/or severity of a subjective state such as anxiety or depression; thus the Dysphorimeter was created to provide an alternate means of communication. The device consists of a tube attached to a base plate. A slot in the tube permits a selector-slide to be moved up and down the tube, which is divided into 10 equidistant marker stops, with the number 1 at the top of the meter and the number 10 at the bottom. In addition, each marker stop produces an audible tone. A neutral tone is produced at the number 1 stop, and an increasingly unpleasant, screeching tone is heard at each successive movement of the selector-slide toward the number 10. The basic instructions are for the subject to move the selector-slide down until it matches the experienced degree of depression (anxiety, fear, etc.). At each assessment occasion, the subject indicates his or her level of discomfort three times in succession, with the mean of the three ratings serving as the outcome datum for that assessment occasion. Measures are then taken repeatedly over time as an evaluation of treatment outcomes. Practitioners who are unable to obtain such a device can easily construct a substitute using cardboard and an elastic band. First, number from 0 to 10 (or any other number serving as the highest value) in equidistant increments on the cardboard. Take the elastic band (doubling the length of the band from the lowest to highest value on the cardboard) and color approximately half the length with a felt-tip pen. Next, cut small slits in the cardboard at the highest and lowest values and insert the elastic band. Fasten each end of the band together on the backside of the cardboard. As in the process described earlier, the subject is asked to move the colored part of the elastic band up or down the increments until the desired level of discomfort is noted. An alternative for younger children is to replace the numbered values with pictorial representations to guide their judgment (e.g., starting with a happy face and moving to a face with a frown, or with intermediate representations of happiness or sadness).

The Peer Nomination Inventory for Depression (PNID; Lefkowitz & Testiny, 1980) is a paper-and-pencil analogue measure consisting of 14 items for depressive behaviors (i.e., Who often plays alone? Who thinks they are bad? Who doesn't try again when they lose? Who often sleeps in class? Who often looks lonely? Who often says they don't feel well? Who says they can't do things? Who often cries? Who worries a lot? Who doesn't play? Who doesn't take part in things? Who doesn't have much fun? Who thinks others

don't like them? Who often looks sad?), 2 items for popularity (i.e., Whom would you like to sit next to in class? Who are the children you would like to have for your best friends?), and 2 items for happiness (i.e., Who often looks happy? Who often smiles?). Using a sociometric peer nomination strategy, all children in a class, for example, rate each other on all 18 items. An individual child's score is his or her number of peer nominations divided by the total number of students in the classroom. Using a similar methodology, the Teacher Nomination Inventory for Depression (TNID; Lefkowitz & Testiny, 1980) provides teacher ratings of all children in a classroom and can be used as a paper-and-pencil situational analogue much like the PNID.

ANALOGUE ASSESSMENT MEASURES FOR BEHAVIORAL CONCERNS

Noncompliance and Aggression

Together, noncompliance and aggression form one of the most common complaints of parents and teachers of young children (Campbell, 1998). Although considered developmental in nature, current research suggests that the emergence of noncompliance and aggression involve a combination of constitutional and environmental factors. Specifically, such behavior patterns appear to occur as a result of the interaction of early negative temperament (e.g., irritability, quickness to anger, low frustration tolerance) with ineffective parenting skills (Barkley, 1998). Such parenting skills often involve the use of unpredictable, noncontingent aversive verbal and physical exchanges, which lead to the child's adopting an aggressive, noncompliant response repertoire as a means of successfully escaping or avoiding the directives of others (Patterson, 1982; Patterson, Reid, & Dishion, 1992). Although less severe forms of such disobedience may be considered developmentally quite normal, more severe displays of noncompliance, aggression, and other similar forms of discord between children and primary caregivers has been shown to be highly associated with the development of adolescent and adult psychological problems (Patterson et al., 1992).

As is the case with emotional problems, the direct assessment of noncompliance and aggression in the natural environment can be difficult. Because such behaviors generally occur at a lower frequency, opportunities to observe them directly may be few. Furthermore, because these behaviors are often maintained by negative reinforcement, such behavior by a child frequently results in the termination of the specific directive or request. Although the practitioner can structure the environment to prompt the occurrence of externalizing behaviors such as aggression and noncompliance, situational analogues provide an acceptable alternative to direct observation.

Examples

In one of the earliest and most frequently cited situational role-play enactment analogues for compliance, Forehand and McMahon (1981) developed the Child's Game and the Parent's Game. In the Child's Game, the parent is instructed to engage in any activity that the child chooses and to allow the child to decide the nature and rules of play in a free play arrangement. In the Parent's Game, the parent is instructed to engage the child in activities for which the rules are determined by the parent. As such, the Parent's Game serves as a role-play command (compliance) situation. Each situation is directly observed for 5 minutes, with interactions recorded systematically. Parent behaviors of interest include (1) approval statements and physical attention, (2) social attention, (3) questioning, (4) commands, (5) warnings, and (6) time-outs. Child behaviors of interest include (1) compliance, (2) noncompliance, and inappropriate behaviors such as (3) whining, (4) yelling, (5) tantrums, (6) aggression, and (7) inappropriate talk.

More recently, Barkley (1997), in a modified version of Forehand and McMahon's situational analogues, developed the Response Class Matrix. Like the Child's Game and the Parent's Game, the Response Class Matrix involves parent–child interaction and systematic observation of a series of parent commands. To start the role-play analogue, both parent and child are taken to a playroom that contains a sofa, coffee table (with magazines laid on top), armchair, several small worktables, an adult's desk chair, a child's desk chair, or similar arrangements. Toys are placed on the worktable for the child to play with. Parent and child enter the room and are given 5 minutes to become accustomed to the surroundings. Then the parent is instructed to issue a series of commands from one of two sets. Table 3.1 presents the commands for each set.

Recording of behaviors occurs in 1-minute blocks. Within each minute, the observer notes the behaviors of interest that occur. New and repeat commands by the parent are noted within each 1-minute block. The child is given 10 seconds to comply with each command or repeat command. Both compliance and noncompliance to commands are noted. In addition, negative child behaviors are recorded any time the child engages in verbal or nonverbal behavior that suggests refusal, anger, or discouragement in direct response to the parent's original or repeat commands. Examples include saying "No!" to a parent's command, whining, hitting, kicking, saying "I don't want to," pushing, throwing things, throwing tantrums, crying, swearing or name-calling at the parent, or displaying other negative reactions directed toward the parent. Similarly, parent negative behaviors are also noted. These include both verbal statements and nonverbal actions suggesting discouragement, nonacceptance, or disapproval of the child's actions. Examples include "You're a bad boy/girl," "That's not right . . . ," "You'd better watch it . . . ,"

TABLE 3.1. Commands for Response Class Matrix

Set 1	Set 2
1. Stand up, please.	1. Come here and let me fix your shirt/blouse.
2. Open the door.	
3. Give me one of those toys.	2. Put these toys away in their boxes.
4. Put all of the toys in their boxes.	3. Empty that wastebasket into the other one near the door.
5. Put the toys and their boxes on the shelves.	4. Fold these clothes neatly and put them in the box (old child-size clothes are provided).
6. Put the chairs under the tables.	
7. Take off your shoes.	5. Put these metal pegs in the holes in this box (child is given a pegboard).
8. Sit at the table and draw copies of these three designs (geometric designs are given).	6. Walk this black line on the floor slowly, heel to toe (black tape line is on floor).
9. Do this sheet of math problems (math problems are given).	7. Stack these magazines neatly on the table.
10. Put your shoes on.	8. Put the toys back on the table.
	9. Wipe off the table with this cloth.
	10. Pick up these papers on the floor.

or spanking, hitting, yanking the child, or raising the hand in a threatening manner. Finally, parent approval statements are also noted. Examples include both verbal praise (e.g., "Okay," "Good job," "I like it when you . . .") and nonverbal gestures (e.g., pat on the back, hug, kiss, clapping for the child's performance, etc.).

For older adolescents, Robin and Foster (1989) have developed the Parent–Adolescent Interaction Coding System (PAICS). In this role-play analogue, the parent and adolescent are asked to engage in a problem-centered discussion of three topic areas: (1) a *neutral* discussion (e.g., where to go on vacation), (2) a discussion of an area of *disagreement* (e.g., curfew time), and (3) a *positive* discussion (e.g., the most positive characteristic of the other person). The discussions may be audio- or videotaped. Following the discussions, data are summarized using simple global behavioral codes (i.e., positive, negative, neutral) for each participant, or in more detail using six mutually exclusive categories (i.e., put-downs/commands, defends/complains, facilitates, problem solves, defines/evaluates, and talks). Both the Response Class Matrix and the PAICS require a considerable amount of observer training for daily practice.

More recently, with advances in functional analysis, researchers have begun to conceptualize noncompliant and aggressive behavior in a manner similar to that used in the seminal work of Iwata and colleagues (Iwata,

Dorsey, Slifer, Bauman, & Richman, 1982; Iwata, Pace, Kalsher, Cowdery, & Cataldo, 1990). For example, Gable, Hendrickson, and Sasso (1995) provide an excellent example of a situational analogue aimed at determining the functional aspects of noncompliant and aggressive behavior. In the first scenario, the examiner and the child together enter a therapy room set up in a similar manner to that described by Barkley (1997). The child is allowed to play alone while the examiner pretends to do paperwork. Each time the child engages in some type of aggressive behavior (e.g., throwing a toy), the examiner provides social attention in the manner of a reprimand or disapproving statement (e.g., "Don't do that"). All other behaviors are ignored (including positive play behaviors). This enactment is designed to ascertain whether social attention maintains or reinforces (increases) inappropriate behavior. The reasoning is that if the inappropriate behavior increases with increased social attention, such behavior is most likely being used by the child to access social approval and will most likely increase. .

In the second enactment, the child is asked to perform a specific task or activity (e.g, writing the alphabet). With each occurrence of inappropriate aggressive behavior, a preferred toy, edible, or desired activity is presented to the child. If the inappropriate aggressive behavior increases, it is very likely that presenting the preferred item or activity is serving to reinforce the inappropriate action.

In the third scenario, the child is asked to complete an activity similar to that in the second enactment. The activity should be something that the child can do, but may find somewhat difficult without assistance. With help from the examiner, the child begins the activity (i.e., a series of somewhat difficult math problems). For each instance of aggression, the task is removed and the examiner walks away in a manner that provides no social attention. Following a brief pause (and when the aggressive behavior ceases), the examiner reintroduces the task. If the inappropriate behavior functions to remove the unwanted activity, aggressive actions will necessarily increase.

In the fourth condition, the examiner and child are placed in a room with no sources of potential reinforcement (e.g., toys or activities). The examiner ignores all behaviors of the child (other versions may place the child alone in the room). All aggressive behaviors are noted. Because no stimulation or reinforcement is given, aggressive behavior is assumed to provide sensory reinforcement to the child. If the child's aggressive actions cease, it can be concluded that the child is not engaging in the behavior for internal arousal.

Finally, the fifth condition places the child and examiner back in the room with the toys and other items of interest. The child is allowed to play alone or with the examiner. However, rather than provide social disapproval for inappropriate behaviors, the examiner gives frequent social praise for the child's behaving appropriately. In this condition, if social reinforcement

serves as a reinforcer, aggressive behaviors should diminish and prosocial co-operative behaviors increase. Specifically, this scenario is designed to act as a control to the other conditions of assessment.

Each assessment condition should be presented for 10 minutes. Preferably, each condition should be presented three times in a random order. Data on inappropriate acts of aggression or noncompliance for each arrangement should be collected via frequency recording (simply counting each episode of aggression or noncompliance). For decision making, the data for each condition across the three trials can be displayed visually on a graph. If one of the conditions is primarily related to increases in inappropriate behavior, the data for that condition should be clearly separate from the other four. An advantage of this type of analogue is that treatments based on results of the assessment are easily determined. For example, if the inappropriate behavior is maintained by escape or avoidance, extinction procedures should be employed; if the inappropriate behavior is maintained by social attention, intervention should be aimed at providing social attention for appropriate behaviors; and so on. Although the literature base is still emerging, such functional analytic procedures are among the most exciting and efficacious treatment procedures available.

ANALOGUE ASSESSMENT MEASURES FOR SOCIAL BEHAVIOR

Social Skills and Competence

The term "social skills" has been defined in a variety of ways. Typically, a distinction is made between "social skills" and "social competence." Social skills are defined as discrete, learned behaviors exhibited by an individual for the purpose of performing a task (Sheridan & Walker, 1999). Children with social skill deficits do not have the necessary social skills in their repertoires, or they may not know a critical step in the performance of a behavioral sequence (Gresham, 1988). For example, a child may not know how to take turns in playing a game, how to introduce him- or herself to others, or how to give a compliment. Social competence, however, is primarily concerned with the evaluative judgments of others (Gresham, 1986). In practice, social competence has generally referred to the global terms and descriptions used by others to describe the behavior of a target child.

The assessment of social skills and competence has received considerable attention in the school psychology literature (Demaray et al., 1995). Research has shown that children who persistently exhibit social skill and competence deficits often experience both short- and long-term negative consequences (Elliott, Sheridan, & Gresham, 1989). For example, peer relationship

problems have been shown to be relatively stable over time (Coie & Dodge, 1983) and to be predictive of later adult psychopathology (Parker & Asher, 1987). In addition, social skill and competence deficits have been linked to poor academic adjustment for children with (McKinney & Speece, 1983) and without disabilities (Hoge & Luce, 1979).

Examples

Historically, one of the most common situational analogue methods for evaluating social competence has been the use of sociometric techniques. Contemporary sociometric techniques generally employ one of two different assessment methods: peer nominations and peer ratings. The basic procedure in using peer nominations is to have children nominate peers according to certain nonbehavioral criteria (Gresham & Elliott, 1984). For example, children are asked to nominate other children as best friends, preferred play partners, work partners, or for their physical attributes. The nomination procedures assess children's attitudes or preferences for engaging in certain activities with specified peers, rather than specific behaviors of the target children (Gresham & Elliott, 1984). Peer nomination can also be used to evaluate negative criteria such as least liked peers or least preferred play or work partners.

One of the most frequently used sociometric models was developed by Coie, Dodge, and Coppotelli (1982). Based on standard scores derived from peer nominations using both positive and negative evaluative statements, children are classified in one of five sociometric status groups: (1) popular, (2) neglected, (3) rejected, (4) controversial, and (5) average. In the model's simplest form, each child in a class is asked to select, from all other children in the class, three peers they like most and three peers they like least. For each student, all peer nominations are summed to yield a liked most (LM) and liked least (LL) score. These scores are then used to calculate social preference (SP) and social impact (SI) scores. Social preference is found by subtracting the liked least score from the liked most score ($SP = LM - LL$). Social impact is derived by adding the liked most score to the liked least score ($SI = LM + LL$).

Interpretation is guided by first standardizing the scores for the entire class on each variable (standardized scores should have a mean of 0 and a standard deviation of 1). This can easily be accomplished with most spreadsheet computer software programs. Once the scores are standardized, an individual child's score can be determined relative to other students in the class. Sociometric status groups are classified according to the following criteria: (1) *popular* includes children receiving SP scores greater than 1.00, LM scores greater than 0, and LL scores of less than 0; (2) *controversial* consists of children who receive SI scores greater than 1.00, and LL and LM scores greater than 0; (3) *neglected* consists of children who receive (SI) scores of less

than −1.00 and absolute LM scores of 0; (4) *rejected* includes children receiving SP scores less than −1.00, LL scores greater than 0, and LM scores less than 0; and (5) *average* refers to children who fall at or around the mean of the social preference (SP) and social impact (SI) dimensions.

In another instance, Bower (1969) described the use of the Class Play. In this assessment technique, children are asked to assign other class members to various roles, both positive and negative, in an imaginary play. For example, children may be asked to cast peers in the parts of different characters— one who is "too bossy," another who is "a born leader," and so forth. In the original scoring, the total number of negative roles assigned to a child is divided by the total number of assigned roles overall. High percentages indicate elevated levels of peer rejection, and lower percentages suggest higher social status.

The "guess who" technique is another sociometric measure whereby brief descriptive personality characteristic statements are provided to a group of children. Each child is then asked to write down the names of other children in the class who fit a description (Merrell, 1999). For example, the children may be asked to list other children who "are the teacher's pets," who "fight with other children," or who "do best in their schoolwork." The content of the descriptive statements can be developed by the teacher or practitioner, based on the specific characteristics they are interested in identifying. Scoring is completed by a simple frequency count for each child on each descriptive statement.

In contrast to peer nomination procedures, peer rating procedures require each child within the class to respond to a sociometric question about all other children in the class. In its most typical form, each child is provided with a class roster and a list of sociometric statements. Each child is then asked to rate all of the other children on each sociometric statement on a 5-point scale (Connolly, 1983). For example, a child may be asked to evaluate the extent to which he or she would like to "play with" or "work with" each other child in the class on a scale ranging from "not at all" to "very much" (Merrell, 1999).

In an extension of peer ratings, teachers are asked to rank order each child in the class according to certain sociometric criteria (Merrell, 1999). For example, all the children in the class may be rank ordered from highest to lowest on attributes such as "popularity" or "disruptiveness." As an alternative, a teacher may first be asked to identify all children who fit a particular social or behavioral description (e.g., disruptiveness) and then to rank order those children from highest to lowest with respect to the particular attribute. In this case, not all children in the class are ranked.

Situational role plays and enactments also lend themselves to the assessment of social skills. In contrast to sociometric measures, role plays and enactments allow practitioners to actually observe the behavior of interest, per-

mit a greater degree of control over selected social stimuli, and, in general, are more acceptable in terms of the manner in which data are collected. With the use of role play measures, a child is presented with a specific interpersonal situation and asked to respond as if the situation were actually occurring. The response of the targeted child is observed and recorded according to a predetermined set of response alternatives. The situations presented to the child are typically representative of those situations in which the child has suggested that he or she has difficulty (Shapiro & Kratochwill, 1988). For example, a role-play test may ask a child to demonstrate how he or she would ask the teacher for help, give a compliment to another child, or accept negative criticism.

In assessing the assertiveness of children, Bornstein, Bellack, and Hersen (1977) developed the Behavioral Assertiveness Test for Children (BAT-C). The BAT-C consists of nine scenes, five involving a same-sex role model and four involving an opposite-sex role model. An attempt was made to include situations that children were likely to engage in daily with other children. Table 3.2 provides the nine scenes of the BAT-C. Following an initial practice scene and a summary of what the role play will entail, the assessment sessions proceed as follows: (1) the narrator presents the scene, (2) the role model delivers a prompt (standard lead-in), (3) the child then responds to the role model.

The authors suggest that the child's responses be videotaped on three separate occasions per week, for four weeks, and rated on three components of assertive behavior and an overall assertiveness score. The first component, *ratio of eye contact to speech duration,* is defined as the total length of time in seconds that the child looked at the role model while he or she (the child) was speaking. A ratio is formed by dividing the total duration of eye contact while speaking by the duration of speech. The second component, *loudness of speech,* is rated on a 5-point scale from 1 (very low) to 5 (appropriately loud). The third component, *requests for new behavior,* is scored when the child showed evidence that he or she wanted the role model to change his or her behavior (e.g., a child had to ask the boy who cut in front of him at the movie to step to the end of the line). Requests for new behavior are scored simply as occurring or not occurring in each scene. Finally, *overall assertiveness* is scored by two outside judges, not familiar with the purposes of the vignettes, to rate the child's overall assertiveness on a 5-point scale, with 1 indicating "very unassertive" and 5 indicating "very assertive."

More recent examples of situational role plays in the area of social skill development can be found in Elliott and Gresham (1991). As an adjunct to their rating scale, the authors have developed a number of role-play analogues in the areas of cooperation, assertion, responsibility, empathy, and self-control. Table 3.3 presents examples of skills assessed in various domains. For each skill area, a number of situational role-play analogues are described.

TABLE 3.2. Role-Play Scenarios for the BAT-C

Female model

- *Narrator:* You're part of a small group in science class. Your group is trying to come up with an idea for a project to present to the class. You start to give your idea, when Amy begins to tell hers also.

  Prompt: "Hey, listen to my idea."

- *Narrator:* Imagine you need to use a pair of scissors for a science project. Betty is using them, but promises to let you have them next. But when Betty is finished, she gives them to Ellen.

  Prompt: "Here's the scissors, Ellen."

- *Narrator:* Pretend you lent your pencil to Joannie. She comes to give it back to you and says that she broke the point.

  Prompt: "I broke the point."

- *Narrator:* Imagine you're about to go to art class when Cindy asks you if she can use your desk while you're gone. You agree to let her use it, but tell her that you'll need it when you get back. When you come back from art class, Cindy says she still needs to use your desk.

  Prompt: "I still need to use your desk."

Male or female model

- *Narrator:* Your class is going to put on a play. Your teacher lists the parts, asking for volunteers. She reads a part you like, and you raise your hand. But (Steve/Sue) raises (his/her) hand after you do and says that (he/she) would like to get the part.

  Prompt: "I want to play this part."

Male model

- *Narrator:* You're playing a game of kickball in the schoolyard and it's your turn at bat. But Bobbie decides he wants to bat first.

  Prompt: "I want to bat first."

- *Narrator:* Imagine you're playing a game of four squares in gym. You make a good serve into Barry's square. But he says that it was out and keeps the ball to serve.

  Prompt: "It's my turn to serve."

- *Narrator:* You're in school and you have taken your chair to another classroom to watch a movie. You go out to get a drink of water. When you come back, Mike is sitting in your seat.

  Prompt: "I'm sitting here."

- *Narrator:* Imagine you're standing in line for lunch. Jon comes over and cuts in front of you.

  Prompt: "Let me cut in front of you."

Data from Bornstein, Bellack, and Hersen (1977).

TABLE 3.3. Examples of Role Plays from the Social Skills Intervention Guide

Cooperation domain

Working and playing subdomain

- Ignoring distractions from classmates when doing classwork
- Making transitions from one classroom activity to another without wasting time or disrupting others

Classroom interaction subdomain

- Paying attention to and following teacher's instructions
- Using time appropriately while waiting for help

Assertion domain

Conversation subdomain

- Giving a compliment to a peer
- Introducing oneself to new people
- Making positive self-statements

Joining and volunteering subdomain

- Volunteering to help peers with classroom tasks
- Inviting others to join activities

Responsibility domain

- Asking an adult for help or assistance
- Refusing unreasonable requests from others
- Answering the telephone
- Questioning rules that may be unfair
- Responding to a compliment from a peer

Empathy domain

Positive feedback subdomain

- Telling adults when they do something for a student that he or she likes or appreciates
- Nonverbally greeting or acknowledging others

Active listening subdomain

- Feeling sorry for others when bad things happen to them
- Listening to adults when they are talking or giving instructions

Self-control domain

Conflict resolution subdomain

- Compromising in conflict situations with peers or adults by changing ideas to reach agreement
- Responding to peer pressure appropriately

Anger control subdomain

- Responding to teasing from peers appropriately
- Responding appropriately when pushed or hit by other children
- Receiving criticism well

Data from Elliot and Gresham (1991).

Situations are presented by the examiner, and the target child is requested to (1) define the skill being prompted, (2) tell why the skill is important, (3) state the skill steps and repeat them with the examiner, and (4) demonstrate the skill within the context of the situational analogue. Although no specific scoring is noted, data can be recorded on each of the four child-prompted requests (i.e., steps 1–4, as noted).

ANALOGUE ASSESSMENT MEASURES OF INTERPERSONAL PROBLEM SOLVING

As in the area of social skills, situational enactments and role plays have had an important part in the treatment of social perception. However, unlike other areas in which situational analogues have been used primarily for assessment, their use in interpersonal problem solving has largely focused on treatment design and intervention. This may be due to the fact that difficulties in interpersonal problem solving and social skill deficits are largely interrelated. That is to say, in many cases, the types of situational enactments and role plays discussed in the area of the assessment of social skills can also be used and adapted for use in interpersonal problem solving.

Although it remains unclear whether the nature of the relationship between emotional/behavior problems and social difficulties is primarily causal, correlational, or simply concomitant (see Gresham, 1988, for a discussion of these types of relationships), the importance of social difficulties among children with such problems is quite clear. Impaired social relationships are highly correlated with suboptimal academic, social, emotional, and occupational outcomes.

Interpersonal problem solving and social–cognitive functioning in children involves their beliefs and perceptions surrounding daily interactions with others, including how successful or unsuccessful they are in given situations, how others perceive their social acumen, and how others experience and react to given situations. The accuracy (or inaccuracy) of these perceptions, and the degree to which they correspond with those of peers, parents, and teachers, appears to play an important role in shaping the social behavior and functioning of children with emotional and behavior problems (Dodge, Pettit, McClaskey, & Brown, 1986; Lochman, Dunn, & Klimes-Dougan, 1993). For example, aggressive children have been shown to misinterpret a peer's intent as hostile during social interactions (Patterson et al., 1992), and children with attention-deficit/hyperactivity disorder (ADHD) appear to consistently overrate their own social acumen and social status (Diener & Milich, 1997; Milich & Okazaki, 1991). Such inaccurate judgments in the context of social relationship development can produce disastrous effects on decisions, choices, and outcomes for these children (see Rach-

lin, 1989, for a cognitive–behavioral discussion of the relationship between judgment, decision, choice, and outcomes).

Examples

Perhaps one of the best examples of the use of situational analogues in the area of interpersonal problem solving comes from the extensive work of Goldstein (1999). Over the course of 20 years, Goldstein has developed a plethora of enactments and role plays for assessment and treatment, focusing on anger control, moral reasoning, stress management, problem solving, and empathy training. The most recent rendition of this work is found in *The Prepare Curriculum* (Goldstein, 1999), which contains a number of situational role plays for use in interpersonal problem solving. In an example of situational perception training entitled "The Right Time and Place," two students and the teacher act out a scene in which one child observes the other stealing money from the teacher's purse while she is out of the room. When the teacher returns to the room, the child who has observed the stealing publicly announces what he saw. The boy accused of stealing is sent to the principal's office. As he leaves the classroom, he makes a fist at the accuser and says, "You are dead today after school. I'm going to kill you. Just wait!" Once the role play has been conducted, the whole class answers questions such as the following: (1) Do you think it was right for the boy to tell the teacher about the other boy's stealing the money? (2) Do you think the accuser chose the right time and place to tell his teacher? and (3) How could the accuser have been more discreet when he told his teacher?

In another instance, students are presented with a scenario in written form and asked to answer a series of questions, first silently to themselves, and then collectively as a group. In one example, a situation is described in which a teacher leaves the class while a math test is being administered. When leaving she tells the students that they are on their honor not to cheat. Once she is out of the room, one boy whispers to another, "Let me see your answers." Questions regarding the situation are first answered individually (e.g., "Should Antonio let Ed copy his answers?" "What if Ed whispers that cheating is no big deal—that he knows plenty of guys who cheat all the time? Then should Antonio let Ed cheat?"), then discussed as a group.

In an example more akin to a situational enactment, Elias and Tobias (1996) describe the "Classroom Constitution." The goal of this situational analogue is to teach students the importance of rules and to give them an experience in group decision making. First, the group leader discusses the United States Constitution in a general manner and suggests that a class constitution would be helpful to the class. Next, the class generates a list of "articles" for appropriate classroom behavior. This list may include both "do's" and "don'ts." Once an initial list is completed, a discussion of each article ensues;

some rules are kept, some amended, and others discarded. The final product contains the "laws" of the class.

Other examples of interpersonal problem solving curricula, which contain numerous models of situational enactments and role plays, include the ACCEPTS program (Walker et al., 1983), the Social Skills in the Classroom program (Stephens, 1992), and the Think Aloud program (Camp & Bash, 1981), to name just a few. Each of these provides numerous examples of role plays that can be used in the treatment of difficulties in interpersonal problem solving.

SUMMARY AND CONCLUSIONS

Analogue assessment techniques comprise a collection of related measurement techniques that allow practitioners to gather important indirect information across a variety of psychological constructs. As can be seen, anxiety, deficiency in social skills, and noncompliant conduct are just a few of the many constructs that can be assessed with the use of analogue procedures. Perhaps the best use of analogue assessment measures is in screening and the monitoring of intervention effectiveness. As a screening tool, analogue measures can quickly help identify behavioral subcomponents of emotional and behavioral disorders, and identify individuals who may be at risk for developing emotional and behavioral difficulties. Furthermore, as part of a comprehensive assessment system, analogue methods lend themselves quite well to the ongoing monitoring of intervention effectiveness. Because analogue methods are often incorporated into various treatment efforts, the distinction between assessment and intervention is often seamless. From a behavioral perspective, such assessment methods are considered the hallmark of sound assessment.

In addition, analogue assessment procedures appear to have some utility in identifying children who may benefit from specialized interventions. However, because of their somewhat limited scope, it is recommended that analogue assessment methods be fortified with other assessment methods (e.g., systematic direct observation, semistructured interviews, informant report). Practitioners should also be mindful, when choosing and developing analogues, to mirror as closely as possible the real world in which the individual will ultimately be asked to function. For example, developing an analogue that asks a child to respond to a situation in which "another child cuts in front of you on the miniature golf course" may have little or no relevance for a child raised and living in an urban setting. Clearly, it is important that practitioners strive to choose and develop analogue methods that are culturally sensitive and reflect those skills and behaviors that are asked of the child in everyday life.

Although analogue assessment procedures offer a number of advan-

tages as compared with other forms of assessment (e.g., direct observation in the natural setting), the methods are not without their shortcomings. Of greatest importance is that because most analogue methods are not standardized, the reliability and validity of the information gathered may be challenged. In comparison with other forms of assessment, the psychometric properties of most analogue procedures are far less well established. Very simply, analogue assessment procedures *should not* be used for making high-stakes diagnosis/classification or placement decisions. Clearly, decisions of this magnitude require the use of assessment techniques that have been proven both reliable and valid in making such decisions. The only possible use of analogue methods in this regard is in confirming or disconfirming other data with known and acceptable psychometric properties.

Second, the generalizability of data gathered through analogue assessment procedures is also in question. That is, to what extent do the data gathered from a highly structured and controlled environment generalize to situations in which there is less control of the environmental arrangements? Although the establishment of control is a desired feature of any assessment and intervention strategy, it is very difficult to duplicate the degree of control possible in analogues within the natural classroom environment. Thus, a major limitation of the types of analogues mentioned in this chapter is their overlap with real-world skills, behaviors, activities, and events.

Overall, analogue measures, like many other forms of assessment, carry with them problems and drawbacks. As compared with systematic direct observation in the natural environment, analogue assessment require a greater deal of inference in drawing conclusions about behavior. However, because of the advantages they offer, practitioners should familiarize themselves with the use of these procedures.

REFERENCES

Albano, A. M., Chorpita, B. F., & Barlow, D. H. (1996). Childhood anxiety disorders. In E. J. Mash & R. A. Barkley (Eds.), *Child psychopathology* (pp. 196–241). New York: Guilford Press.

Barkley, R. A. (1997). *Defiant children* (2nd ed.): *A clinician's manual for assessment and parent training* New York: Guilford Press.

Barkley, R. A. (1998). *Attention-deficit hyperactivity disorder: A handbook for diagnosis and treatment* (2nd ed.). New York: Guilford Press.

Bellak, L., Kay, S. R., & Murrill, L. M. (1989). The Dysphorimeter: An objective analogue for the assessment of depression, anxiety, pain, and other dysphoric states. *American Journal of Psychotherapy, 43,* 260–268.

Bell-Dolan, D., & Brazeal, T. J. (1993). Separation anxiety disorder, overanxious disorder, and school refusal. *Child and Adolescent Psychiatric Clinics of North America, 2,* 563–580.

Bornstein, M. R., Bellack, A. S., & Hersen, M. (1977). Social-skills training for unassertive children: A multiple-baseline analysis. *Journal of Applied Behavior Analysis, 10,* 183–195.

Bower, E. (1969). *Early identification of emotionally handicapped children in school* (3rd ed.). Springfield, IL: Thomas.

Butler, L., Miezitis, S., Friedman, R., & Cole, E. (1980). The effect of two school-based intervention programs on depressive symptoms in preadolescents. *American Educational Research Journal, 17,* 111–119.

Camp, B. W., & Bash, M. A. (1981). *Think aloud.* Champaign, IL: Research Press.

Campbell, S. B. (1998). Developmental perspectives. In T. H. Ollendick & M. Hersen (Eds.), *Handbook of child psychopathology* (3rd ed, pp. 3–35). New York: Plenum Press.

Coie, J. D., & Dodge, K. A. (1983). Continuities and changes in children's social status: A five-year longitudinal study. *Merrill-Palmer Quarterly, 29,* 261–282.

Coie, J. D., Dodge, K. A., & Coppotelli, H. (1982). Dimensions and types of social status: A cross-age perspective. *Developmental Psychology, 18,* 557–570.

Connolly, J. A. (1983). A review of sociometric procedures in the assessment of social competencies in children. *Applied Research in Mental Retardation, 4,* 315–327.

Demary, M. K., Ruffalo, S. L., Carlson, J., Busse, R. T., Olson, A. E., McManus, S., & Leventhal, A. (1995). Social skills assessment: A comparative evaluation of six published rating scales. *School Psychology Review, 24,* 648–671.

Diener, M. B., & Milich, R. (1997). Effects of positive feedback on the social interactions of boys with attention deficit hyperactivity disorder: A test of the self-protective hypothesis. *Journal of Clinical Child Psychology, 26,* 256–265.

Dodge, K. A., Pettit, G. S., McClaskey, C. L., & Brown, M. M. (1986). Social competence in children. *Monographs of the Society for Research in Child Development, 51* (2, Serial No. 213).

Eckert, T. L., Dunn, E. K., Guiney, K. M., & Codding, R. S. (2000). Self-reports: Theory and practice in interviewing children. In E. S. Shapiro & T. R. Kratochwill (Eds.), *Behavioral assessment in schools* (2nd ed.): *Theory, research, and clinical foundations* (pp. 288–322). New York: Guilford Press.

Elias, M. J., & Tobias, S. E. (1996). *Social problem solving: Interventions in the schools.* New York: Guilford Press.

Elliott, S. N., & Gresham, F. M. (1991). *Social skills intervention guide: Practical strategies for social skills training.* Circle Pines, MN: American Guidance Services.

Elliott, S. N., Sheridan, S. M., & Gresham, F. M. (1989). Assessing and treating social skills deficits: A case study for the scientist-practitioner. *Journal of School Psychology, 27,* 197–222.

Esveldt-Dawson, K., Wisner, K. L., Unis, A. S., Matson, J. L., & Kazdin, A. E. (1982). Treatment of phobias in a hospitalized child. *Journal of Behavior Therapy & Experimental Psychiatry, 13,* 77–83.

Forehand, R. L., & McMahon, R. J. (1981). *Helping the noncompliant child: A clinician's guide to parent training.* New York: Guilford Press.

Gable, R. A., Hendrickson, J. M., & Sasso, G. M. (1995). Toward a more functional analysis of aggression. *Education and Treatment of Children, 18,* 226–242.

Gettinger, M. (1988). Analogue assessment: Evaluating academic abilities. In E. S. Shapiro & T. R. Kratochwill (Eds.), *Behavioral assessment in schools: Conceptual foundations and practical applications* (pp. 247–289). New York: Guilford Press.

Goldstein, A. P. (1999). *The prepare curriculum* (rev. ed.). Champaign, IL: Research Press.

Gresham, F. M. (1986). Conceptual issues in the assessment of social competence in children. In P. S. Strain, M. J. Guralnick, & H. M. Walker (Eds.), *Children's social behavior: Development, assessment, and modification* (pp. 143–179). New York: Academic Press.

Gresham, F. M. (1988). Social skills: Conceptual and applied aspects of assessment, training, and social validation. In J. C. Witt, S. N. Elliott, & F. M. Gresham (Eds.), *Handbook of behavior therapy in education* (pp. 523–546). New York: Plenum Press.

Gresham, F. M., & Elliott, S. N. (1984). Assessment and classification of children's social skills: A review of methods and issues. *School Psychology Review, 13*, 292–301.

Hamilton, D. I., & King, N. J. (1991). Reliability of a behavioral avoidance test for the assessment of dog phobic children. *Psychological Reports, 69*, 18.

Hintze, J. M., & Shapiro, E. S. (1995). Systematic observation of classroom behavior. In A. Thomas & J. Grimes (Eds.), *Best practices in school psychology–III* (pp. 651–660). Washington, DC: National Association of School Psychologists.

Hintze, J. M., Stoner, G., & Bull, M. H. (2000). Analogue assessment: Research and practice in evaluating emotional and behavioral problems. In E. S. Shapiro & T. R. Kratochwill (Eds.), *Behavioral assessment in schools* (2nd ed.): *Theory, research, and clinical foundations* (pp. 104–138). New York: Guilford Press.

Hoge, R. D., & Luce, S. (1979). Predicting academic achievement from classroom behavior. *Review of Educational Research, 49*, 479–496.

Iwata, B., Dorsey, M., Slifer, K., Bauman, K., & Richman, G. (1982). Toward a functional analysis of self-injury. *Analysis and Intervention in Developmental Disabilities, 2*, 3–20.

Iwata, B., Pace, G., Kalsher, M., Cowdery, G., & Cataldo, M. (1990). Experimental analysis and extinction of self-injurious escape behavior. *Journal of Applied Behavior Analysis, 23*, 11–27.

Kashani, J. H., Orvaschel, H. (1988). Anxiety disorders in midadolescence: A community sample. *American Journal of Psychiatry, 145*, 960–964.

King, N. J., & Ollendick, T. H. (1989). Children's anxiety and phobic disorders in school settings: Classification, assessment, and intervention issues. *Review of Educational Research, 59*, 431–470.

Kratochwill, T. R., Sheridan, S. M., Carlson, J., & Lasecki, K. L. (1999). Advances in behavioral assessment. In C. R. Reynolds & T. B. Gutkin (Eds.), *The handbook of school psychology* (pp. 350–382). New York: Wiley.

Lang, P. J., & Lazovik, A. D. (1963). Experimental desensitization of a phobia. *Journal of Abnormal and Social Psychology, 66*, 519–525.

Lefkowitz, M. M., & Testiny, E. P. (1980). Assessment of childhood depression. *Journal of Consulting and Clinical Psychology, 48*, 43–50.

Lochman, J. E., Dunn, S. E., & Klimes-Dougan, B. (1993). An intervention and consultation model from a social cognitive perspective: A description of the Anger Coping Program. *School Psychology Review, 22*, 458–471.

McFall, R. M. (1977). Analogue methods in behavioral assessment: Issues and prospects. In J. D. Cone & R. P. Hawkins (Eds.), *Behavioral assessment: New directions* (pp. 152–177). New York: Brunner/Mazel.

McKinney, J. D., & Speece, D. C. (1983). Classroom behavior and the academic progress of learning disabled students. *Journal of Applied Developmental Psychology, 4*, 149–161.

Merrell, K. W. (1999). *Behavioral, social, and emotional assessment of children and adolescents.* Mahwah, NJ: Erlbaum.

Milich, R., & Okazaki, M. (1991). An examination of learned helplessness among attention deficit hyperactivity disordered boys. *Journal of Abnormal Child Psychology, 19*, 607–623.

Nay, W. R. (1977). Analogue measures. In A. R. Ciminero, K. S. Calhoun, & H. E. Adams (Eds.), *Handbook of behavioral assessment* (pp. 233–277). New York: Wiley.

Parker, J. G., & Asher, S. R. (1987). Peer relations and later personal adjustment: Are low-accepted children at risk? *Psychological Bulletin, 102*, 357–389.

Patterson, G. R. (1982). *Coercive family process.* Eugene, OR: Castalia.

Patterson, G. R., Reid, J. B., & Dishion, T. J. (1992). *Antisocial boys: A social interactional approach.* Eugene, OR: Castalia.

Prout, H. T., & Ferber, S. M. (1988). Analouge assessment: Traditional personality assessment measures in behavioral assessment. In E. S. Shapiro & T. R. Kratochwill (Eds.), *Behavioral assessment in schools: Conceptual foundations and practical applications* (pp. 322–350). New York: Guilford Press.

Rachlin, H. (1989). *Judgment, decision, and choice: A cognitive/behavioral synthesis.* New York: W. H. Freeman.

Robin A. L., & Foster, S. L. (1989). *Negotiating parent–adolescent conflict: A behavioral–family systems approach.* New York: Guilford Press.

Shapiro, E. S., & Kratochwill, T. R. (1988). Analogue assessment: Methods for assessing emotional and behavioral problems. In E. S. Shapiro & T. R. Kratochwill (Eds.), *Behavioral assessment in schools: Conceptual foundations and practical applications* (pp. 290–321). New York: Guilford Press.

Sheridan, S. M., & Walker, D. (1999). Social skills in context: Considerations for assessment, intervention, and generalization. In C. R. Reynolds & T. B. Gutkin (Eds.), *The handbook of school psychology* (3rd ed., pp. 686–708). New York: Wiley.

Stephens, T. M. (1992). *Social skills in the classroom.* Columbus, OH: Cedars Press.

Sulzer-Azaroff, B., & Mayer, G. R. (1991). *Behavior analysis for lasting change.* New York: Harcourt Brace.

Van Hasselt, V. B., Hersen, M., Bellack, A. S., Rosenblum, N. D., & Lamparski, D. (1979). Tripartite assessment of the effects of systematic desensitization in a multi-phobic child: An experimental analysis. *Journal of Behavior Therapy & Experimental Psychiatry, 10*, 51–55.

Walker, H. M., McConnell, S. R., Holmes, D., Todis, B., Walker, J., & Golden, H. (1983). *The Walker social skills curriculum: The ACCEPTS program.* Austin, TX: Pro-Ed.

CHAPTER 4

◆◆◆

Functional Analysis

◆

JENNIFER J. McCOMAS
HANNAH HOCH
F. CHARLES MACE

Teachers are faced with the task of ensuring that students acquire skills that will contribute to their ability to be independent and to lead full and productive lives. This must be accomplished despite the fact that resources are shrinking and students arrive in classrooms with an ever-increasing diversity of strengths and needs. An area that poses particular difficulties for teachers in their efforts to provide effective instruction is severe and persistent problem behavior. Although most students do not present serious behavior problems, the small number who do can be very disruptive to the learning environment, which can affect everyone in the classroom (Smith & Rivera, 1994). During the course of the average day, students may engage in a wide variety of disruptive behaviors, including refusal to follow directions, swearing, property destruction, aggression toward peers or teachers, and self-injurious behavior. Student misbehavior has several negative effects. First, valuable instructional time is lost while the teacher attempts to interrupt, intervene, and remedy the situation. Second, peers may fail to form friendships with students who engage in disruptive behavior. Third, teachers may be less enthusiastic about working with a student who causes severe disruptions to the learning environment. Although these effects may be temporary, the quality and quantity of future peer–student, teacher–student, and instructional interactions may be compromised. Thus, an effective technology for managing problem behavior is a crucial need of all teachers (Schloss & Smith, 1998).

The continued occurrence of serious problem behavior in schools has resulted in an ever-growing body of available behaviorally oriented technologies for managing problem behavior. Much research has been conducted on

the effects of interventions such as token economies, time-out, extinction, planned ignoring, contingent exercise, overcorrection, and restitution. Typically, interventions are selected on the basis of what has "worked" in the past for a particular teacher, what has seemed to be effective with other students displaying similar behavior, what the school district endorses, or other nonindividualized criteria. When a particular intervention fails, other interventions are selected and attempted, typically becoming increasingly intrusive and punishing. This "cookbook" approach to treatment selection seldom results in meaningful changes in behavior that are maintained over time.

Although there are numerous interventions for severe and persistent problem behavior, how can an effective intervention be selected? Unlike treatments for some medical problems that are selected according to the form of the malady (e.g., aspirin for a headache), contemporary practice calls for selection of interventions for problem behavior based on the function of the individual's behavior. For example, we do not treat all cases of loud verbal outbursts with planned ignoring; planned ignoring may effectively reduce the frequency of such outbursts in some individuals, but not in many others, including those for whom loud verbal outbursts are related to physiological states (e.g., painful ear infections) or specific disorders (e.g., Tourette's syndrome). Furthermore, in those individuals whose verbal outbursts are maintained by social contingencies, but are treated without regard to function, more severe forms of problem behavior may emerge. Therefore, pretreatment assessment of the social contingencies (i.e., function) of behavior is necessary for the identification of effective intervention.

Functional analysis methodology is a pretreatment assessment that consists of manipulating environmental events to provide information regarding the functional relationship between those events and problem behavior. This methodology can be especially useful to classroom teachers because it is applicable across many forms of problem behavior (disruptive classroom behavior, aggression, property destruction, inappropriate verbalizations, tantrums, self-injury, and reluctant speech) and can result in effective interventions for all groups of children (those with mild, moderate, and severe mental retardation; average abilities; emotional disabilities; autism; learning disorders).

Reliance on "one size fits all" or cookbook models of treatment selection may not produce reliable and durable changes in problem behavior of individuals. Instead, effective interventions for any given individual are based on the function of the target behavior (Iwata, Pace, Kalsher, Cowdery, & Cataldo, 1990; Wacker, Northup, & Cooper, 1991) that is identified via direct observations of changes in the student's behavior in response to manipulations of experimentally controlled environmental conditions (Iwata, Dorsey, Slifer, Bauman, & Richman, 1982/1994). Moreover, the Individuals with Disabilities Education Act (IDEA) Amendments of 1997 (Public Law 105-17) require by law that functional behavioral assessment be conducted and be-

havioral intervention be implemented for children with disabilities, including behavior disorders, prior to any disciplinary action. Thus, if the purpose of pretreatment assessment is to prescribe treatment (Hayes, Nelson, & Jarrett, 1987), the use of direct observation and experimental analyses is recommended over psychometric or indirect measures (Wacker, Northup, & Lambert, 1997).

Pretreatment assessment, such as functional assessment, is a process of gathering information on the events and other variables associated with the occurrence of a target behavior. The information is used to suggest general directions for treatment. A functional analysis involves systematic manipulation of events within a single-case design and results in the identification of the behavior–environmental relations, or behavioral mechanisms, that maintain the problem behavior. Knowledge of these mechanisms permits the specification and individualization of interventions for severe and persistent behavior problems.

The purpose of this chapter is to provide an overview of the behavioral mechanisms typically involved in maintaining problem behavior, to present guidelines for conducting functional analyses in school settings, and to illustrate clinical applications of functional assessment methods employed by practitioners. Two case examples are included to highlight the methods of conducting a comprehensive functional analysis and intervention for problem behavior in an applied setting.

VARIABLES MAINTAINING PROBLEM BEHAVIOR

The functional analysis approach to treating problem behavior begins by identifying the maintaining contingencies for problem behavior. Through the direct and systematic manipulation of environmental variables, relationships between behavior and the environment are specified. Problem behavior is typically maintained by one of four general classes of reinforcement: (1) attention, (2) access to materials or activities, (3) escape or avoidance of demand conditions, (4) sensory (automatic) reinforcement.

Positive reinforcement in the form of attention can maintain problem behavior in a number of ways. The reaction of adults and other children to a student's problem behavior may inadvertently increase the future likelihood of undesirable behavior. Specifically, misbehavior may result in an increased rate, quality, or duration of attention. Moreover, it may be easier to access attention through misbehavior than through desirable behavior. For example, if a child engages in a dangerous behavior, such as dangling heavy objects out of the second-floor classroom window, a host of reactions are probable. First, the student's peers may squeal, laugh, or come running to the window to see what is happening. The teacher may immediately stop what he is doing and

rush over to the student to prevent her from dropping the object. The teacher may then hold a lengthy, serious discussion with the student in private to emphasize why that behavior is dangerous and unacceptable. If these types of reactions (peer excitement; immediate, animated, and lengthy periods of one-to-one teacher attention) are not easily available for desirable behavior (e.g., compliant behavior, academic excellence), several aspects of this scenario can potentially result in an increase in the future probability of similar disruptive behavior.

Access to materials or activities is another form of positive reinforcement that maintains problem behavior. Self-injurious, aggressive, or other disruptive behavior may result in adults or children providing access to materials or activities that are not otherwise accessible. For example, a student who engages in high rates of head hitting may be given a toy to occupy his hands. This consequence of self-injury may temporarily interrupt the undesirable behavior, but may also result in an increased future likelihood of self-injury because the student learns that self-injury results in access to materials.

Negative reinforcement, in the form of escape or avoidance of unpleasant tasks, is a common maintaining variable for problem behavior. Inappropriate behavior can naturally result in the interruption, delay, or termination of a task. For example, a student who tears up her worksheet may postpone having to complete that worksheet. The delivery of a replacement worksheet may be delayed, or the replacement may be not as unpleasant (e.g., difficult, boring) as the original. Similarly, a student who frequently scratches his teacher with enough force to break her skin when she presents a task, may delay having to complete a task while the teacher leaves to clean and dress her wounds. When the teacher returns, there may not be sufficient time to resume the task, or the teacher may be reticent to present tasks for fear of further injury. As problem behavior continues to result in interruption, delays, or termination of tasks, the likelihood of future problem behavior increases.

Finally, problem behavior may be maintained by sensory consequences that occur automatically following a behavior. Sensory reinforcement can involve positive reinforcement (e.g., visual stimulation, auditory stimulation) or negative reinforcement (e.g., pain attenuation). Although problem behavior primarily maintained by sensory reinforcement is not a function of social contingencies, sensory stimuli can be isolated and manipulated within analogue conditions of a functional analysis (e.g., Piazza et al., 1998).

STEPS INVOLVED IN CONDUCTING A FUNCTIONAL ANALYSIS

Although there are four general classes of variables that maintain problem behavior, the specific variables that may be selected for evaluation are nu-

merous, and it is pragmatically impossible to systematically assess all potential events that may influence behavior. In the classroom there are a number of continually changing variables (e.g., varying levels of adult attention, peer-related activities, task demands) that make it difficult to isolate the effect of one or more factors. To allow an approximation of controlling variables, analogue conditions are constructed. These analogue conditions incorporate variables (i.e., stimuli and materials) that represent "real-life" situations but tightly control the presence or absence of those variables to determine the effects of specified stimuli or events on the target behavior.

A comprehensive functional analysis methodology for the assessment of specified behavior problems includes the following steps:

1. Information gathering and descriptive analysis under natural conditions in which the problem behavior occurs (e.g., the classroom)
2. Hypothesis formation regarding the environmental variables that maintain problem behavior
3. Direct assessment of hypothesized maintaining variables under analogue conditions (via single-case design)
4. Developing and implementing intervention
5. Evaluating maintenance and generalization of intervention effects

Gather Information

Before any information is gathered, it is important to specify the target behavior. The behavior of concern should be defined in such a way that the care providers in the natural setting agree on the form and dimensions of the behavior. For example, if the target behavior is aggression, is it defined as *any* touching of another person? If not, what type of physical contact is considered aggression? Does aggression include throwing or destroying objects in the classroom? Without a clearly specified target behavior, the results of the functional analysis may be erroneous. Once a definition is agreed upon, information about the behavior can be gathered directly or indirectly.

Indirect

Information gathered from historical records, interviews, rating scales, and checklists (Aberrant Behavior Checklist [Aman & Singh, 1986, 1994], the Child Behavior Checklist [Achenbach & Edelbrook, 1981], the Conners Teacher Rating Scale [Conners, 1997b], the Conners Parent Rating Scale [Conners, 1997a], and the Parent Attitude Test [Cowen, Huser, Beach, & Rappoport, 1970]) constitutes indirect information. (See Merrell, Chapter 8, and McConaughy, Chapter 7, this volume for further discussion). The information contained in these chapters pertains to the form, frequency, intensity,

and conditions under which the behavior is likely to occur, *as reported by care providers*. Such reports can offer valuable information that can be used in generating hypotheses about the behavior–environmental relations, but are not generally sufficient for the prescription of interventions. When gathering indirect information, the assessor seeks specific "clues" as to the potential events maintaining the problem behavior (e.g., specific antecedents and consequences, physical and social environments, activities, physiological conditions). (See Appendix 4.1 for a sample interview form.)

Direct

Anecdotal recordkeeping, antecedent–behavior–consequence (A-B-C) assessments (Bijou, Petersen, Ault; 1968; O'Neill, Horner, Albin, Storey, & Sprague, 1990), scatterplots (Touchette, MacDonald, & Langer, 1985), and descriptive assessments (Lalli & Goh, 1993; Sasso et al., 1992) are all conducted by directly observing the behavior as it occurs in the natural environment. Examples of some of these are provided in Appendix 4.2. The investigator simultaneously observes and records behavioral events as they occur. The behavior may be objectively described in an anecdotal record, or a description of the behavior and the events preceding and following it may be documented, as is done in A-B-C assessments. Patterns of responding throughout the day can be identified with the use of a scatterplot by recording occurrences of the target behavior on a grid of time slots across successive days. This method of recording, or plotting the occurrence of the problem behavior, allows a visual analysis of possible correlations between the occurrence of the problem behavior and time of day or specific activities. In addition, a descriptive assessment may be conducted in which occurrences of the target behavior and environmental events are recorded during observation sessions. The occurrences of the target behavior, other undesirable behavior, and even desirable behavior are recorded as they occur in relation to ongoing antecedent and consequent events. Conditional probabilities of the occurrence of each behavioral response recorded are then calculated under the specific environmental conditions that were observed and recorded (see Mace & Lalli, 1991, for methods of calculating conditional probabilities based on descriptive assessments). These probabilities, like the information derived from the other methods of direct observation, are used to generate a hypothesis about the environmental conditions in which the problem behavior is most likely to occur. In other words, descriptive assessments help to specify the environmental events that may be correlated with the occurrence of problem behavior.

An assessment strategy that appears to be useful for specifying variables is to employ indirect information gathering and direct observation in the naturally occurring situation to describe the interactions between behavior and

environmental events. This approach to naturalistic observation without manipulating the variables that are associated with a problem behavior has been termed "descriptive assessment" (Bijou et al., 1968; Mace & Lalli, 1991) and is used to identify variables that appear to influence the behavior (i.e., are correlated with the behavior). Those variables are then tested within a more precise functional analysis in which environmental events are systematically manipulated and examined. Descriptive assessments provide direct observational data on the student's behavior in relation to naturally occurring events in the environment. In addition, preliminary observations and caregiver reports often serve to focus the subsequent functional analysis by providing information suggesting that the occurrence of a behavior is related to particular environmental conditions. Thus, information gathered from a wide variety of sources, combined with a descriptive assessment, (1) allows for data-based hypothesis development and (2) provides for direct analogue assessment of maintaining contingencies and intervention development (Lalli & Goh, 1993). This information also specifies the naturally occurring conditions under which the behavior will be expected to be maintained and generalized. However, information gathered without the systematic isolation and manipulation of environmental variables is only suggestive of functional relations that must be further tested in a functional analysis via a single-case design.

Formulate Hypotheses

Based on the information gathered from both indirect and direct sources, one or more hypotheses about the maintaining contingencies for problem behavior are generated. The information may indicate that the behavior occurs at different frequencies in different situations, suggesting that it is probably maintained by specific environmental events. Hypotheses may involve situations in which a social consequence typically follows the problem behavior. For example, if a verbal outburst by a high school student typically results in attention from his peers, one hypothesis is that the verbal outbursts are maintained by positive reinforcement in the form of peer attention. Similarly, if verbal outbursts are reliably followed by an exclusionary time-out, one hypothesis is that the verbal outbursts are maintained by negative reinforcement in the form of escape from the classroom or avoidance of academic or other demands present in the classroom.

Behavior Maintained by Social Consequences

Two fundamental assumptions common to this approach to intervention are that (1) behavior occurs within a context of antecedent and consequent events and (2) behavior occurs directly as a function of the consequent

events. The vast majority of the relevant consequent events are *social* in nature; that is, they are consequences provided by others in the environment. These consequent events can be grouped in two main categories: positive reinforcement (social attention or access to materials) and negative reinforcement (escape or avoidance of unpleasant situations). For example, if the behavior seems to occur predominantly when adult attention is diverted to another activity, or is divided between two or more students, the behavior may be maintained by positive reinforcement in the form of attention. If direct observation data reveal that the problem behavior typically results in peer attention or some type of adult attention, including reprimands, there is further evidence to suggest that the behavior may be maintained by attention. Alternately, observations of problem behavior that occurs when preferred items or activities are restricted, or of problem behavior that frequently results in access to materials (e.g., toys, leisure activities, food), suggests that the behavior may be maintained by positive reinforcement in the form of tangible items. Conversely, negative reinforcement (escape from unpleasant tasks) is the hypothesized reinforcer for problem behavior that is observed to occur when a task is presented. If the problem behavior results in a discontinuation of the task, then there is further evidence to suggest that escape from or avoidance of task performance maintains the behavior. The behavior may not occur every time a task is presented; it may occur only when novel demands are placed on a student, difficult tasks are assigned, easy tasks are required, boring tasks are presented, or some other aspect of the task is unpleasant.

Behavior Maintained by Sensory Consequences

If a behavior occurs at relatively high rates across most environmental situations, it may not be maintained by social consequences, but instead by sensory consequences. Like social consequences, sensory consequences (i.e., automatic reinforcement) can be grouped in two main categories: positive reinforcement (e.g., sensory stimulation) and negative reinforcement (e.g., sensory reduction, pain attenuation). Positive reinforcement in the form of sensory stimulation can reinforce behavior that produces sensory feedback, such as visual stimulation or auditory stimulation. Conversely, a behavior may function to alleviate unpleasant sensations or attenuate pain. A cautionary note: There are some "stereotypic" behavioral responses that occur at high rates (i.e., are repetitive) and are nonfunctional, thus appearing to be "automatically reinforced." However, it is impossible to tell for certain whether these responses are maintained by sensory or social consequences unless a functional analysis is conducted. For example, repetitive eye pressing or chin rubbing (Hoch, McComas, & McDonald, 1998) may appear to be maintained by sensory consequences, yet may, in fact, be maintained by social consequences.

Finally, it must be remembered that descriptive assessments are merely correlational; therefore, they must be followed by a functional analysis. Often, the information gathered will suggest one maintaining variable, but when environmental variables are isolated and manipulated in analogue conditions, a different variable or combination of variables emerge as the maintaining variable(s). The occurrence of problem behavior maintained by more than one variable or a combination of variables has been documented (Horner, Day, & Day, 1997; Richman, Wacker, Asmus, & Casey, 1998; Smith, Iwata, Vollmer, & Zarcone, 1993), further supporting the necessity of a comprehensive functional analysis for the identification of an appropriate intervention.

Test Hypothesis

The purpose of the next phase of the comprehensive assessment is to isolate the influences of particular variables on the child's target behavior. Brief (5 to 10 minute) conditions are arranged that are simulations of the naturally occurring conditions, but which control for extraneous variables. Specifically, analogue conditions are arranged in which the variable being tested is directly manipulated while all other variables are held constant. The occurrences of problem behavior are then compared across a number of sessions under each condition to examine the effects of specific environmental variables on the problem behavior. In these analogue conditions, the effects of any or all of the described social consequences can be tested, but at least two conditions are needed: control and test.

In the control condition, the environment is arranged to minimize the probability of the problem behavior's occurring. This typically involves giving the child frequent access to preferred activities and attention, with no demands presented. The types of activities and attention are determined on an individual basis, according to the information previously gathered. That is, situations that involve access to the type of attention and preferred activities identified on an individual basis should be replicated in the control condition. It is important that no consequences be provided for the target problem behavior in the control condition.

Test conditions involve the systematic isolation and examination of variables that are hypothesized to influence the occurrence of the problem behavior. In distinct conditions, positive or negative reinforcement contingencies are individually delivered, contingent on the problem behavior, on either a continuous or intermittent schedule.

If the primary hypothesis is that the problem behavior is negatively reinforced, the test condition involves presentation of a task and removal of the task contingent on the occurrence of the problem behavior. At the beginning of the 5- to 10-minute analogue session, the task is presented. The type of

task will depend on the information previously gathered. Contingent on the occurrence of the problem behavior, the task is removed and the student is allowed to briefly "escape" the task. After 20 to 30 seconds, the teacher re-presents the task. The contingency is repeated until the end of the session.

To evaluate the effects of attention on a problem behavior, the session may begin with the teacher indicating to the student that she will be busy with another activity and that the student should play quietly. To isolate the role of attention, the student is permitted to play with preferred materials and no tasks are presented. Contingent on the occurrence of the problem be-havior, attention is given to the student for a brief period of time. The type of attention is based on the previously gathered information. The teacher then returns to her activity and leaves the student to play quietly. The contingency is repeated until the end of the session.

To evaluate the effects of preferred activities and materials on a prob-lem behavior, the session begins after the student has been allowed to engage in a preferred activity for a reasonable period of time. The teacher then re-stricts access to the preferred activity by indicating to the student that it is no longer time to have those materials. Depending on the information previous-ly gathered, the materials may be shared with another student or simply put away. To isolate the role of the materials, attention is continuously available and no tasks are presented. Contingent on the occurrence of the problem be-havior, the teacher briefly returns the preferred materials to the student. Then the teacher again restricts access to the materials or offers a substitute, and the contingency is repeated until the end of the session.

Frequencies of the problem behavior are graphically displayed for each session and are compared across conditions to determine the relationships between the target behavior and the environmental variables tested. Test conditions in which the problem behavior occurs most frequently and consis-tently are considered to be the maintaining variable(s) for problem behavior.

Select and Implement Appropriate Intervention

After the maintaining variable(s) for problem behavior is (are) identified, in-tervention selection can begin. Interventions should relate directly to the re-sponse–reinforcer relation specified in the functional analysis (Iwata, Pace, Cowdery, & Miltenberger, 1994; Iwata et al., 1990). Three distinct approach-es to intervention are commonly considered: extinction, alternative reinforce-ment, and antecedent interventions. These three intervention types can be combined in any number of ways. They can also be adjusted systematically to increase their effectiveness for a given child. Careful consideration should be given to the feasibility, advantages, and disadvantages of any intervention before selection and implementation. The purpose of this section is to pro-vide a sample of the types of interventions available; it is beyond the scope of

this chapter to provide a detailed description of the advantages and disadvantages of the various interventions.

Extinction involves the termination of the relationship between the reinforcer and the problem behavior. Specifically, the response no longer results in the reinforcer (e.g., attention is no longer provided in response to problem behavior, access to materials is no longer available as a result of problem behavior, or task demands are not interrupted when problem behavior occurs). Because extinction involves the termination of the response–reinforcer contingency, it is critical to have identified the maintaining reinforcer via a functional analysis. For example, withholding attention following a negatively reinforced problem behavior would not be expected to have a therapeutic effect (Iwata, Pace, et al., 1994).

Alternative reinforcement involves the presentation of the maintaining reinforcer on some schedule that is not contingent on problem behavior. Specific arrangements of alternative reinforcement vary widely. Reinforcement can be provided contingent on an *appropriate behavior* (e.g., Vollmer & Iwata, 1992) or a *communicative behavior* (e.g., Steege et al., 1990; Wacker et al., 1990); contingent on the *omission of the target problem behavior* for specified periods of time (e.g., Mazeleski, Iwata, Vollmer, Zarcone, & Smith, 1993); or *noncontingently*, that is, regardless of any behavior exhibited by the individual (e.g., Lalli, Casey, & Kates, 1997; Vollmer, Iwata, Zarcone, Smith, & Mazaleski, 1993).

In many cases, it is desirable to provide reinforcement contingent on an appropriate alternative response. This type of alternative reinforcement can be arranged in numerous ways. Perhaps the most common of the differential reinforcement procedures is delivery of reinforcement contingent on a specific alternative behavior (DRA). With DRA, the teacher selects an appropriate alternative behavior and consistently provides reinforcement when the student displays that response. Examples of appropriate alternative responses include compliance, raising one's hand, keeping one's hands to oneself, and other appropriate replacement responses. Similarly, reinforcement can be delivered contingent on a communicative gesture (DRC). This is actually a specific case of DRA. In this case, the teacher identifies an appropriate method of requesting a specific reinforcer and consistently provides reinforcement when the individual appropriately makes the request. Common communicative gestures include manual signs, picture-exchange cards, prerecorded messages, and the use of a vocal output device. Finally, alternative reinforcement can be delivered contingent on the omission of the problem behavior for a specified period of time (DRO). With DRO procedures, the instructor identifies a length of time (interval) that the individual is required to go without engaging in the problem behavior. This interval should be carefully selected. If it is too long, the individual will not meet the response requirements and, therefore, will not earn reinforcement. Conversely, if the interval is too short, it will be cumbersome and difficult for the instructor to consistently monitor

the student's behavior and deliver reinforcement. In addition, if the interval is too short and reinforcement very frequently delivered, the student may become satiated with the reinforcer and it may lose its effectiveness. Again, the functional reinforcer must be identified in a functional analysis in order to increase the likelihood of successful intervention. For example, teaching a student whose problem behavior is maintained by attention, to ask for snacks (DRC) would not be expected to have a therapeutic effect.

An alternative to providing contingent reinforcement involves arranging noncontingent delivery of the reinforcer maintaining the problem behavior. Specifically, the delivery of reinforcers is based on the passage of a fixed (FT) or variable (VT) amount of time, regardless of the individual's behavior. With noncontingent reinforcement, the teacher sets a timer for the selected length of time. When the timer sounds, the teacher delivers the identified reinforcer, no matter what the individual is doing at the time. Time-based schedules of reinforcement like this may operate to decrease the individual's motivation to engage in problem behavior, because the problem behavior no longer has to be produced to obtain the reinforcer (i.e., the reinforcer is "free"). FT or VT schedules may also operate to decrease behavior because the reinforcer is available in the absence of the behavior, thus the response–reinforcer relationship is weakened and ultimately eliminated. Thus, if attention-maintained problem behavior occurs when the teacher has been working on another activity for long periods of time, brief but frequent noncontingent positive comments to the student may decrease the occurrence of attention-maintained problem behavior.

Yet interventions for problem behavior are not limited to consequences; treatment can be directed at the antecedent events. Like consequent-based interventions, antecedent interventions are also most effective if they are related to the maintaining variables for problem behavior (Wacker, Berg, Asmus, Harding, & Cooper, 1998). The environmental events that occur prior to problem behavior and are related to the maintaining contingencies for the behavior can be altered to decrease the likelihood of future occurrences of problem behavior. A wide variety of interventions, including but not limited to curricular modifications (Dunlap, Kern-Dunlap, Clarke, & Robbins, 1991), high-probability request sequences (Davis & Reichle, 1996; Mace et al., 1988), and stimulus fading (Zarcone et al., 1993) are available.

Like consequent-based interventions, antecedent interventions should be matched to the underlying behavioral mechanisms maintaining an individual's problem behavior (McComas & Progar, 1998). Specifically, after the maintaining contingency is known, proactive interventions can be arranged to decrease the likelihood of the occurrence of the problem behavior. For example, if negatively reinforced problem behavior occurs when difficult tasks are presented, instructional strategies may be provided to the student to give assistance in successful task completion, thus decreasing the unpleasantness

of the task and the motivation to avoid or escape it (McComas, Hoch, Goddard, & Vintere, 1998). Similarly, if problem behavior occurs when access to preferred materials is restricted, arrangements can be made for the student to have ready access to attractive alternative materials. Alternatively, some sort of signal can be provided to specify to the student exactly when the preferred materials will be available. Regardless of which of the many available antecedent- and consequent-based interventions is selected, continued data collection and assessment are necessary to evaluate the effectiveness of the intervention.

Evaluate the Effectiveness, Maintenance, and Generalization of the Intervention

The effectiveness of an intervention is typically evaluated over time and in a variety of school settings. Ongoing data collection is necessary to accomplish this, for several reasons. First, with interventions like those described earlier, the problem behavior may actually increase before it decreases. This is an expected effect of these types of behavior-change procedures. However, this pattern of behavior change can be frustrating to professionals who are unprepared or do not anticipate it, and can lead to premature or inaccurate interpretation of the effects of the intervention and, ultimately, to the abandonment of an effective intervention. Continued data collection and graphic display of data will allow professionals to objectively assess the effects of the intervention. Second, ongoing data collection facilitates integrity of the treatment and, therefore, the maintenance of behavior change. Specifically, if the problem behavior returns, the data can be examined to determine what variables in the environment may have changed to produce the problem behavior. If the teacher has "relaxed" the procedures somewhat, the intervention can be "tightened up" to reestablish the effectiveness of the intervention. If the data indicate that the previous rate of reinforcement has decreased, adjustments can be made to increase the rate of reinforcement or to teach more efficient means to access reinforcement. Third, ongoing data collection allows for the systematic fading of reinforcement from frequent provision to a more practical schedule with little risk of its fading too quickly or losing effectiveness altogether. Thus, ongoing data collection is critical for maintenance of behavior change.

Generalization of behavior change to situations other than those in which the intervention has been intensively implemented is an important objective. Stokes and Baer (1977) prescribed seven methods for actively programming generalized behavior change: introducing response to natural maintaining contingencies, training sufficient exemplars, training loosely, using indiscriminable contingencies, programming common stimuli, mediating generalization, and training to generalize. These methods may be best imple-

mented when combined with information gathered regarding the occurrence of the problem behavior in a wide variety of situations. For example, information obtained from teacher or parent interviews, rating scales, or checklists, and direct descriptive assessment may identify additional situations in which the problem behavior may occur (e.g., in school assemblies, at recess, during long writing assignments). Generalization can be enhanced by introducing the intervention or a variation of it in these potentially problematic situations.

PROCEDURAL VARIATIONS OF FUNCTIONAL ANALYSIS

Situations may be encountered in which conducting extended multisession analogue assessment is not feasible. In such cases, variations of the functional analysis procedures described here may be considered. In any variation, only one of the five steps is changed. All analyses require that information is gathered and used to generate a hypothesis, direct observation data are collected, a single-case design is conducted to analyze relationships between the target response and environmental events, an intervention is selected based on the results of the analysis, and an evaluation of maintenance and generalization of the effects of the intervention is conducted. What varies is either (1) the environmental events included in the analysis or (2) the number of sessions conducted within the analysis. Specifically, analyses may identify antecedent–response relationships rather than response–reinforcer relationships, or they may be conducted in a brief format within very few sessions.

An evaluation of the response–reinforcer relationship maintaining the target behavior provides the most direct assessment of behavioral function (Wacker et al., 1998). As we have indicated, functional analysis procedures that involve the systematic isolation and evaluation of consequences of behavior allow the professional to both identify the reason (i.e., reinforcers) that the problem behavior is occurring and match an intervention to the results of the analysis. However, antecedent variables also influence behavior, and knowledge of these influences can be useful in the design of effective interventions. Thus, analysis of antecedent–response relationships is sometimes warranted (see Wacker et al., 1998). In this type of antecedent analysis, the consequences for problem behavior are held constant across conditions and specified antecedent variables are systematically isolated and evaluated in analogue conditions within a single-case experimental design. These analyses, sometimes referred to as "structural analyses" (Axelrod, 1987), can produce highly individual changes in problem behavior (Carr & Durand, 1985; Dunlap, Kern-Dunlap, Clarke, & Robbins, 1991; Mace, Yankanich, & West, 1988).

A second variation involves a reduction in the overall number of sessions conducted. Such analyses, initially developed to meet the time restrictions imposed in outpatient clinics, were used for children with behavior disorders (Cooper, Wacker, Sasso, Reimers, & Donn, 1990; Northup et al., 1991). These brief analyses are typically conducted in two phases: (1) initial analogue assessment of two or more conditions (e.g., attention and escape), and (2) replication, in which the "best" and "worst" conditions are repeated. Control over behavior is established when marked differences in the rate of target behavior are apparent across analogue conditions and are replicated within a "mini-reversal" design (Cooper et al., 1992). These designs have also been used to assess combinations of antecedents and consequences related to problem behavior and the effects of preliminary treatment recommendations (Harding, Wacker, Cooper, Millard, & Jensen-Kovalan, 1994; Millard et al., 1993). Although these brief experimental analyses allow for replication of effects and produce differentiated outcomes approximately half the time, they do not permit an evaluation of stability within conditions (Derby et al., 1992).

APPLICATIONS OF FUNCTIONAL ANALYSIS

Evelyn was an 8-year-old girl with developmental disabilities. She scored an IQ of 60 on the Stanford–Binet LM, and she had limited receptive and expressive language skills, using four to five-word utterances to communicate. She was referred to the child study team at her school for an evaluation of destructive behavior, defined as biting and tearing her shirt, that resulted in destruction of several shirts each week. Interviews with her teachers and A-B-C data collected in her special education classroom suggested that the destructive behavior occurred mainly during two types of situations: (1) when she was required to complete tasks and (2) when she was told that it was time to stop playing. Evelyn's teachers typically reacted to the behavior by physically redirecting her hands; when Evelyn bit or attempted to tear her shirt, a teacher typically pulled the shirt out of Evelyn's mouth, placed her hands in her lap, away from her shirt, and reminded her to keep her shirt out of her mouth. A scatterplot suggested that occurrences of the problem behavior were correlated with times of day when Evelyn was working on academic tasks. Given this information, it was hypothesized that destructive behavior was maintained by negative reinforcement, although the role of positive reinforcement (attention and access to preferred activities) was unclear. Completed samples of a Functional Analysis Interview Form (O'Neill et al., 1990) and the scatterplot (Touchette et al., 1985) are included in Appendix 4.3.

The functional analysis was conducted by an instructor in Evelyn's classroom where teacher's assistants and Evelyn's peers were present. Occurrences of her destructive behavior were compared across control, escape, at-

tention, and tangible conditions. All sessions were 10 minutes long and were videotaped so that the data could be scored at a later time. Data were scored using a 10-second partial-interval recording system and calculated as a percentage of intervals with destructive behavior. A sample of the direct observation data recording form is located in Appendix 4.3.

The data indicated that destructive behavior was differentially elevated in escape conditions, supporting the hypothesis that the behavior was maintained by negative reinforcement (i.e., escape from tasks). The intervention selected involved extinction. Specifically, the teachers no longer reacted by physically redirecting Evelyn's attempts to bite and tear her shirt. Instead, they persisted with task instruction. Results of the functional analysis and intervention appear in Figure 4.1. This intervention resulted in a decrease and eventual elimination of destructive behavior that was demonstrated to be maintained over time and across teachers.

Jason was a 12-year-old boy diagnosed with autism. His expressive language was limited to fewer than a dozen comprehensible words. He was referred to the child study team in his school for an evaluation of self-injurious behavior that involved hitting his head and chest with an open hand or closed fist. Interviews with his teachers and A-B-C data collected at school suggest-

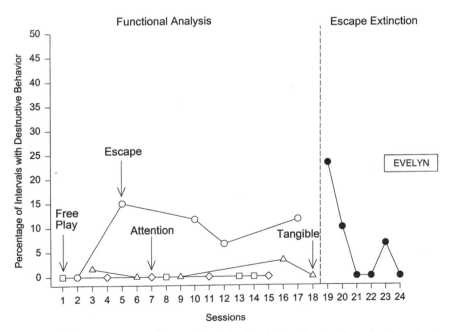

FIGURE 4.1. Percentage of intervals with shirt biting during functional analysis and intervention for Evelyn.

ed that the destructive behavior occurred during tasks, when teacher attention was diverted to another student, and when access to edibles was restricted. Jason's teachers typically ignored the self-injury. The scatterplot did not
reveal an interpretable visual pattern. Completed copies of a Functional
Analysis Interview Form (O'Neill et al., 1990), a scatterplot (Touchette et al.,
1985), and A-B-C data collection forms are included in Appendix 4.4.

   During the descriptive assessment, Jason's teachers videotaped him during four different activities: independent work, snack time, gym, and recreation. Observers scored the videotapes for the occurrence of self-injury and a
number of naturally occurring environmental variables, including restricted
access to food, diverted teacher attention, and presentation of task demands.
The results are displayed in Figure 4.2. The data indicated that Jason was
most likely to display self-injury in situations where food was present but un-
available. Diverted attention was never observed in any condition. This information suggested that Jason's self-injury may have been maintained by positive reinforcement (access to food).

   A brief functional analysis was conducted by an instructor in Jason's
classroom where teacher's assistants and his peers were present. Occurrences

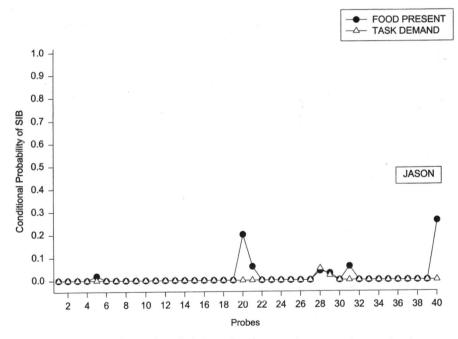

FIGURE 4.2. Conditional probability of self-injury for Jason during the descriptive assessment.

of his self-injury were compared across tangible, escape, and control conditions. There was little evidence to suggest that attention was a maintaining variable; therefore, the analysis could be shortened by omitting that condition. All sessions were 10 minutes long and were videotaped so that the data could be scored at a later time. Data were scored using a 10-second partial-interval recording system and calculated as a percentage of intervals with destructive behavior. A copy of the completed scatterplot, A-B-C, descriptive assessment, and functional analysis data recording forms are included in Appendix 4.4.

Results of the functional analysis appear in Figure 4.3. The data indicated that Jason's self-injury was differentially elevated in the tangible condition, supporting the hypothesis that the behavior was maintained by access to tangibles (i.e., edibles). The intervention selected involved DRO. Specifically, Jason was given tokens for every 60 seconds that passed in which he did not engage in self-injury. When he earned 10 tokens (approximately every 10 minutes), he traded in his tokens for a small snack (e.g., popcorn). The effects of the intervention are depicted in Figure 4.4. The data show a gradual descending trend in self-injury, with rates at or near zero in the final five sessions. After these results were obtained, the DRO interval and number of to-

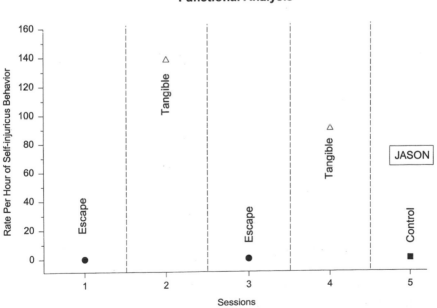

Functional Analysis

FIGURE 4.3. Rate per hour of self-injury for Jason during the functional analysis.

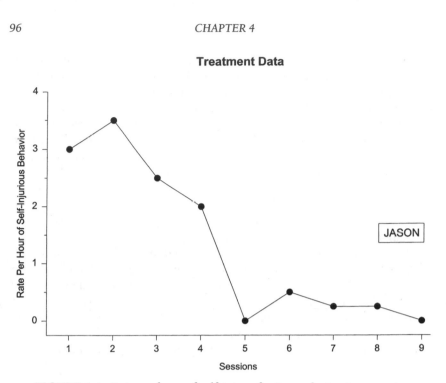

FIGURE 4.4. Rate per hour of self-injury for Jason during intervention.

kens required to earn the snack were gradually faded over time so that Jason earned a midmorning snack, dessert at lunch, and a midafternoon snack.

CONSIDERATIONS

The comprehensive functional assessment we have presented requires considerable investment of professional resources. However, it is an investment that can avoid costly and restrictive interventions in the future if the child's behavior problems continue and worsen. Every consideration should be given to adopting practices that will prevent the majority of behavior problems (Taylor-Greene et al., 1997; Walker et al., 1996). Preventative efforts are far less expensive than efforts aimed at reparation. Severe and persistent problem behavior that occurs despite preventative practices warrants allocation of special resources. Those resources are best spent on a comprehensive assessment that can lead directly to the identification of a class of interventions that are likely to be effective. Implementing an intervention without first identifying the function of the problem behavior may decrease the likelihood of behavior change (Iwata, Pace, et al., 1994). It is sometimes tempting to

skip certain steps in the process, such as the descriptive assessment. However, descriptive assessment is a valuable tool in specifying idiosyncratic variables that are involved in an individual's problem behavior and can contribute to a more effective, expedient functional analysis.

In addition, some children engage in very serious but low-frequency problem behavior. Low-frequency, high-intensity behavior problems may be difficult to capture in an analogue functional analysis. In these cases, a descriptive assessment may lead to the identification of chains of behavior that occasionally escalate to high-intensity, severe problem behavior. Hypotheses regarding the function of the behaviors observed earlier in the chain may be tested directly in a functional analysis (Lalli, Mace, Wohn, & Livezey, 1995) or indirectly through an evaluation of the effects of an intervention (Repp & Karsh, 1994).

CONCLUSIONS

The comprehensive functional analysis methodology described in this chapter has many benefits. First, it focuses assessment and intervention on the behavior–environmental relations that maintain problem behavior rather than on the individual traits, characteristics, or diagnosis of an individual child, thus increasing the likelihood of effective intervention. Second, it allows for the individualized treatment of problem behavior, also increasing the likelihood of effective intervention. Finally, effective interventions will increase opportunities for positive student–student, teacher–student, and instructional interactions. Functional analyses are not necessary for every problem behavior; preventative efforts should be employed to reduce the overall number of behavior problems in schools. However, for those severe and persistent problems that occur despite efforts at prevention, a comprehensive functional analysis can provide an excellent return for the investment.

ACKNOWLEDGMENT

We wish to thank the teachers who conducted the analysis contained in this chapter, as well as Evelyn and Jason.

REFERENCES

Achenback, T. M., & Edelbrook, C. S. (1981). *Behavioral problems and competences reported by parents of normal and disturbed chidlren aged four through sixteen.* Monograph on Social Research in Child Development, 46 (1, Serial No. 188).

Aman, M. G., & Singh, N. N. (1986). *The Aberrant Behavior Checklist and Manual.* East Aurora, NY: Slosson.

Aman, M. G., & Singh, N. N. (1994). *The Aberrant Behavior Checklist: Community.* East Aurora, NY: Slosson.

Axelrod, S. (1987). Functional and structural analyses of behavior: Approaches leading to reduced use of punishment procedures? *Research in Developmental Disabilities, 8,* 165–178.

Bijou, S. W., Petersen, R. F., & Ault, M. F. (1968). A method to integrate descriptive and experimental field studies at the level of data and empirical concepts. *Journal of Applied Behavior Analysis, 1,* 175–191.

Carr, E. G., & Durand, V. M. (1985). Reducing behavior problems through functional communication training. *Journal of Applied Behavior Analysis, 18,* 111–126.

Conners, K. C. (1997a). *Conners Parent Rating Scale—Revised (S).* North Tonawanda, NY: Multi-Health Systems, Inc.

Conners, K. C. (1997b). *Conners Teacher Rating Scale—Revised (S).* North Tonawanda, NY: Multi-Health Systems, Inc.

Cooper, L. J., Wacker, D. P., Sasso, G. M., Reimers, T., & Donn, L. (1990). Using parents as therapists to evaluate appropriate behavior of their children: Application to a tertiary clinic. *Journal of Applied Behavior Analysis, 23,* 285–296.

Cooper, L. J., Wacker, D. P., Thursby, D., Plagmann, L. A., Harding, J., Millard, T., & Derby, M. (1992). Analysis of the effects of task preferences, task demands, and adult attention on child behavior in outpatient and classroom. *Journal of Applied Behavior Analysis, 25,* 823–840.

Cowen, E. L., Huser, J., Beach, D. R., & Rappaport, J. (1970). Parent perceptions of young children and their relation to indexes of development. *Journal of Consulting and Clinical Psychology, 34,* 97–103.

Davis, C. A., & Reichle, J. (1996). Variant and invariant high-probability requests: Increasing appropriate behaviors in children with emotional-behavioral disorders. *Journal of Applied Behavior Analysis, 29,* 471–482.

Derby, K. M., Wacker, D. P., Sasso, G., Steege, M., Northup, J., Cigrand, K., & Asmus, J. (1992). Brief functional assessment techniques to evaluate aberrant behavior in an outpatient setting: A summary of 79 cases. *Journal of Applied Behavior Analysis, 25,* 713–722.

Dunlap, G., Kern-Dunlap, L., Clarke, S., & Robbins, F. R. (1991). Functional assessment, curricular revision, and severe behavior problems. *Journal of Applied Behavior Analysis, 24,* 387–397.

Harding, J., Wacker, D. P., Cooper, L. J., Millard, T., & Jensen-Kovalan, P. (1994). Brief hierarchical assessment of potential treatment components with children in an outpatient clinic. *Journal of Applied Behavior Analysis, 27,* 291–300.

Hayes, S. C., Nelson, R. O., Jarrett, R. B. (1987). The treatment utility of assessment: A functional approach to evaluating assessment quality. *American Psychologist, 42,* 963–974.

Hoch, H., McComas, J. J., & McDonald, M. (1998). *An experimental analysis of chin rubbing and prevention of other related behavior.* Paper presented at the annual conference of the Association for Behavior Analysis, Orlando, FL.

Horner, R. H., Day, M. H., & Day, J. R. (1997). Using neutralizing routines to reduce problem behaviors. *Journal of Applied Behavior Analysis, 30,* 601–613.

Iwata, B. A., Dorsey, M. F., Slifer, K. J., Bauman, K. E., & Richman, C. S. (1994). Toward a functional analysis of self-injury. *Journal of Applied Behavior Analysis, 27,* 197–209. (Reprinted from *Analysis and Intervention in Developmental Disabilities, 2,* 3–20, 1982).

Iwata, B. A., Pace, G. M., Cowdery, G. E., & Miltenberger, R. G. (1994). What makes extinction work: An analysis of procedural form and function. *Journal of Applied Behavior Analysis, 27,* 131–144.

Iwata, B. A., Pace, G. M., Kalsher, M. J., Cowdery, G. E., & Cataldo, M. F. (1990). Experimental analysis and extinction of self-injurious escape behavior. *Journal of Applied Behavior Analysis, 23,* 11–27.

Lalli, J. S., Casey, S. D., & Kates, K. (1997). Noncontingent reinforcement as treatment for severe problem behavior: Some procedural variations. *Journal of Applied Behavior Analysis, 30,* 127–138.

Lalli, J. S., & Goh, H. (1993). Naturalistic observations in community settings. In J. Reichle & D. Wacker (Eds.), *Communicative alternatives to challenging behavior: Integrating functional assessment and intervention strategies* (pp. 11–39). Baltimore: Brookes.

Lalli, J. S., Mace, F. C., Wohn, T., & Livezey, K. (1995). Identification and modification of a response-class hierarchy. *Journal of Applied Behavior Analysis, 28,* 551–559.

Mace, F. C., Hock, M. L., Lalli, J. S., West, B. J., Belfiore, P., Pinter, E., & Brown, D. K. (1988). Behavioral momentum in the treatment of noncompliance. *Journal of Applied Behavior Analysis, 21,* 123–142.

Mace, F. C., & Lalli, J. S. (1991). Linking descriptive and experimental analyses in the treatment of bizarre speech. *Journal of Applied Behavior Analysis, 24,* 553–562.

Mace, F. C., Yankanich, M. A., & West, B. J. (1988). Toward a methodology of experimental analysis and treatment of aberrant classroom behaviors. *Special Services in the Schools, 4(3/4),* 71–87.

Mazeleski, J. L., Iwata, B. A., Vollmer, T. R., Zarcone, J. R., & Smith, R. G. (1993). Analysis of the reinforcement and extinction components in DRO contingencies with self-injury. *Journal of Applied Behavior Analysis, 26,* 143–156.

McComas, J. J., Hoch, H., Goddard, C., & Vintere, P. (1998). *Escape behavior during academic tasks: A preliminary analysis of establishing operations.* Paper presented at the annual conference of the Association for Behavior Analysis, Orlando, FL.

McComas, J. J., & Progar, P. (1998). Interventions for noncompliance based on instructional control. In J. K. Luiselli & M. J. Cameron (Eds.), *Antecedent control: Innovative approaches to behavioral support.* Baltimore, MD: Brookes.

Millard, T., Wacker, D. P., Cooper, L. J., Harding, J., Drew, J., Plagmann, L. A., Asmus, J., McComas, J., & Jensen-Kovalan, P. (1993). A brief component analysis of potential treatment packages in an outpatient clinic setting with young children. *Journal of Applied Behavior Analysis, 26,* 475–476.

Northup, J., Wacker, D., Sasso, G., Steege, M., Cigrand, K., Cook, J., & DeRaad, A. (1991). A brief functional analysis of aggressive and alternative behavior in an outclinic setting. *Journal of Applied Behavior Analysis, 24,* 509–522.

O'Neill, R. E., Horner, R. H., Albin, R. W., Storey, K., & Sprague, J. (1990). *Functional analysis of problem behavior: A practical assessment guide.* Sycamore, IL: Sycamore Press.

Piazza, C. C., Fisher, W. W., Hanley, G. P., LeBlanc, L. A., Worsdell, A. S., Lindauer,

S. E., & Keeney, K. M. (1998). Treatment of pica through multiple analyses of its reinforcing functions. *Journal of Applied Behavior Analysis, 31,* 165–188.

Repp, A. C., & Karsh, K. G. (1994). Hypothesis-based interventions for tantrum behaviors of persons with developmental disabilities in school settings. *Journal of Applied Behavior Analysis, 27,* 21–31.

Richman, D. M., Wacker, D. P., Asmus, J. A., & Casey, S. D. (1998). Functional analysis and extinction of different behavior problems exhibited by the same individual. *Journal of Applied Behavior Analysis, 31,* 475–478.

Sasso, G. M., Reimers, T. M., Cooper, L. J., Wacker, D. P., Berg, W., Steege, M., Kelly, L., & Allaire, A. (1992). Use of descriptive and experimental analyses to identify the functional properties of aberrant behavior in school settings. *Journal of Applied Behavior Analysis, 25,* 809–822.

Schloss, P. J., & Smith, M. A. (1998). *Applied behavior analysis in the classroom.* Boston: Allyn & Bacon.

Smith, D. D., & Rivera, D. P. (1994). Discipline in special education and general education settings. *Focus on Exceptional Children, 27,* 1–14.

Smith, R. G., Iwata, B. A., Vollmer, T. R., & Zarcone, J. R. (1993). Experimental analysis and treatment of multiply controlled self-injury. *Journal of Applied Behavior Analysis, 26,* 183–195.

Steege, M. W., Wacker, D. P., Cigrand, K.C., Berg, W. K., Novak, C. G., Reimers, T. M., Sasso, G. M., & DeRaad, A. (1990). Use of negative reinforcement in the treatment of self-injurious behavior. *Journal of Applied Behavior Analysis, 23,* 459–467.

Stokes, T. F., & Baer, D. M. (1977). An implicit technology of generalization. *Journal of Applied Behavior Analysis, 10,* 349–367.

Taylor-Greene, S., Brown, D., Nelson, L., Longton, J., Gassman, T., Cohen, J., Swartz, J., Horner, R. H., Sugai, G., & Hall, S. (1997). School-wide behavioral support: Starting the year off right. *Journal of Behavioral Education, 7,* 99–112.

Touchette, P. E., MacDonald, R. F., & Langer, S. N. (1985). A scatter plot for identifying stimulus control of problem behavior. *Journal of Applied Behavior Analysis, 18,* 343–351.

Vollmer, T. R., & Iwata, B. A. (1992). Differential reinforcement as treatment for severe behavior disorders: Procedural and functional variations. *Research in Developmental Disabilities, 13,* 393–417.

Vollmer, T. R., Iwata, B. A., Zarcone, J. R., Smith, R. G., & Mazaleski, J. L. (1993). The role of attention in the treatment of attention-maintained self-injurious behavior: Noncontingent reinforcement and differential reinforcement of other behavior. *Journal of Applied Behavior Analysis, 22,* 9–21.

Wacker, D. P., Berg, W. K., Asmus, J. A., Harding, J. W., & Cooper, L. J. (1998). Experimental analysis of antecedent influences on challenging behavior. In J. K. Luiselli & M. J. Cameron (Eds.), *Antecedent control: Innovative approaches to behavioral support* (pp. 67–86). Baltimore: Brookes.

Wacker, D. P., Northup, J., & Cooper, L. (1991). Behavioral assessment. In D. Greydanus & M. Wolraich (Eds.), *Behavioral pediatrics* (pp. 57–68). New York: Springer-Verlag.

Wacker, D., Northup, J., & Lambert, L. (1997). Self-injury. In N. Singh (Ed.), *Prevention*

and treatment of severe behavior problems: Models and methods in developmental disabilities (pp. 179–198). Pacific Grove, CA: Brooks/Cole.

Wacker, D. P., Steege, M. W., Northup, J., Sasso, G., Berg, W., Reimers, T., Cooper, L., Cigrand, K., & Donn, L. (1990). A component analysis of functional communication training across three topographies of severe behavior problems. *Journal of Applied Behavior Analysis, 23*, 417–429.

Walker, H. M., Horner, R. H., Sugai, G., Bullis, M., Sprague, J. R., Bricker, D., & Kaufman, M. J. (1996). Integrated approaches to preventing antisocial behavior patterns among school-aged children and youth. *Journal of Emotional and Behavioral Disorders, 4*, 194–209.

Zarcone, J. R., Iwata, B. A., Vollmer, T. R., Jagtiani, S., Smith, R. G., & Mazaleski, J. L. (1993). Extinction of self-injurious escape behavior with and without instructional fading. *Journal of Applied Behavior Analysis, 26*, 353–360.

APPENDIX 4.1

Functional Analysis Interview Form

Person with Challenging Behavior: _____   Age: ____   Sex: M F

Interviewer: _____   Date of Interview: _____

A. *Describe the Behavior of Concern:*

What is the behavior of concern? Define the topography (how it is performed), frequency (how often it occurs per week, day, or month), duration (how long it lasts when it occurs), and intensity (low, medium, or high).

1. Behavior: _____
2. Topography: _____
3. Frequency: _____
4. Duration: _____
5. Intensity: _____

B. *Define Events and Situations That Predict Occurrences of the Behavior:*

1. *Time of Day:* When is the behavior
   a. Most likely: _____
   b. Least likely: _____
2. *Setting:* Where is the behavior
   a. Most likely: _____
   b. Least likely: _____
3. *Social Control:* With whom is the behavior
   a. Most likely: _____
   b. Least likely: _____
4. *Activity:* What activity is most/least likely to occasion the behavior?
   a. Most likely: _____
   b. Least likely: _____
5. What could you do that would be most/least likely to make the behavior occur?
   a. Most likely: _____
   b. Least likely: _____

Note. Based on O'Neill, Horner, Albin, Storey, and Sprague (1990). Copyright 1990.

C. *Identify the Function of the Problem Behavior:*
   1. What function do you believe the behavior serves for the person (i.e., what does he/she get and/or avoid by engaging in the behavior)?
   2. Describe the person's most typical response (i.e., if the behavior is more likely to occur, less likely to occur, or unaffected) in the following situations:

Situation	More Likely	Less Likely	Unaffected
Present student with a task			
Interrupt a preferred activity (i.e., watching TV)			
Deliver a strong request/command/ reprimand			
You are present but ignore the student for 15 minutes			
Changes in routine			
Something the student wants is present but unavailable to him			

D. *Provide a history of programs that have attempted previously to decrease the behavior:*
   1. _____
   2. _____
   3. _____

APPENDIX 4.2

Scatterplot

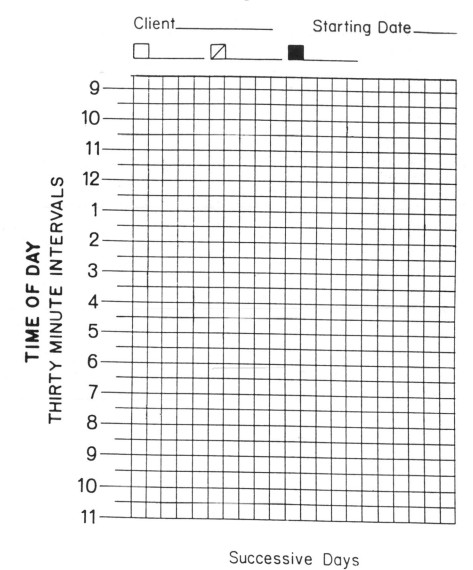

Note. From Touchette, MacDonald, and Langer (1985, p. 344). Copyright 1985 by the Society for the Experimental Analysis of Behavior, Inc. Reprinted by permission.

Student:_____ Observer:_____

Date	Time	Antecedent	Behavior	Consequence	Comments

Child's Name: _____ Date: _____ Tape #: _____

Condition: _____ Counter Numbers: _____ Session #: _____

Scored By: _____ Agreement Scorer: _____ Primary ❑ Agreement ❑

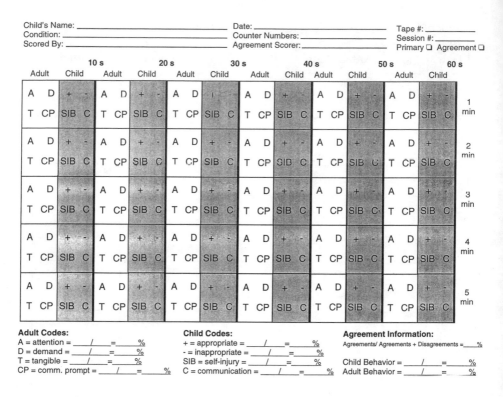

Adult Codes:
A = attention = ____/____ = ____%
D = demand = ____/____ = ____%
T = tangible = ____/____ = ____%
CP = comm. prompt = ____/____ = ____%

Child Codes:
+ = appropriate = ____/____ = ____%
- = inappropriate = ____/____ = ____%
SIB = self-injury = ____/____ = ____%
C = communication = ____/____ = ____%

Agreement Information:
Agreements/ Agreements + Disagreements = ____%

Child Behavior = ____/____ = ____%
Adult Behavior = ____/____ = ____%

Note. Reprinted with permission of Stephanie Peck, PhD, Utah State University.

Participant:_____ Date:_____ Time:_____ Session Number:_____

Observer:_____ Observer Type:_____ Condition:_____

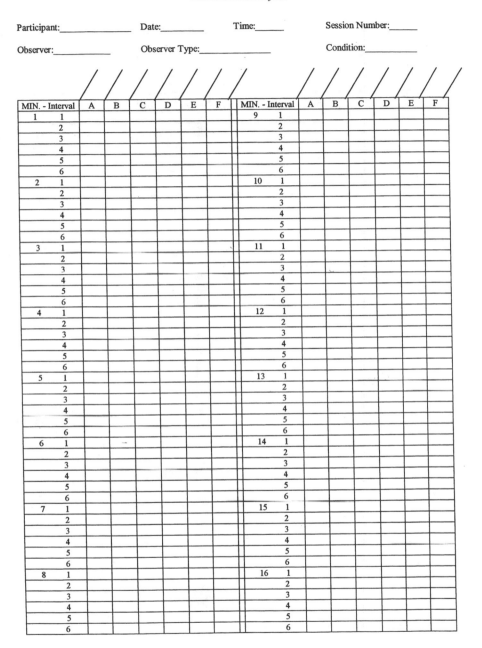

MIN. - Interval		A	B	C	D	E	F	MIN. - Interval		A	B	C	D	E	F
1	1							9	1						
	2								2						
	3								3						
	4								4						
	5								5						
	6								6						
2	1							10	1						
	2								2						
	3								3						
	4								4						
	5								5						
	6								6						
3	1							11	1						
	2								2						
	3								3						
	4								4						
	5								5						
	6								6						
4	1							12	1						
	2								2						
	3								3						
	4								4						
	5								5						
	6								6						
5	1							13	1						
	2								2						
	3								3						
	4								4						
	5								5						
	6								6						
6	1							14	1						
	2								2						
	3								3						
	4								4						
	5								5						
	6								6						
7	1							15	1						
	2								2						
	3								3						
	4								4						
	5								5						
	6								6						
8	1							16	1						
	2								2						
	3								3						
	4								4						
	5								5						
	6								6						

Participant: _____   Date: _____ Time: _____ Session: _____   Pg.:_____

Observer: _____   IOA: _____   Counter Beg.: _____ End: _____

INTERVAL		Pref. Food Pres.	RA	Access	Div. Att'n	Att'n	Prompt	Task Dem	ENG		VOC	JUMP	SIB	REQ	Hits Alt. O/C	INT	
1	1															1	1
	2																2
	3																3
	4																4
	5																5
	6																6
2	1															2	1
	2																2
	3																3
	4																4
	5																5
	6																6
3	1															3	1
	2																2
	3																3
	4																4
	5																5
	6																6
4	1															4	1
	2																2
	3																3
	4																4
	5																5
	6																6
5	1															5	1
	2																2
	3																3
	4																4
	5																5
	6																6
6	1															6	1
	2																2
	3																3
	4																4
	5																5
	6																6
7	1															7	1
	2																2
	3																3
	4																4
	5																5
	6																6

INTERVAL		Pref. Food Pres.	RA	Access	Div. Att'n	Att'n	Prompt	Task Dem	ENG		VOC	JUMP	SIB	REQ	Hits Alt. O/C	INT	
8	1															8	1
	2																2
	3																3
	4																4
	5																5
	6																6
9	1															9	1
	2																2
	3																3
	4																4
	5																5
	6																6
10	1															10	1
	2																2
	3																3
	4																4
	5																5
	6																6
TOTALS																	

APPENDIX 4.3

Completed Functional Analysis Interview Form, Scatterplot, and Direct Observation Interval Recording for Evelyn

Person with Challenging Behavior: ___EVELYN___   Age: _8_   Sex: M Ⓕ

Interviewer: ___LAUREN___   Date of Interview: ___11/20___

A. *Describe the Behavior of Concern:*

What is the behavior of concern? Define the topography (how it is performed), frequency (how often it occurs per week, day, or month), duration (how long it lasts when it occurs), and intensity (low, medium, or high).

1. Behavior: _destructive behavior_
2. Topography: _biting, tearing shirt_
3. Frequency: _> 12×/day_
4. Duration: _1 sec.–10 min._
5. Intensity: _med–high; often tears/bites holes in shirt!_

B. *Define Events and Situations That Predict Occurrences of the Behavior:*

1. *Time of Day:* When is the behavior
   a. Most likely: _tasks, work breaks while playing_
   b. Least likely: _mealtimes, gym, transitions_
2. *Setting:* Where is the behavior
   a. Most likely: _classroom_
   b. Least likely: _gym, cafeteria, halls, bathroom_
3. *Social Control:* With whom is the behavior
   a. Most likely: _teachers, parents_
   b. Least likely: _peers_
4. *Activity:* What activity is most/least likely to occasion the behavior?
   a. Most likely: _tasks, (math, spelling) (paper-pencil)_
   b. Least likely: _small group verbal tasks_
5. What could you do that would be most/least likely to make the behavior occur?
   a. Most likely: _give tasks_
   b. Least likely: _walk, snack, gross motor activities_

C. *Identify the Function of the Problem Behavior:*
1. What function do you believe the behavior serves for the person (i.e., what does he/she get and/or avoid by engaging in the behavior)? *escape, tangible (toys)*
2. Describe the person's most typical response (i.e., if the behavior is more likely to occur, less likely to occur, or unaffected) in the following situations:

Situation	More Likely	Less Likely	Unaffected
Present student with a task	✓		
Interrupt a preferred activity (i.e., watching TV)	✓		
Deliver a strong request/command/reprimand	✓		
You are present but ignore the student for 15 minutes			✓
Changes in routine		✓	
Something the student wants is present but unavailable to him		✓	

D. *Provide a history of programs that have attempted previously to decrease the behavior:*
1. _Block/redirect_
2. _verbal reprimand (mild)_
3. _tokens—for "quiet mouth" (no shirt in mouth) trade in for edibles_

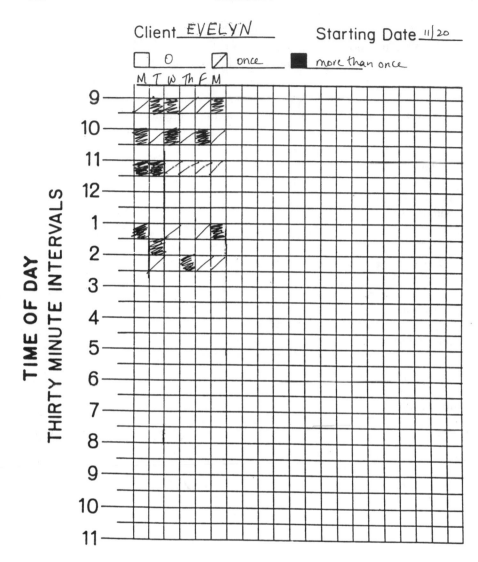

FUNCTIONAL ANALYSIS

Participant: **EVELYN**   Date: **11/26**   Time: **11 am**   Session Number: **10**

Observer: **HH**   Observer Type: **PRIMARY**   Condition: **ESCAPE**

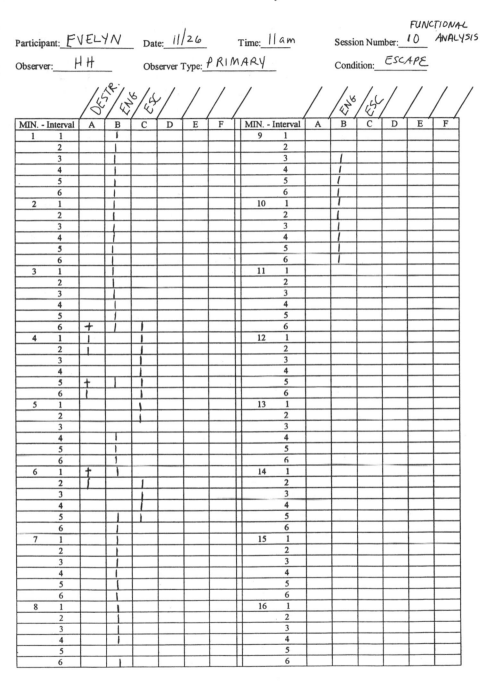

Column headers (left block): A = DESTR., B = ENG, C = ESC

MIN. - Interval	A	B	C	D	E	F	MIN. - Interval	A	B	C	D	E	F
1 1		I					9 1						
2		I					2						
3		I					3		I				
4		I					4		I				
5		I					5		I				
6		I					6		I				
2 1		I					10 1		I				
2		I					2		I				
3		I					3		I				
4		I					4		I				
5		I					5		I				
6		I					6		I				
3 1		I					11 1						
2		I					2						
3		I					3						
4		I					4						
5		I					5						
6	+	I	I				6						
4 1	I		I				12 1						
2	I		I				2						
3			I				3						
4			I				4						
5	+	I	I				5						
6	I		I				6						
5 1			\				13 1						
2			I				2						
3							3						
4		I					4						
5		I					5						
6		I					6						
6 1	+	I					14 1						
2	I		I				2						
3			I				3						
4			I				4						
5		I	I				5						
6		I					6						
7 1		I					15 1						
2		I					2						
3		I					3						
4		I					4						
5		I					5						
6		I					6						
8 1		I					16 1						
2		I					2						
3		I					3						
4		I					4						
5							5						
6		I					6						

APPENDIX 4.4

Completed Functional Analysis Interview Form, Scatterplot, A-B-C Data Form, Direct Observation Descriptive Assessment Recording Form, and Direct Observation Functional Analysis Recording Form for Jason

Person with Challenging Behavior: __JASON__   Age: _12_   Sex:(M) F

Interviewer: __KELLY__   Date of Interview: __3/20__

A. *Describe the Behavior of Concern:*

What is the behavior of concern? Define the topography (how it is performed), frequency (how often it occurs per week, day, or month), duration (how long it lasts when it occurs), and intensity (low, medium, or high).

1. Behavior: _self-injurious behavior [SIB]_
2. Topography: _hitting head & face_
3. Frequency: _↑ 20×/day_
4. Duration: _2–5 slaps will occur consecutively_
5. Intensity: _medium → high_

B. *Define Events and Situations That Predict Occurrences of the Behavior:*

1. *Time of Day:* When is the behavior
   a. Most likely: _afternoons_
   b. Least likely: _____

2. *Setting:* Where is the behavior
   a. Most likely: _home, during meals or free time_
   b. Least likely: _while doing work at school_

3. *Social Control:* With whom is the behavior
   a. Most likely: _Mom_
   b. Least likely: _____

4. *Activity:* What activity is most/least likely to occasion the behavior?
   a. Most likely: _before/during/after meals_
   b. Least likely: _when doing puzzles_

5. What could you do that would be most/least likely to make the behavior occur?
   a. Most likely: _take away his food, interrupt his routine_
   b. Least likely: _give him lots of snacks_

C. *Identify the Function of the Problem Behavior:*
   1. What function do you believe the behavior serves for the person (i.e., what does he/she get and/or avoid by engaging in the behavior)? *Escape or tangible*
   2. Describe the person's most typical response (i.e., if the behavior is more likely to occur, less likely to occur, or unaffected) in the following situations:

Situation	More Likely	Less Likely	Unaffected
Present student with a task		✓	
Interrupt a preferred activity (i.e., watching TV)	✓		
Deliver a strong request/command/reprimand	✓		
You are present but ignore the student for 15 minutes			✓
Changes in routine	✓		
Something the student wants is present but unavailable to him	✓		

D. *Provide a history of programs that have attempted previously to decrease the behavior:*
   1. *DRO schedule*
   2. *verbal reprimand*
   3. _____

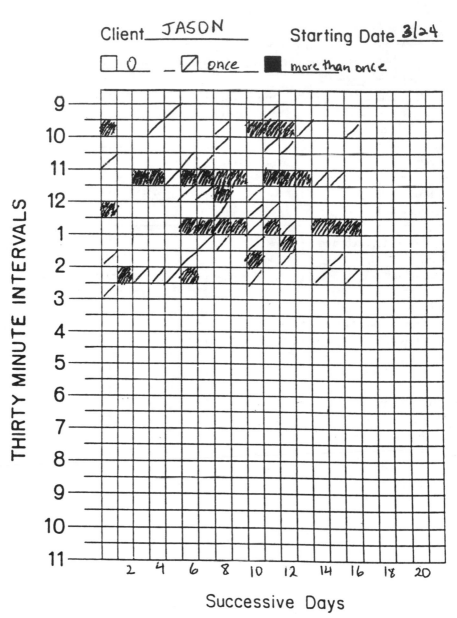

Student: ___JASON___   Observer: ___KELLY___

Date	Time	Antecedent	Behavior	Consequence	Comments
4/2	10:00	Eating snack	Hit head 3×	Teacher ignored it	Continued eating
	11:00	Jason was playing on a break	Hit face 2×	Teacher called him back to his desk	Hitting stopped when left play area
	11:30	Playing on a break	Hit head 3×	Teacher sent him back to his desk	No more hitting at desk
	12:45	Waiting for lunch at the table	Hit his head 5×	Teacher ignored it	Received his lunch two minutes later
	12:55	Finished his lunch, waiting for friends to finish	Hit his head 5×	Teacher gave him some snack from his friend	Hitting stopped when received the snack
	1:30	Working on math sheet at his desk	Hit his face 4×	Teacher prompted him to do his work sheet	When sat quietly, received last token and got a snack
	2:30	Waiting for his turn to run in gym	Hit his face 6×	Teacher prompted him to wait quietly	Peers were receiving snacks for waiting quietly

DESCRIPTIVE ASSESSMENT

Participant: **JASON**   Date: **6/24** Time: **11 am** Session: **16-SNACK**   Pg.: **1**

Observer: **HH**   IOA: **GW**   Counter Beg.: _____ End: _____

H = Hit Table

INTERVAL		Pref. Food Pres.	RA	Access	Div. Att'n	Att'n	Prompt	Task Dem	ENG		VOC	JUMP	SIB	REQ	Hits Alt. O/C	INT	
1	1	I							I						I	1	1
	2	I							I								2
	3	i							I								3
	4	I							i								4
	5	I	'						I								5
	6	I	II						I		III			1			6
2	1	I							I		1				IIH*	2	1
	2	I	II						I					1			2
	3	I							I								3
	4	I							I		I				IH		4
	5	I		II					I					I			5
	6	I		I					I		II	III			2H		6
3	1	I							I		IIII					3	1
	2	I							I		II				1H		2
	3	I					II		I			I					3
	4	I							I		i				IIH		4
	5	I		II					I					I			5
	6	I		I					I								6
4	1	I		I					I		I					4	1
	2	I							I		II						2
	3	I							I						}		3
	4	I							I		II				I, "'H		4
	5	I							I		I	II					5
	6	I							I		I				I		6
5	1	I							I			I			H	5	1
	2	I							I								2
	3	I	II						I		I			I			3
	4	I	II	HH					I		II\			I IIII\			4
	5	I		I					i		I						5
	6	I							I						IH		6
6	1	I							I		I				IH	6	1
	2	I									1	II					2
	3	I													IH		3
	4	I							I								4
	5	I				I			I		III				IIH		5
	6	\							I		I				IIH		6
7	1	I	II						I					I		7	1
	2	I															2
	3	I					II		I		I						3
	4	I							i						IH		4
	5	I		II					i					I			5
	6	I		I					I								6

INTERVAL		Pref. Food Pres.	RA	Access	Div. Att'n	Att'n	Prompt	Task Dem	ENG		VOC	JUMP	SIB	REQ	Hits Alt. O/C	INT	
8	1	/						/			/				// H	8	1
	2	/															2
	3	/						/							/ H		3
	4	/									/						4
	5	/															5
	6	/									/	//					6
9	1	/									/					9	1
	2	/						/			/						2
	3	/						/							/ H		3
	4	/										/			/ H		4
	5	/								/							5
	6	/		//						/				/	/ H		6
10	1	/		/						/						10	1
	2	/		/						/	/						2
	3	/								/	/						3
	4	/								/	/						4
	5	/								/	/						5
	6	/								/				/			6
TOTALS																	

Participant: JASON   Date: 8/12   Time: 11am   Session Number: 4   FUNCTIONAL ANALYSIS

Observer: HH   Observer Type: PRIMARY   Condition: TANGIBLE

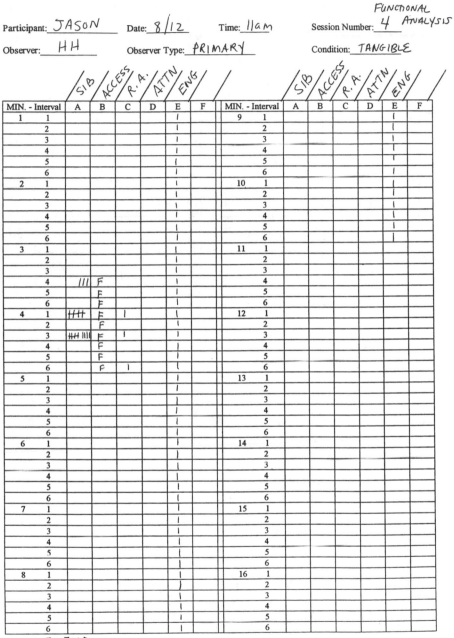

MIN. - Interval		A	B	C	D	E	F	MIN. - Interval		A	B	C	D	E	F
1	1					I		9	1					(	
	2					I			2					I	
	3					I			3					I	
	4					I			4					I	
	5					(			5					I	
	6					I			6					I	
2	1					\		10	1					(	
	2					\			2					(	
	3					\			3					\	
	4					I			4					\	
	5					I			5					\	
	6					I			6					I	
3	1					I		11	1						
	2					I			2						
	3					(			3						
	4	III	F			\			4						
	5		F			I			5						
	6		F			\			6						
4	1	₩₩	F	I		\		12	1						
	2		F			\			2						
	3	₩ IIII	F	I		I			3						
	4		F			I			4						
	5		F			I			5						
	6		F	I		(			6						
5	1					I		13	1						
	2					I			2						
	3					\			3						
	4					I			4						
	5					(			5						
	6					I			6						
6	1					I		14	1						
	2					)			2						
	3					\			3						
	4					\			4						
	5					I			5						
	6					(			6						
7	1					I		15	1						
	2					I			2						
	3					I			3						
	4					I			4						
	5					(			5						
	6					I			6						
8	1					I		16	1						
	2					)			2						
	3					\			3						
	4					I			4						
	5					I			5						
	6					I			6						

F = FOOD

CHAPTER 5

♦♦♦

Self-Monitoring

♦

CHRISTINE L. COLE
TAMARA MARDER
LORI McCANN

Jim is the school psychologist at Monroe Elementary School. He frequently consults with teachers regarding students who are having academic or behavior problems. In almost every case, Jim and the teacher decide it would be helpful to collect some information about aspects of the child's behavior. Typically, the initial purpose of this data collection is to determine how severe the problem really is, and later, when an intervention has been implemented, it can help to track student progress. Most of the time, the teacher assumes responsibility for recording the data inasmuch as he or she is able to observe the student throughout the day. Unfortunately, Jim is frequently disappointed to find that the teacher has not followed through with the data collection. Reasons commonly given by teachers include not having enough time to collect data or just simply forgetting to write down the information as it happens. Jim understands there are tremendous demands on teachers; in fact, his own busy schedule often prevents him from observing in the classroom as much as he would like. Given the reality of these time constraints, Jim is interested in finding an easier, more time-efficient way to collect information on student behavior.

Marion has taught seventh grade at Allen Junior High for 17 years. She reports seeing a disturbing trend suggesting that students are less independent and responsible than they used to be. The specific problems she encounters on a daily basis include students coming to class without necessary books and materials, students exhibiting limited organizational skills, and students consistently failing to complete homework assignments. She believes that too often we assume children and adolescents will automatically develop independent, responsible behaviors but that, in truth, these behaviors must be actively taught. Marion would like to see efforts made in her school to encourage these types of student behaviors.

Jim and Marion have identified typical concerns of school-based practitioners related to both assessment and intervention for problem behaviors. Jim
would like to find a more efficient approach to assessing student behavior.
Marion would like a strategy to promote more independent, responsible student behavior. Each of these concerns has many possible solutions. However,
one strategy that may be useful for both assessment and intervention purposes is self-monitoring.

OVERVIEW OF SELF-MONITORING

Description

Self-monitoring is a procedure that students can be taught, whereby they observe and record specific aspects of their own behavior. *Observation* involves
both becoming aware of one's actions and knowing whether or not a behavior of interest has occurred. *Recording* involves noting the occurrence of the
observed behavior, typically via a paper-and-pencil method. For example, a
student who engages in disruptive talking during independent seat work may
be asked to notice each time he talks to a peer during this time. The student
may then record each instance of talking-out behavior by placing a check-
mark on an index card taped to his desk.

Uses of Self-Monitoring

Self-monitoring may be used in school settings as an assessment or intervention procedure. When self-monitoring is used for *assessment* purposes, a student may be asked to collect data on a particular behavior of interest. This
application may be part of the functional assessment process designed to obtain an initial behavior level or to determine specific antecedents and consequences of a behavior. Self-monitoring can also be used for more extended
periods as an outcome measure to determine the effects of intervention procedures or instructional activities over time. The most obvious benefit of using a self-monitoring approach for data collection is that child-collected data
are more convenient to obtain than data collected by adult observers such as
a teacher or school psychologist. Students can record data even when these
adults are not present or are attending to other instructional duties. Moreover, a self-monitoring approach that shifts responsibility for data collection
from the teacher to the student typically reduces demands on the teacher's
time and avoids problems such as those encountered by Jim, as described
earlier.
        However, a major concern in using self-monitoring for assessment pur-
poses is the accuracy of the data collected. Most children and adolescents

with varying cognitive, social, emotional, and behavioral characteristics are capable of self-monitoring accurately (e.g., Blick & Test, 1987; McCarl, Svobodny, & Beare, 1991). However, sometimes students' accuracy of self-monitoring is moderate to low (e.g., Lloyd & Hilliard, 1989; Marshall, Lloyd, & Hallahan, 1993). A number of factors that may account for this variability in accuracy, as well as procedures for enhancing the accuracy of student self-monitoring, are described later in this chapter. However, it is important to acknowledge that limited or inconsistent accuracy can be a major limitation of using self-monitoring for assessment purposes.

In addition to being a valuable assessment procedure, self-monitoring may also be used as an *intervention* strategy to encourage behavior change. It is well known that the self-monitoring activities of observing and recording one's behavior often result in positive changes in the behavior being self-monitored. These changes are called reactivity, or reactive effects. Although reactivity does not always result from self-monitoring, it does occur frequently enough to support its usefulness as an intervention. In fact, self-monitoring has most often been used for intervention purposes with children and adolescents in school-based settings. If, for example, Marion (described earlier) has her junior high school students self-monitor target behaviors such as completing assignments or bringing materials to class, without any additional contingencies, she may see an improvement in these target areas. The specific mechanisms responsible for the reactivity of self-monitoring remain a matter of speculation. Two basic theoretical explanations, one emphasizing covert, mediational variables (Kanfer, 1970, 1977) and the other focusing on external controlling variables (Nelson & Hayes, 1981; Rachlin, 1974), have been offered. Although there is empirical support for each of these positions, it is possible that both cognitive and environmental influences interact to produce reactive effects. Whatever the theoretical explanation for reactivity, the simplicity and ease of use of self-monitoring has made it a commonly employed intervention in school settings.

Even though positive changes in student behavior are usually welcomed by practitioners, these changes may create difficulties when self-monitoring is being used for assessment purposes. For example, the reactive effects associated with self-monitoring may make it impossible to obtain a clear picture of initial behavioral levels when self-monitoring is used as the sole assessment method. Therefore, the usefulness of self-monitoring as an assessment procedure is dependent on both the accuracy with which students are able to monitor their behavior and the degree to which reactivity occurs.

Benefits of Self-Monitoring

As mentioned earlier, self-monitoring can free teachers from having to spend time on routine tasks such as observing and recording behavior, thus allowing

them to devote more time to actual instruction. It can also be useful as a simple intervention strategy for academic or behavior problems. But there are several other important benefits of self-monitoring. First may be the elimination of the need for immediate external contingencies that characterize typical classroom management (Kern, Marder, Boyajian, Elliot, & McElhattan, 1997). In many cases, self-monitoring may prevent undesired behavior from occurring in the first place and eliminate the need for a more structured consequence-based intervention.

A related benefit is that decreasing reliance on external control may increase the likelihood that students will actually learn to independently control their behavior over time and across settings (Kern et al., 1997; Lonnecker, Brady, McPherson, & Hawkins, 1994). For example, a student who self-monitors her on-task behavior during math class may, as a result, become more attentive in spelling, even though she is not self-recording during spelling.

Finally, self-monitoring is consistent with the philosophy that it is important and desirable to increase the active involvement of students in the planning and implementation of their programming. If independence is an overall goal of education, many would argue that we should be actively teaching and encouraging self-management behaviors such as self-monitoring (Kern et al., 1997; Shapiro & Cole, 1994).

Limitations of Self-Monitoring

Despite the potential uses and benefits of self-monitoring, there are several limitations to this strategy. First, like most interventions, self-monitoring is not appropriate for all students. There may be certain individuals who, because of personal characteristics, such as distractibility, are unable to carry out the steps involved in self-monitoring. For some, having to stop what they are doing to observe and record their behavior is such a time-consuming and arduous task that it actually interferes with desired responding.

A related limitation of self-monitoring is the requirement for student cooperation. If students are resistant to intervention efforts, they may simply refuse to participate in self-monitoring. Unlike interventions that involve externally delivered reinforcement or punishment contingencies, regardless of initial student motivation, self-monitoring requires the active involvement and participation of students. Students who are not motivated to participate can easily sabotage the intervention efforts. This may be a particularly relevant concern for those working with older students or students who have a history of oppositional, noncompliant behavior.

Finally, in some cases involving seriously challenging behavior, or complex problems, it may be unreasonable to expect that self-monitoring alone can be used successfully for either assessment or intervention purposes.

Rather, it may be more useful to include self-monitoring as one component of a comprehensive intervention package that includes other strategies such as functional assessment, skill training procedures, and external contingencies. Given the benefits and limitations of self-monitoring, we now turn to a discussion of how practitioners can go about teaching children to self-monitor their behavior in school-based settings.

TEACHING STUDENTS TO SELF-MONITOR

Student Characteristics

Almost any student can be a candidate for self-monitoring. Self-monitoring has been used successfully with a diversity of populations. It has been used in general and special education settings with students who have developmental disabilities (Hughes, Korinek, & Gorman, 1991), learning disabilities (Dunlap & Dunlap, 1989), autism (Koegel & Koegel, 1990), and emotional/behavioral disorders (Hughes, Ruhl, & Misra, 1989). In addition, students with no exceptionality have also successfully used self-monitoring in nonspecial education settings (e.g., Wood, Murdock, Cronin, Dawson, & Kirby, 1998). Children of all ages, from preschool to high school, can learn to use and benefit from self-monitoring. It is evident that this procedure may be useful with the entire range of children served in school-based settings.

Types of Behaviors Self-Monitored

A variety of academic and nonacademic behaviors can be self-monitored by students in school-based settings. Examples include self-monitoring of teachers' expectancies by middle school students with learning disabilities (Clees, 1994), self-monitoring in-class transition behaviors by preschoolers with developmental delays (Connell, Carta, Lutz, Randall, & Wilson, 1993), self-monitoring spelling study behavior by elementary-age students with severe behavior disorders (McDougall & Brady, 1995), and self-monitoring attending behavior by elementary students with attention-deficit/hyperactivity disorder (Mathes & Bender, 1997). Almost any relevant target behavior may be successfully self-monitored by children and adolescents in school settings.

Designing a Self-Monitoring Procedure

There are a number of factors to consider in designing a self-monitoring procedure for a particular student or group of students (see the Preparation Worksheet in Figure 5.1). Obviously, the goal is to ensure that students will, in fact, self-monitor their behavior and that such monitoring will be accurate.

1. What is the target behavior(s)?

_____

2. What is the desired outcome?

_____

3. In what setting(s) will the student self-monitor?

_____

4. What type of prompt is most appropriate for the setting?

_____

5. Which recording device is most appropriate?

_____

6. At what intervals will the student self-monitor?

_____

7. Will accuracy checks be used? If so, how often?

_____

8. Will external reinforcement be used? If so, what kind and how often?

_____

9. Will additional staff be required to implement self-monitoring?

_____

10. How and how often will outcomes be evaluated?

_____

FIGURE 5.1. Self-Monitoring Preparation Worksheet.

To achieve this outcome, the procedure should be appropriate for the behavior(s) being recorded and as easy to use as possible. To be feasible for use in a school setting, the procedure should also be inexpensive and relatively unobtrusive. Using these guidelines, the practitioner must make a number of specific decisions regarding the type of prompting, recording device, schedule for self-monitoring, and accuracy checks that will be used.

Prompts to Self-Monitor

Many different types of prompts may be used to signal students to self-monitor their behavior. In school settings, this tactic has most often involved the use of external prompts. *External prompts* can be either verbal or nonverbal, and can be delivered by another person (e.g., teacher, aide, support person) or by a mechanical device (e.g., tone on a prerecorded tape, kitchen timer). Verbal prompting, which may be useful when an entire class is self-monitoring, can involve a simple reminder from the teacher to self-monitor at the end of each class period. In other cases in which only one or a few students are self-

monitoring, it may be more feasible to use nonverbal prompts such as having the teacher periodically signal or tap the individual students on the shoulder when it is time to self-monitor their behavior. A prerecorded tone is one of the most commonly used prompts, because it requires a limited amount of teacher time and can be used with an individual or an entire class (e.g., Di-Gangi, Maag, & Rutherford, 1991).

Another type of prompting that has been successfully used in school-based settings is self-prompting. With *self-prompting,* students are typically instructed to note on their own, from time to time during the designated self-monitoring period, whether or not they were engaging in the target behavior. This type of self-prompting, which has been used most often with self-monitoring attending, or on-task, behavior, is described in more detailed in a later section.

Recording Devices

A variety of recording devices are available for use in self-monitoring. The most popular recording devices in school settings are paper-and-pencil procedures (e.g., Harris, Graham, Reid, McElroy, & Hamby, 1994). Paper-and-pencil recording forms vary, ranging from an index card or slip of paper on which the child makes a tally mark at each cue, to a more detailed individualized form (see Figure 5.2 for examples). The recording form may be taped to the child's desk (e.g., Piersel, 1985), placed on the wall next to the child's desk (e.g., Workman, Helton, & Watson, 1982), included in the child's packet of work materials (e.g., Schunk, 1982), or carried by an adolescent throughout the day (e.g., Clees, 1994).

More unconventional strategies have also been used for "recording" following children's self-monitoring. One example involved preschoolers who used a thumbs up or thumbs down signal when teachers asked them to monitor their behavior following transition, free play, and small-group instruction times (Miller, Strain, Boyd, Jarzynka, & McFetridge, 1993). In another novel interpretation of self-recording, teenagers with autism removed a token from a back pocket and placed it in a front pocket to self-monitor each transition to a new activity (Newman et al., 1995).

Schedule of Self-Monitoring

Another factor to consider is the schedule of self-monitoring, or how often a student will be asked to monitor his or her behavior. This issue will depend, to some extent, on the nature of the target behavior and the environmental setting in which self-monitoring will occur. A popular procedure used with self-monitoring of attending behavior is spot-checking, also called momentary time sampling (e.g., Prater, Hogan, & Miller, 1992). Using this proce-

WAS I PAYING ATTENTION WHEN I HEARD THE TONE?

Mark Y for yes and N for no.

SELF-RECORDING FORM

Name _____ Date _____

I worked quietly or raised my hand to ask a question.

Yes	No

CLASS PREPARATION CHECKLIST

Student _____ Class _____

☐ Sharp pencil on desk

☐ Notebook open to clean page

☐ Check board for page number

☐ Book open to correct page

☐ All other materials put away

☐ Eyes on teacher

☐ Sitting quietly

FIGURE 5.2. Examples of paper-and-pencil recording forms used in self-monitoring.

dure, children are signaled (i.e., usually by an auditory tone) to self-monitor several times throughout a class period following short intervals of time, such as every 5 minutes. The children are instructed to decide, at each tone, whether they were attending or not attending, and to mark a + or − on their recording sheets. The results are typically summarized as percentage on-task, calculated by dividing the number of on-task occurrences by the total number of times the signal was given and multiplying by 100.

For academic productivity behaviors such as the completion of math problems, students may be asked to record the number of problems completed and number of problems completed correctly at the end of each independent work period. In this case, data are summarized as percentage of problems completed and percentage completed correctly.

In the case of problem behaviors, students may be asked to record each occurrence of the target behavior, usually at the time of occurrence. For example, a student may be asked to record each instance of talking out in class or out-of-seat behavior. This procedure is feasible only when the frequency of the target behavior is relatively low, the occurrence is of short duration, and the behavior is discrete (i.e., it has a definite beginning and end). Data are summarized as total frequency during each period or, if self-monitoring sessions vary in length, as rate of occurrence. Behavior rate is calculated by dividing the total number of occurrences by the total observation time.

Accuracy Checks

A final consideration is the procedure for determining the accuracy of students' self-monitoring. The most commonly used procedure is to compare recordings made by the child with those made simultaneously by another observer, usually an adult such as the teacher (e.g., Dunlap & Dunlap, 1989). The extent to which a student is able to match an observer's recordings of a particular behavior will determine the accuracy of self-monitoring.

Self-Monitoring Training

The specific methods used in teaching children and adolescents to self-monitor their behavior are related to the characteristics of the particular student (e.g., age, cognitive level) as well as the type of self-monitoring procedure being used. The overriding concern in training should be to ensure that the child or adolescent understands what is expected and has the skills to implement the self-monitoring procedure being taught. Training may take place in the setting in which self-monitoring will occur or in a separate room, and training procedures can range from simple verbal instructions to detailed training programs involving multiple components. The components included

in most self-monitoring training programs are verbal instruction, modeling and behavior rehearsal, and praise and performance feedback.

Verbal Instruction

Self-monitoring training typically begins with a general description of the self-monitoring activity and situations in which it may be useful to the student. This introduction sets the stage for the training session and attempts to generate student interest and motivation for participation. The specific steps involved in self-monitoring are described in a way students can understand. For example, the instructor may say, "Today we're going to talk about a new program that will help you work better in math class. It's called self-monitoring. Self-monitoring is a way to help students improve their work habits and get better grades. Occasionally during math class, you're going to hear a beep. That's a signal for you to ask yourself whether or not you were working at the moment the beep sounded. Then you'll record your behavior by checking the correct box on a self-recording sheet like this. It's that simple! I think you'll have fun with self-monitoring!"

Modeling and Behavior Rehearsal

Next, the instructor models self-monitoring of relevant desired and undesired behaviors for the student. For example, the instructor may ask the child to watch while he simulates a classroom situation. The instructor may then engage in on-task behavior and, at the tone, ask himself the question, "Was I paying attention or not paying attention?" This is followed by demonstrating the self-recording of on-task behavior.

After several desired and undesired behaviors have been modeled by the instructor, the student may be asked to label and record the instructor's behavior. Finally, behavior rehearsal is used to practice self-monitoring in situations that are made as realistic as possible. Students are encouraged to role-play both desired and undesired behaviors at various times during the practice sessions, and to accurately self-monitor these behaviors. At this point in the training, emphasis is on accuracy of self-monitoring rather than on engaging in desired behavior.

Praise and Performance Feedback

Following each self-monitoring interval, the student is given praise and specific performance feedback. Praise is given for participation in the training and for accurate self-monitoring. Performance feedback focuses on specific behaviors that may have influenced the accuracy of self-monitoring during preceding intervals.

Evaluating Training Success

The success of self-monitoring training can be evaluated both during and following the training sessions. For example, instructors may set an initial criterion for accuracy of self-monitoring (e.g., 10 consecutive matches with the instructor) that students must meet prior to using self-monitoring in the natural setting. Then, students may be required to maintain a designated level of accuracy following training (e.g., no more than one session per week with less than 80% accuracy). If this level is not maintained, booster sessions may be provided in which behavior definitions and self-monitoring steps are reviewed and practiced.

APPLICATIONS OF SELF-MONITORING

As noted earlier, students with diverse characteristics have been taught to self-monitor a variety of target behaviors. However, applications of self-monitoring in school-based settings have generally targeted on-task behavior or academic performance.

Self-Monitoring On-Task Behavior

Paying attention is an essential classroom behavior, and it is well recognized that problems of attention are associated with poor academic performance (DeHaas-Warner, 1991; Ross, 1981). As a result of its importance, attention to task, or on-task behavior, has been a popular target of school-based self-monitoring interventions. Attentional behavior of students with learning disabilities (e.g., Maag, Rutherford, & DiGangi, 1992), emotional/behavioral disorders (e.g., Lloyd & Hilliard, 1989), attention-deficit disorders (e.g., Mathes & Bender, 1997), or cognitive deficits (e.g., Boyle & Hughes, 1994) may be improved by self-monitoring on-task behavior. As mentioned earlier, self-monitoring on-task behavior has also been used as an intervention strategy to remediate attentional difficulties of children and adolescents, rather than solely as an assessment strategy.

Procedures for Self-Monitoring On-Task Behavior

The prototypical procedure for self-monitoring on-task behavior in the classroom was developed by Hallahan and his colleagues (Hallahan, Lloyd, & Stoller, 1982). The procedure uses time sampling, in which the class period is divided into equal time intervals and students record on-task or off-task behavior during each of the separate intervals. Students are taught to ask themselves the question, "Was I paying attention when I heard the tone?" The

most commonly used recording device is a paper-and-pencil recording sheet (see Figure 5.2). For example, in one case, three highly distractible girls with mild to moderate mental handicaps, ages 9 to 11, were taught to self-record at the sound of a tone (McCarl et al., 1991). The girls were instructed to place a Y or an N in each square, on a sheet of paper with three rows of 10 squares, to indicate whether or not they were working at the sound of each tone. All three girls demonstrated an increase in on-task behavior using this procedure.

TYPES OF SELF-MONITORING PROMPTS

External cueing (such as produced by a tone) may be particularly useful with young children or with children who have significant disabilities because it serves as a reminder to monitor their behavior. On the other hand, external cues may be detrimental to some students' performance if the cues distract them from the task or disrupt their concentration. In these cases, it may be better to use noncued self-monitoring of attention to task (e.g., Heins, Lloyd, & Hallahan, 1986). As described earlier, in noncued self-monitoring students are given a self-recording sheet and directed to record their behavior whenever they think about it during the class session. A recording sheet like the one at the top of Figure 5.2 may be used simply by modifying the instruction to read, "Mark a + or – whenever you think about it."

In a study that compared cued and noncued self-recording of attention to task, four boys with learning disabilities were trained to self-monitor using both procedures (Heins et al., 1986). One procedure was in effect for the first half of each period and the other for the second half, with the order randomly determined. Although the students did learn to self-monitor using both procedures, their monitoring was inconsistent in the noncued condition and fewer reactive effects were reported for this condition than for cued self-monitoring. This outcome suggests that it may be more beneficial to use a cued prompting procedure with some students who exhibit significant impairment in their ability to attend.

SELF-MONITORING INTERVAL

There is no set standard length of intervals for self-monitoring on-task behavior, and intervals have varied widely in the literature, from self-monitoring every 15 seconds to every 120 seconds. Typically, the interval will depend on the characteristics of the students involved, such as their age, type of disability, or attentional problems. Obviously, younger students and students with more severe cognitive and attentional difficulties are candidates for shorter self-monitoring intervals. In many cases, it may be beneficial to vary the length of intervals to avoid having students predict the point at which the

self-monitoring cue will be delivered and pay attention only at that time (e.g., Maag et al., 1992).

In addition, increasingly longer self-monitoring intervals may be used with students in an effort to reduce their reliance on external cueing over time. In one example, two different audiotapes were used with five elementary students with moderate mental retardation who self-monitored on-task behavior during biweekly prevocational workshop sessions (Boyle & Hughes, 1994). Tones on the first audiotape were emitted on average every 45 seconds, and children were to ask themselves, "Am I working?" During fading conditions, a second tape was used that emitted tones at consecutive intervals of 2 minutes, 4 minutes, and 6 minutes during the work period.

In a second example, this time with older children, a series of four different 40-minute audiotapes were used with a group of 12 high school students with mild disabilities (Blick & Test, 1987). Two different cues could be heard on each of these tapes—one signaling the teacher to record student behavior (chime) and the other cueing students to self-monitor (a voice stating "record"). Initially, students were cued to self-monitor every 5 minutes, then this interval was increased to every 10 minutes, and then to every 20 minutes in subsequent tapes. In the final phase, students were no longer required to self-record their behavior so their cue was eliminated, although the audiotape continued to chime every 5 minutes to prompt teacher recording of their behavior.

Some teachers may find the use of multiple tapes too cumbersome, or it may not be necessary to gradually increase the self-monitoring interval. For example, some students may be capable, from the onset, of self-monitoring on-task behavior following rather lengthy intervals (e.g., at the end of the class period). In a recent example, four charter middle school students who were considered to be at risk for school failure were taught to self-monitor on-task behavior following each of three academic periods—language arts, computer class, and reading class (Wood et al., 1998). The students were instructed to self-monitor five specific on-task behaviors at the end of each of these 50-minute class periods. Self-recording sheets were placed on the students' desks before they entered the classroom and remained on their desks throughout the class period. This self-monitoring procedure was reportedly easy to use, and the lengthy self-monitoring intervals required no extra teacher time, effort, or prompting.

TRAINING PROCEDURES USED

In most cases, the training procedures described earlier can be used successfully to teach students to self-monitor on-task behavior. However, with very young children or students with more severe disabilities, a slightly different training strategy may be necessary. A novel training procedure was used suc-

cessfully with preschoolers who had poor on-task behavior during independent prereadiness tasks (De Haas-Warner, 1992). The training revolved around a story about a preschooler who had difficulty completing tasks without talking, looking around the room, or getting out of his seat. Drawings that depicted appropriate and inappropriate on-task behavior, corresponding to the story, were used. Children were then asked to repeat the story and the self-monitoring procedure that the story child used. Finally, the trainer modeled the self-monitoring procedure, allowed the children to rehearse that procedure until they displayed mastery of the technique, and provided the children positive feedback and a sticker.

ACCURACY OF SELF-MONITORING ON-TASK BEHAVIOR

It is well established that children and adolescents with various learning, behavioral, and cognitive characteristics may be capable of accurately self-monitoring on-task behavior (e.g., Blick & Test, 1987). In the example described earlier in which middle school students self-monitored five on-task behaviors at the end of each 50-minute class period, students' self-monitoring accuracy was verified by an independent observer and averaged 98% (range 80–100%) (Wood et al., 1998). This outcome suggests that many students are capable of accurately identifying and recording the presence or absence of multiple behaviors.

However, not all students self-monitor accurately; in fact, some have very low or inconsistent accuracy in self-monitoring on-task behavior. This may be due to factors such as a limited ability to attend to and correctly discriminate the occurrence of behavior, or simply a limited motivation to monitor accurately. In one example, mixed levels of self-monitoring accuracy were found across three elementary-age boys with severe emotional disturbance (McDougall & Brady, 1995). Whereas one boy self-monitored accurately during an average of 83% of the observations, the other two had lower mean accuracy levels of 70% and 30%, respectively. In addition, the accuracy of the participants ranged from 0% to 100% across sessions.

Not surprisingly, accuracy in self-monitoring on-task behavior can increase when children are trained to self-monitoring accurately (Shapiro, McGonigle, & Ollendick, 1981). However, even training for accuracy may not always prove successful. This was the case for four upper-elementary students with learning disabilities who were trained to self-monitor on-task behavior (Marshall et al., 1993). Results suggested that accuracy training produced only small and inconsistent improvements in students' accuracy of self-monitoring. It may be that training is insufficient for students who are the most inaccurate recorders. Perhaps these students may need additional measures to bolster their accuracy.

A rather straightforward strategy for enhancing the accuracy of self-

monitoring is to positively reinforce children or adolescents for being accurate. For example, in one case, initial low levels of accuracy were observed when five students in a self-contained special education classroom for students with emotional disturbance were asked to self-monitor on-task behavior during math class (Lloyd & Hilliard, 1989). When 50 cents was provided for accurate student recording, regardless of actual on-task behavior, accuracy was high. This finding suggests that reinforcement for accurate self-monitoring may be useful for increasing accuracy in some students.

A further option for increasing accuracy in self-monitoring is to make children or adolescents aware that their monitoring is being checked by an external observer. This task is typically accomplished by using a form of matching in which a student's self-recordings are compared with another observer's simultaneously recorded observations. Students may then also be reinforced for accurate self-monitoring. In one instance, a noncued self-monitoring and matching procedure was used with two adolescent males enrolled in a suburban middle school (Hertz & McLaughlin, 1990). Students were instructed to mark a + for on-task or a − for off-task behavior whenever they thought about it during class (although the teacher encouraged them to note on-task and off-task behavior about every 5 minutes). She also showed the students the card on which she would be simultaneously recording on-task and off-task behavior. At the end of each class period, if their tallies were within two marks in either direction of the teacher's, the students received a ticket. Tickets were redeemable for supplies, postcards, books, magazines, and edibles on a monthly basis. Because of its simplicity and unstructured nature, this strategy may be useful in many school-based settings. The case study of Wesley illustrates the use of a matching procedure to increase the accuracy of self-monitoring on-task behavior.

CASE STUDY: WESLEY

Wesley was a 7-year-old boy of average intellectual functioning who exhibited attentional difficulties in his first-grade classroom. The teacher noted that, especially during group activities, Wesley frequently watched and talked with other students, gazed or stared into space, and even turned his back to the speaker. Because his attention appeared to deteriorate throughout the course of the day, she decided to implement self-monitoring during the afternoon group lessons. To avoid any stigma that might be associated with singling out Wesley, she also decided to use a classwide self-monitoring procedure.

All children in the class were given an index card marked with 25 squares (see Figure 5.2) and were told that a tone would occasionally sound during their group lessons. Each time they heard the tone they were to stop and ask themselves, "Was I paying attention?" and answer by marking a Y for yes or an N for no. Initially, following each tone, the teacher matched with

a few randomly selected students to provide feedback on their accuracy. Thus, the students were uncertain as to who would be picked to match. Those students who accurately self-monitored received a special sticker placed at the bottom of their index cards. The accuracy of self-monitoring on-task behavior by Wesley and the other children in the class quickly rose to near 100% with the use of this matching procedure. In addition, Wesley's on-task behavior increased from an average of 35% before self-monitoring to almost 90% using this procedure.

Self-Monitoring Academic Performance

A second popular application of self-monitoring in school-based settings is the monitoring of academic performance. This strategy involves having students observe and record discrete behaviors related to some aspect of their own academic work. For example, they may self-monitor completion of problems on a worksheet, accuracy in answering math problems, number of words written in an essay, or number of words spelled correctly on a spelling test.

Self-monitoring academic performance is typically used with students who are having academic difficulties. However, beyond this broad criterion, student characteristics can vary and may include learning disabilities (e.g., Maag, Reid, & DiGangi, 1993), developmental disabilities (e.g., McCarl et al., 1991), and emotional/behavioral disorders (e.g., Carr & Punzo, 1993). Although self-monitoring academic performance can be used for assessment purposes, in school-based settings it is generally used as an intervention strategy inasmuch as students tend to show improvements in their academic behavior as a result of the monitoring process. These positive effects are consistent and evident across age groups, types of tasks, and student populations with which the procedures have been implemented.

Procedures for Self-Monitoring Academic Performance

Like self-monitoring on-task behavior, self-monitoring academic performance is straightforward and typically involves the use of pencil-and-paper recording after brief training sessions. Periodically during the class, or at the end of each academic period, students check their work to determine the number of responses completed and the number correct, and then record that information on a previously developed recording sheet (e.g., Reid & Harris, 1993). Types of self-monitoring prompts can vary but are essentially the same as those described for self-monitoring on-task behavior (e.g., audio cues, teacher signals).

Self-monitoring academic performance is frequently used during independent seat work periods when students are completing practice worksheets

or other independent assignments. At designated intervals or at the end of each independent work period, students may be asked to count and record the number of worksheet problems they completed and, using an answer key, record the number of problems they completed correctly. An example of a recording form used to self-monitor the completion and accuracy of math problems is provided in Figure 5.3. In some cases, students also record daily scores on graphs or charts as an additional assessment or incentive procedure (e.g., Carr & Punzo, 1993; DiGangi et al., 1991).

The academic behaviors targeted for self-monitoring usually involve either the production of an academic response (i.e., productivity) or the correctness of the academic performance (i.e., accuracy). A third, less common, strategy involves having students self-monitor the steps or actions involved in completing the task itself (i.e., process).

SELF-MONITORING PRODUCTIVITY

When the focus is on productivity, a self-recorded response simply provides evidence that the student has completed the required academic task, irre-

SELF-CHECK RECORD FOR _____

Interval	# Problems completed	# Problems correct	% Problems correct
1			
2			
3			
4			
5			
6			
7			
8			
9			
10			

FIGURE 5.3. Math self-check record.

spective of its accuracy. This may be the strategy of choice for a student whose primary difficulty is a slow work rate, but who generally completes the work accurately. In one example, as a measure of their performance students were asked to record the number of words they had written in stories they had composed, regardless of spelling accuracy (Harris et al., 1994). In another example, fourth-grade students with learning disabilities who were working on math assignments were instructed to record the number of problems completed at the moment the audible tone was heard (Maag et al., 1993). The tones sounded at various intervals, and students were instructed to count the number of problems completed since the last tone and record this on their self-monitoring sheets.

In a third example, elementary-age students with mild mental retardation were taught to record the number of numerals they had written during an independent math worksheet assignment (McCarl et al., 1991). In each of these examples, a specific academic behavior was identified, such as completing math problems or answering questions on an answer sheet, and the students were instructed to count the items and record the production of their responses, without regard to their accuracy. The case of Barry further illustrates self-monitoring academic productivity.

Case Study: Barry. Barry, a third-grader, was having difficulty completing his math assignments during the independent work period. Although Barry was capable of performing at grade level in math, he worked very slowly and, as a result, frequently did not finish his work during the allotted time period. In this case, a self-monitoring procedure was implemented to encourage Barry to increase his productivity during independent seat work. Specifically, Barry was taught to self-monitor the number of math problems he completed during the period. At the end of the independent work period, Barry simply counted the number of problems completed and recorded this number on a daily graph. Each week, Barry and his teacher identified a goal for the number of daily problems he needed to complete. On Friday, if he had reached his goal each day that week, Barry earned computer time at the end of the school day. By the end of the second week of self-monitoring, Barry's math productivity had increased from a low of two problems completed the first day to eight problems completed on the tenth day, a level the teacher considered acceptable. To ensure ongoing success, the program was continued for the remaining weeks of the school year.

SELF-MONITORING ACADEMIC ACCURACY

Often, it may also be beneficial to have students self-monitor the accuracy of their academic responses. This tactic may be especially beneficial for students who have academic skill deficits in addition to motivational difficulties. In self-monitoring academic accuracy, students are instructed to record the

number of *correct* responses they produce. For example, in one case fourth- to sixth-grade students with learning disabilities were instructed to record the number of words written correctly from weekly spelling lists during practice sessions (Harris et al., 1994). They were then taught to graph the results of their self-monitoring.

In another example, adolescents with emotional/behavior disorders recorded the accuracy of math problems they had completed whenever they heard an audible tone played at random intervals in the classroom (Lam, Cole, Shapiro, & Bambara, 1994). The students were taught to compare their responses with those on an answer sheet, mark those that were correct, count and record the number of problems correct, and, at the end of the work session, graph the results. Many similar examples can be found in which self-monitoring academic accuracy has been used successfully in school settings (e.g., Carr & Punzo, 1993; Maag et al., 1992). The cases of Carlos and Susan illustrate the use of two different strategies for self-monitoring academic accuracy.

Case Study: Carlos. Carlos, a fourth-grader, was a poor speller. In fact, a curriculum-based assessment revealed that he was functioning at a second-grade level in spelling. His teacher noted that Carlos's written work usually contained a large number of misspelled words, even words included on previous spelling lists. In addition, he often failed the weekly spelling tests because of poor accuracy and lack of speed. Although Carlos appeared to be attentive during the spelling lesson, he was easily frustrated when attempting to complete his spelling assignments.

In this case, a self-monitoring strategy was used in an effort to increase Carlos's spelling accuracy. The teacher first created an audiotape of the weekly spelling list. On the tape, each word was pronounced, followed by a several-second delay, and then the word was spelled correctly. After the tape was created, Carlos was given a prepared sheet for use during spelling practice sessions. Carlos began each session by turning on the practice tape. He was instructed to turn off the taperecorder when he heard the word, and to write the word in a column labeled "My Spelling." He then turned on the taperecorder and wrote the correct spelling of the word in the next column, "Correct Spelling," as it was presented on the tape. Carlos then turned off the taperecorder and checked his initial spelling of the word against the taperecorded spelling. If his initial spelling was correct, he marked Y in the third column. If his initial spelling was incorrect, he marked N and practiced the correct spelling in the next three columns, "Correct #1, 2, & 3." Carlos repeated these steps with each word on the list. Once he was able to complete the entire list with 100% accuracy, he was tested on the spelling list.

An obvious benefit of this procedure was that it allowed Carlos to progress through the academic material at an individualized pace. In addition, he was motivated to learn the words on his own and had increased op-

portunities for practice to spell the words correctly. In cases in which a teacher does not have time to make the spelling tapes, other student "tutors" or the student him- or herself can make the practice tapes. This procedure can also be applied to the practice of basic math facts or to more complex tasks such as learning vocabulary from science textbooks. Although the content of the material would change, the strategy for self-monitoring academic accuracy would remain essentially the same. In the following case, Susan used a slightly different self-monitoring strategy.

Case Study: Susan. Susan, a first-grade student, had difficulty adding single-digit numbers. During independent work periods, when the class was required to complete math worksheets, Susan frequently engaged in off-task behaviors, presumably because she was struggling with the academic material. Although the teacher had taught her to use a number line strategy, she was still unable to complete the worksheets accurately and within the time period allotted. She was also receiving unacceptable grades on weekly math tests.

For Susan, a Cover, Copy, and Compare procedure (Skinner, Turco, Beatty, & Rasavage, 1989) was implemented to increase her accuracy on math worksheets. At the beginning of each session she was given a recording sheet with specific math problems and their answers listed in the left column (see Figure 5.4). Susan was instructed to look at the first problem and its answer, cover the first column with a piece of construction paper, and write the math problem and answer she just saw. Next, she uncovered the original problem and copied it in the third column. Finally, she compared the "Cover" and "Copy" columns and placed a + or − in the "Compare" column on the right.

This practice procedure has a number of advantages. It provides students with immediate, corrective feedback following each response. The activity is completely self-directed, requiring no ongoing teacher involvement. Furthermore, the technique can easily be applied to almost any academic subject area. A modified version of this strategy that also enables students to check their own accuracy is simply to provide students access to an answer key after completing each worksheet. This procedure also enables students to see which problems they got wrong and correct them immediately. Having students check their own work can be useful in learning vocabulary words, answering comprehension questions, or any other type of worksheet activity.

SELF-MONITORING ACADEMIC PROCESS

A third, less common, form of self-monitoring academic performance involves monitoring, not the outcome of the academic task, but the steps or

Look	Cover	Copy	Compare
5 +3 8			
4 +2 6			
6 +1 7			
2 +5 7			
3 +3 6			
4 +3 7			
8 +1 9			
2 +2 4			
1 +5 6			

FIGURE 5.4. Cover, Copy, and Compare recording sheet.

process required to correctly reach the conclusion. For example, in one case students self-monitored their performance regarding whether or not they had completed each step of a self-instruction procedure that was designed to teach regrouping skills (Miller, Miller, Wheeler, & Selinger, 1989). These students with behavior disorders were taught to record their use of each step of the procedure.

In another example, students with learning disabilities used individualized self-monitoring checklists during completion of their subtraction assignments (Dunlap & Dunlap, 1989). Based on analyses of their typical errors in subtraction, individualized checklists were constructed. Each error was represented on a student's list as a "reminder," written in a first-person format, that the student would refer to and check off after each problem (e.g., "I regrouped when I needed to," "I crossed out only the number next to the underlined number and made it one less"). This self-monitoring procedure resulted in immediate gains in correct responding for each student.

Self-Monitoring Other Behaviors

As emphasized in previous sections of this chapter, self-monitoring has frequently been used to target attentional and academic difficulties in school settings. However, this strategy has also been applied to a range of other targets of interest, such as disruptive behaviors (e.g., Houghton, 1991), social or interpersonal skills (e.g., Ninness, Fuerst, Rutherford, & Glenn, 1991), inappropriate verbalizations (e.g., Kern et al., 1997), and daily calendar use (e.g., Flores, Schloss, & Alper, 1995). Applications can be grouped into two main categories: self-monitoring challenging behavior and self-monitoring desired behaviors, such as schedule following.

Like self-monitoring of on-task behavior and academic performance, self-monitoring of other behaviors has been used primarily for the purpose of improving behavior, rather than for assessment purposes, in school-based settings. The ease of implementing self-monitoring procedures for these types of behaviors provides educators with a practical, positive, and minimally intrusive option for modifying target behaviors.

Procedures for Self-Monitoring Other Behaviors

Many of the self-monitoring procedures described earlier can be applied to other target behaviors with only minor modifications. However, the following issues should also be considered:

1. *Positive reinforcement for desired responding may be necessary.* For some students with particularly challenging behavior, self-monitoring alone may fail to produce accuracy in monitoring and the desired change in behavior. However, adding external positive reinforcement contingencies for accurate self-monitoring and/or reductions in challenging behaviors may help to establish the desired responding.

2. *Adding a self-evaluation component may be useful.* Some of the most successful approaches have included a self-evaluation component whereby students are asked to rate their behavior on a 0- to 5-point scale periodically during a

class period. This added dimension may be necessary to produce behavior change in some students with challenging behavior.

3. *Involving students early in the process may be beneficial.* As an added incentive for participation in self-monitoring, a student may be encouraged to assist in the development of a self-monitoring method, as well as in the selection of behaviors to be monitored.

4. *Desired behaviors should be targeted.* To help students maintain a clear focus on the target goal, it may be beneficial to have them self-monitor appropriate, desired behaviors rather than undesired actions. This may increase the likelihood of positive reactive effects of self-monitoring.

5. *Various recording methods can be used.* The characteristics of the target behavior, the setting, and the student will determine the type of recording device used. Examples include the use of schedules, sticker charts, checklists, calendars, and more concrete methods (e.g., transferring a token from one pocket to another).

SELF-MONITORING CHALLENGING BEHAVIORS

Self-monitoring can be applied to a variety of disruptive, acting-out behaviors of children of all ages in school settings. Even children in preschool may be candidates for this type of self-monitoring. For example, in one case four disruptive preschool boys were taught to self-monitor during transition, free play, and small group instruction (Miller et al., 1993). The procedure involved having the teacher lead the children through a series of questions during and following activities (e.g., "Robert, did you start to clean up at the bell?" "Are you cleaning up right now?"). Students were asked to indicate by a thumbs-up or a thumbs-down whether they thought they had performed each behavior during the activity. Students whose results matched with the teacher's assessment were reinforced with stamps or stickers. The use of this self-monitoring procedure, which focused on the desired actions, decreased the off-task and competing behaviors of these students.

For older, more aggressive students, self-monitoring is typically used as one component of a multicomponent treatment package. For example, students may be initially involved in a social skills training program designed to teach specific appropriate behaviors, and then may be asked to self-monitor their newly acquired skills in natural settings (e.g., Ninness et al., 1991). For example, two junior high school students with emotional/behavioral disorders who attended a self-contained special education class were initially provided formal social skills instruction (Ninness, Fuerst, & Rutherford, 1995). The students then assessed their own socially appropriate behavior during each social skills session and at prescribed intervals throughout the entire academic day. Positive behavior change was maintained, even without adult supervision, with the use of this self-monitoring procedure. The following

case of Peter further illustrates the use of self-monitoring to decrease disruptive behavior in a classroom setting.

Case Study: Peter. Peter was a fifth-grade general education student with average intelligence who exhibited disruptive classroom behaviors (e.g., calling out in class, throwing pens and pencils, getting out of his seat). His behaviors annoyed the teacher, interfered with instructional time, and hindered his classmates. Several interventions had been tried without success, including verbal reprimands, time-out, loss of recess, and detention. As the disruptive behaviors required an increasing amount of the teacher's time and energy, she considered referring Peter for special services. However, because he was completing grade-level work, removal from the classroom was a last resort.

In an effort to maintain Peter in his current placement, the teacher decided to try implementing a self-monitoring procedure. Three target behaviors were identified for self-monitoring, including Peter's sitting in his seat, raising his hand before speaking, and using materials appropriately (i.e., no throwing). Preliminary observation before self-monitoring had determined that Peter was most likely to engage in disruptive behaviors during independent seat work periods.

Because Peter was the only student who would be self-monitoring and other students in the classroom might be disturbed by an auditory cue, the teacher decided to cue Peter to self-monitor by tapping the corner of his desk at various times during each work period. The tap occurred at random times to prevent Peter from predicting when he should record, but, on average, every 3 minutes. At each cue, Peter was to check as to whether or not he had engaged in each of the behaviors since the last cue (see Figure 5.5). In addition, a matching procedure was implemented, and following only brief training, Peter was able to self-monitor accurately. Within a few weeks the target behaviors had increased to acceptable levels even though the teacher had increased the self-monitoring interval to an average of only once every 10 minutes. This procedure was continued for the next few months, although the

Goal behaviors	Spot checks						Total
	1	2	3	4	5	6	
1. Was I sitting in my seat?							
2. Did I raise my hand before speaking?							
3. Did I use materials appropriately?							

FIGURE 5.5. Peter's self-monitoring chart.

long-term goal was for Peter to eventually self-record whenever he thought of it.

SELF-MONITORING SCHEDULE FOLLOWING

Another application of self-monitoring is to encourage schedule following. With this strategy, students are typically provided a daily schedule of activities or expectations and asked to record the completion of each activity. One example involved the use of a personal calendar by secondary students with mild to moderate mental retardation (Flores et al., 1995). Students were taught to carry and use their personal calendars, which was associated with an increase in accomplishing personal responsibilities.

A second example involved self-recording teachers' daily expectancies by middle school students with learning disabilities or behavioral disorders (Clees, 1994). Students were given a schedule that identified specific behaviors that teachers expected for each class or locker visit. The activity of self-monitoring whether or not these expectancies were met resulted in an increase in the target behaviors. The use of self-monitoring with Jane further illustrates this type of self-monitoring.

Case Study: Jane. Jane was a seventh-grade student whom teachers described as extremely disorganized. She appeared disheveled and often had difficulty finding books, notebooks, and writing instruments for class. Jane frequently failed to hand in homework assignments, claiming she did not know about the assignment or forgot to complete it. The work she did complete was generally at or above grade level.

Jane's science teacher decided to initiate self-monitoring in his class. He identified five expectations (e.g., "Brought materials to class," "Handed in homework," "Completed class work") and listed these on a self-monitoring card (see Figure 5.6). Then he had Jane tape the card to the inside of her science notebook, and every day as Jane entered the science classroom, he reminded her to check her card. At the end of each class, the teacher checked Jane's card and provided praise for self-monitoring and positive feedback on aspects of her academic performance that day. Jane's behavior improved so much with this simple self-monitoring strategy that her other teachers began using it for math, English, and social studies classes.

SUMMARY

Self-monitoring is a simple and practical procedure that has proven useful in school-based settings. Although it has potential utility as an assessment strategy, the positive reactive effects typically found with self-monitoring by chil-

MONDAY	☐ Brought all materials to class ☐ Handed in homework ☐ Completed all class work
TUESDAY	☐ Brought all materials to class ☐ Handed in homework ☐ Completed all class work
WEDNESDAY	☐ Brought all materials to class ☐ Handed in homework ☐ Completed all class work
THURSDAY	☐ Brought all materials to class ☐ Handed in homework ☐ Completed all class work
FRIDAY	☐ Brought all materials to class ☐ Handed in homework ☐ Completed all class work

FIGURE 5.6. Jane's science class checklist.

dren and adolescents have resulted in its use mainly as an intervention strategy. These reactive effects have been found across age groups, for both academic and nonacademic problems, and across many different types of student characteristics. For school-based practitioners, it may not make sense to use self-monitoring solely as an assessment tool, given its potential power for producing positive outcomes as an intervention.

With the fundamental shift toward inclusion of students with disabilities in general education, there is a recognition that students should be provided more experiences that encourage skills for independent functioning. Self-monitoring is one of the independence skills that can be taught relatively quickly and easily, and that students can use in a variety of settings. It may, for example, create an opportunity for some students with exceptional characteristics to participate or function more adaptively in general education settings. At a minimum, self-monitoring serves to involve the student in some aspect of his or her learning and behavior. This represents a clear departure from more traditional teacher-directed instruction and should be encouraged.

REFERENCES

Blick, D. W., & Test, D. W. (1987). Effects of self-recording on high-school students' on-task behavior. *Learning Disability Quarterly, 10*, 203–213.

Boyle, J. R., & Hughes, C. A. (1994). Effects of self-monitoring and subsequent fading of external prompts on the on-task behavior and task productivity of elementary students with moderate mental retardation. *Journal of Behavioral Education, 4*, 439–457.

Carr, S. C., & Punzo, R. P. (1993). The effects of self-monitoring of academic accuracy and productivity on the performance of students with behavioral disorders. *Behavioral Disorders, 18*, 241–250.

Clees, T. J. (1994). Self-recording of students' daily schedules of teachers' expectancies: Perspectives on reactivity, stimulus control, and generalization. *Exceptionality, 5*, 113–129.

Connell, M. C., Carta, J. J., Lutz, S., Randall, C., & Wilson, J. (1993). Building independence during in-class transitions: Teaching in-class transition skills to preschoolers with developmental delays through choral-response-based self-assessment and contingent praise. *Education and Treatment of Children, 16*, 160–174.

DeHaas-Warner, S. J. (1991). Effects of self-monitoring on preschoolers' on-task behavior: A pilot study. *Topics in Early Childhood Special Education, 11*, 59–73.

DeHaas-Warner, S. (1992). The utility of self-monitoring for preschool on-task behavior. *Topics in Early Childhood Special Education, 12*, 478–495.

DiGangi, S. A., Maag, J. W., & Rutherford, R. B. (1991). Self-graphing of on-task behavior: Enhancing the reactive effects of self-monitoring on on-task behavior and academic performance. *Learning Disability Quarterly, 14*, 221–230.

Dunlap, L. K., & Dunlap, G. (1989). A self-monitoring package for teaching subtraction with regrouping to students with learning disabilities. *Journal of Applied Behavior Analysis, 22*, 309–314.

Flores, D. M., Schloss, P. J., & Alper, S. (1995). The use of a daily calendar to increase responsibilities fulfilled by secondary students with special needs. *Remedial and Special Education, 16*, 38–43.

Hallahan, D. P., Lloyd, J. W., & Stoller, L. (1982). *Improving attention with self-monitoring: A manual for teachers.* Charlottesville: University of Virginia.

Harris, K. R., Graham, S., Reid, R., McElroy, K., & Hamby, R. S. (1994). Self-monitoring of attention versus self-monitoring of performance: Replication and cross-task comparison studies. *Learning Disability Quarterly, 17*, 121–139.

Heins, E. D., Lloyd, J. W., & Hallahan, D. P. (1986). Cued and noncued self-recording of attention to task. *Behavior Modification, 10*, 235–254.

Hertz, V., & McLaughlin, T. F. (1990). Self-recording: Effects for on-task behavior of mildly handicapped adolescents. *Child and Family Behavior Therapy, 12*, 1–11.

Houghton, S. J. (1991). Promoting generalisation of appropriate behaviour across special and mainstream settings: A case study. *Educational Psychology in Practice, 7*, 47–54.

Hughes, C. A., Korinek, L., & Gorman, J. (1991). Self-management for students with mental retardation in public school settings: A research review. *Education and Training in Mental Retardation, 26*, 271–291.

Hughes, C. A., Ruhl, K. L., & Misra, A. (1989). Self-management with behaviorally disordered students in school settings: A promise unfulfilled? *Behavioral Disorders, 14*, 250–262.

Kanfer, F. H. (1970). Self-monitoring: Methodological limitations and clinical applications. *Journal of Consulting and Clinical Psychology, 35*, 143–152.

Kanfer, F. H. (1977). The many faces of self-control. In R. B. Stuart (Ed.), *Behavioral self-management: Strategies, techniques, and outcomes.* New York: Brunner/Mazel.

Kern, L., Marder, T. J., Boyajian, A. E., Elliot, C. M., & McElhattan, D. (1997). Augmenting the independence of self-management procedures by teaching self-initiation across settings and activities. *School Psychology Quarterly, 12,* 23–32.

Koegel, R. L., & Koegel, L. K. (1990). Extended reductions in stereotypic behavior of students with autism through a self-management treatment package. *Journal of Applied Behavior Analysis, 23,* 119–127.

Lam, A. L., Cole, C. L., Shapiro, E. S., & Bambara, L. M. (1994). Relative effects of self-monitoring on-task behavior, academic accuracy, and disruptive behavior in students with behavior disorders. *School Psychology Review, 23,* 44–58.

Lloyd, M. E., & Hilliard, A. M. (1989). Accuracy of self-recording as a function of repeated experience with different self-control contingencies. *Child and Family Behavior Therapy, 11,* 1–14.

Lonnecker, C., Brady, M. P., McPherson, R., & Hawkins, J. (1994). Video self-modeling and cooperative classroom behavior in children with learning and behavior problems: Training and generalization effects. *Behavioral Disorders, 20,* 24–34.

Maag, J. W., Reid, R., & DiGangi, S. A. (1993). Differential effects of self-monitoring attention, accuracy, and productivity. *Journal of Applied Behavior Analysis, 26,* 329–344.

Maag, J. W., Rutherford, R. B., & DiGangi, S. A. (1992). Effects of self-monitoring and contingent reinforcement on on-task behavior and academic productivity of learning-disabled students: A social validation study. *Psychology in the Schools, 29,* 157–172.

Marshall, K. J., Lloyd, J. W., & Hallahan, D. P. (1993). Effects of training to increase self-monitoring accuracy. *Journal of Behavioral Education, 3,* 445–459.

Mathes, M. Y., & Bender, W. N. (1997). The effects of self-monitoring on children with attention-deficit/hyperactivity disorder who are receiving pharmacological interventions. *Remedial and Special Education, 18,* 121–128.

McCarl, J. J., Svobodny, L., & Beare, P. L. (1991). Self-recording in a classroom for students with mild to moderate mental handicaps: Effects on productivity and on-task behavior. *Education and Training in Mental Retardation, 26,* 79–88.

McDougall, D., & Brady, M. P. (1995). Using audio-cued self-monitoring for students with severe behavior disorders. *Journal of Educational Research, 88,* 309–317.

Miller, L. J., Strain, P. S., Boyd, K., Jarzynka, J., & McFetridge, M. (1993). The effects of classwide self-assessment on preschool children's engagement in transition, free play, and small group instruction. *Early Education and Development, 4,* 162–181.

Miller, M., Miller, S. R., Wheeler, J. J., & Selinger, J. (1989). Can a single-classroom treatment approach change academic performance and behavioral characteristics in severely behaviorally disordered adolescents?: An experimental inquiry. *Behavioral Disorders, 14,* 215–225.

Nelson, R. O., & Hayes, S. C. (1981). Theoretical explanations of reactivity in self-monitoring. *Behavior Modification, 5,* 3–14.

Newman, B., Buffington, D. M., O'Grady, M. A., McDonald, M. E., Poulson, C. L., & Hemmes, N. S. (1995). Self-management of schedule following in three teenagers with autism. *Behavioral Disorders, 20,* 190–196.

Ninness, H. A. C., Fuerst, J., & Rutherford, R. (1995). A descriptive analysis of disruptive behavior during pre- and post-unsupervised self-management by students with serious emotional disturbance: A within-study replication. *Journal of Emotional and Behavioral Disorders, 3,* 230–240.

Ninness, H. A. C., Fuerst, J., Rutherford, R. D., & Glenn, S. S. (1991). Effects of self-management training and reinforcement on the transfer of improved conduct in the absence of supervision. *Journal of Applied Behavior Analysis, 24,* 499–508.

Piersel, W. C. (1985). Self-observation and completion of school assignments: The influence of a physical recording device and expectancy characteristics. *Psychology in the Schools, 22,* 331–336.

Rachlin, H. (1974). Self-control. *Behaviorism, 2,* 94–107.

Reid, R., & Harris, K. R. (1993). Self-monitoring of attention versus self-monitoring of performance: Effects on attention and academic performance. *Exceptional Children, 60,* 29–40.

Ross, A. O. (1981). Deficits in attention. In A. O. Ross (Ed.), *Child behavior therapy* (pp. 88–104). New York: Wiley.

Schunk, D. H. (1982). Progress self-monitoring: Effects on children's self-efficacy and achievement. *Journal of Experimental Education, 51,* 89–93.

Shapiro, E. S., & Cole, C.L. (1994). *Behavior change in the classroom: Self-management interventions.* New York: Guilford Press.

Shapiro, E. S., McGonigle, J. J., & Ollendick, T. H. (1981). Analysis of self-assessment and self-reinforcement in a self-managed token economy with mentally retarded children. *Applied Research in Mental Retardation, 1,* 227–240.

Skinner, C. H., Turco, T., Beatty, K., & Rasavage, C. (1989). Cover, Copy, and Compare: A method for increasing multiplication performance. *School Psychology Review, 18,* 412–420.

Wood, S. J., Murdock, J. Y., Cronin, M. E., Dawson, N. M., & Kirby, P. C. (1998). Effects of self-monitoring on on-task behaviors of at-risk middle school students. *Journal of Behavioral Education, 8,* 263–279.

Workman, E. A., Helton, G. B., & Watson, P. J. (1982). Self-monitoring effects in a four-year-old child: An ecological behavior analysis. *Journal of School Psychology, 20,* 57–64.

CHAPTER 6

◆◆◆

Self-Report: Rating Scale Measures

◆

TANYA L. ECKERT
ERIN K. DUNN
ROBIN S. CODDING
KATIE M. GUINEY

The purpose of this chapter is to provide school-based applications for the use of child and adolescent self-report measures within the context of a multimethod behavioral assessment (Eckert, Dunn, Guiney, & Codding, 2000). Recently developed self-report measures are reviewed and highlighted across a number of important domains, including behavior dimensions assessed, relevant clinical subscales, and unique measurement features. Following this introduction, the chapter focuses on a decision-making framework for using self-report measures in the assessment of children's and adolescents' emotional and behavioral functioning. General characteristics of the assessment process are described, and the components of the decision-making framework are outlined in detail. Attention is focused on describing how self-report measures can be used to identify potential comorbid conditions. Finally, the chapter concludes with a case example illustrating this method of behavioral assessment.

SELF-REPORT MEASURES FOR ASSESSING CHILDREN'S EMOTIONAL AND BEHAVIORAL FUNCTIONING

Quantitative and qualitative data obtained from self-report measures constitute an indirect form of behavioral assessment (Cone, 1978). These data represent an individual's perceptions of behavior across varying dimensions of time, setting, or context relative to the assessment condition (Kratochwill &

Shapiro, 1988). Although the accuracy of data obtained from self-report measures may be biased or unreliable (Martens, 1993), the information can be used to complement other sources of information within the context of a multimethod behavioral assessment (Elliott, Busse, & Gresham, 1993). That is, child and adolescent self-reports can be used in conjunction with informant reports (i.e., reports of parents, teachers, peers), semistructured interviews, and observations in natural settings. However, only self-report measures with adequate psychometric properties should be used within this context (Breen, Eckert, & DuPaul, 1996; Martens, 1993; McConaughy & Ritter, 1995).

A number of self-report rating scales have been developed for measuring the emotional and behavioral functioning of children and adolescents. Broad-band rating scales and narrow-band rating scales are two categories of self-report measures (Eckert & DuPaul, 1996). Broad-band rating scales, such as the Youth Self-Report (YSR; Achenbach, 1991), assess a wide area of behavior. Narrow-band rating scales, such as the Reynolds Child Depression Scale (RCDS; Reynolds, 1989), assess a specific area of behavior. Combining these two distinct categories of self-report measures allows information to be collected regarding a child's perceived level of functioning in relation to broad categories of behavior (i.e., broad-band measures) and specific dimensions of behavior (i.e., narrow-band measures). This results in a comprehensive assessment of potential behavior problems that concludes with a detailed examination of specific emotional or behavioral functioning.

USING SELF-REPORT MEASURES TO ASSESS BROAD DOMAINS OF BEHAVIOR

A number of broad-band self-report measures have been developed to measure children's and adolescents' emotional or behavioral functioning across broad domains of behavior. As reviewed in our chapter on self-report measures (Eckert et al., 2000), three self-report measures that assess broad domains of behavior include the YSR, the Self-Report of Personality (SRP) of the Behavior Assessment System for Children (BASC; Reynolds & Kamphaus, 1992), and the Internalizing Symptoms Scale for Children (ISSC; Merrell & Walters, 1996). Although these three scales share some common features (i.e., assess a wide range of syndromes), they also differ across a number of dimensions, such as clinical subscales. In an attempt to facilitate comparisons across relevant domains of these measures, we have compiled a more specific overview of the YSR, SRP, and ISSC. Specifically, we have reviewed these instruments across the following dimensions in tabular form: type of behavior problem assessed, age range, item format, number of items, behavior dimensions assessed, and clinical subscales (see Table 6.1). This in-

TABLE 6.1. General Characteristics of Self-Report Measures Used with Children and Adolescents

Measure	Behavior assessed	Age range	Item format	Number of items	Behavior dimensions assessed	Composite scores
Internalizing Symptoms Scale for Children (Merrell & Walters, 1996)	General internalizing symptoms	Grades 3–6	True/false	48	Anxiety Depression Social withdrawal Somatic complaints	Negative affect/general distress Positive affect
Self-Report of Personality of the Behavior Assessment System for Children (Reynolds & Kamphaus, 1992)	General internalizing and externalizing symptoms	8–11 years (SRP-C) 12–18 years (SRP-A)	Binary scale (i.e., true/false)	152 (SRP-C) 186 (SRP-A)	Anxiety Attitude to school Attitude to teacher Atypicality Depression Interpersonal relations Locus of control Relations with parents Self-esteem Self-reliance Sensation seeking (SRP-A) Sense of inadequacy Social stress Somatization (SRP-A)	School maladjustment Clinical maladjustment Personal adjustment Emotional Symptoms Index
Youth Self-Report (Achenbach, 1991)	General internalizing and externalizing symptoms	11–18 years	3-point Likert-type scale	136	Aggressive behavior Anxious/depressed Attention problems Delinquent behavior Social problems Somatic complaints Thought problems Withdrawn	Total Problem Behavior Scale Internalizing Problem Behavior Scale Externalizing Problem Behavior Scale Total Competence Scale

Instrument	Domain	Age range	Response format	Items	Subscales	Additional scales
Adolescent Behavior Checklist (Adams, Kelley, & McCarthy, 1997)	Externalizing symptoms; dimensions of ADHD	11–17 years	4-point Likert-type scale	44	Conduct problems Emotional liability Inattention Impulsivity/hyperactivity Poor work habits Social problems	Total scale score
Assessment of Interpersonal Relations (Bracken & Kelley, 1993)	Internalizing symptoms; dimensions of interpersonal relations	9–19 years	4-point Likert-type scale	105	Acceptance Affect Companionship Conflict Emotional comfort Emotional support Empathy Guidance Identity Intimacy Reliance Respect Shared values Trust Understanding	Mother Father Male peers Female peers Teachers Total Relationship Index
Children's Depression Inventory (Kovacs, 1992)	Internalizing symptoms; depression symptoms	7–17 years	Multiple choice	27	Anhedonia Ineffectiveness Interpersonal problems Negative mood Negative self-esteem	
Multidimensional Anxiety Scale for Children (March, 1997)	Internalizing symptoms; anxiety symptoms	8–19 years	4-point Likert-type scale	39	Anxiety Anxious coping Humiliation fears Perfectionism Performance fears Somatic symptoms Tense symptoms	Anxiety Disorders Index Harm Avoidance Scale Inconsistencies Index Physical Symptoms Scale Social Anxiety Scale Total Anxiety Scale

(continued)

TABLE 6.1. *Continued*

Measure	Behavior assessed	Age range	Item format	Number of items	Behavior dimensions assessed	Composite scores
Multidimensional Self-Concept Scale (Bracken, 1992)	Internalizing symptoms; dimensions of self-concept	9–19 years	4-point Likert-type scale	150	Academic Affect Competence Family Physical Social	Global self-concept
Piers–Harris Children's Self-Concept Scale (Piers, 1984)	Internalizing symptoms; dimensions of self-concept	8–18 years	Binary scale (i.e., yes/no)	80	Anxiety Behavior Happiness/satisfaction Intellectual/school status Physical appearance Popularity	Global self-concept
Reynolds Child Depression Scale (Reynolds, 1989)	Internalizing symptoms; depressive symptoms	8–12 years	4-point Likert-type scale	30	Anhedonia Generalized demoralization Despondency–worry Dysphoric mood Somatic–vegetative	Total scale score
Reynolds Adolescent Depression Scale (Reynolds, 1989)	Internalizing symptoms; depressive symptoms	13–18 years	4-point Likert-type scale	30	Anhedonia Despondency–worry Generalized demoralization Somatic–vegetative Self-worth	Total scale score
Social Skills Rating System—Student Form (Gresham & Elliott, 1990)	Externalizing symptoms; social skills	5–18 years	3-point Likert-type scale	55	Assertion Cooperation Empathy Self-control	Total social skills

formation may be particularly useful when school-based practitioners are examining the applicability of various self-report measures. However, school-based practitioners should also consider developmental issues, environmental influences, type of population assessed, variance in self-report measures, and ethical concerns when selecting self-report measures (Eckert et al., 2000).

The use of self-report measures to assess broad domains of behavior should be guided by the need to obtain general information regarding emotional and behavioral functioning. As such, the assessment process begins with the selection of a broad-band self-report measure. Because several broad-band instruments are available, it is important for the school-based practitioner to review the general characteristics of each scale. The selection of a broad-band self-report measure should be based on the range of behaviors assessed by the scale, as well as the relevance of the scale to the nature of the referring problem(s). In the next sections, we describe how the general characteristics of the YSR, SRP, and ISSC can be used in assessing the emotional and behavioral functioning of children and adolescents.

Broad-Band Measures of Internalizing and Externalizing Disorders

The YSR is an example of a broad-band self-report measure of internalizing and externalizing behavior problems. Administration of the YSR yields eight problem behavior dimensions, including aggressive behavior, anxious/depressed, attention problems, delinquent behavior; social problems, somatic complaints, thought problems, and withdrawal. In addition, four composite scores can be computed with the following scales: Total Competence Scale, Total Problem Behavior Scale, Total Externalizing Problem Behavior Scale, and Total Internalizing Problem Behavior Scale. One of the key aspects of the YSR is the inclusion of clinical syndromes based on empirical studies of clinical and nonclinical samples of children and adolescents (Achenbach & McConaughy, 1992). In assessing the emotional and behavioral functioning of students, school-based practitioners may find that the YSR provides relevant clinical information along the continuum of internalizing and externalizing disorders. This aspect is particularly important when school-based practitioners are involved with classification or eligibility decisions.

Another self-report measure that assesses internalizing and externalizing disorders is the SRP of the BASC. The SRP contains 14 clinical scales: Anxiety, Attitude to School, Attitude to Teachers, Atypicality, Depression, Interpersonal Relations, Locus of Control, Relations with Parents, Self-Esteem, Self-Reliance, Sensation Seeking, Sense of Inadequacy, Social Stress, and Somatization. In addition, four composite scores can be computed: Clinical Maladjustment, Emotional Symptoms Index, Personal Adjustment, and School Maladjustment. School-based practitioners using the BASC will find

that a range of information can be collected. That is, data can be obtained documenting the presence of clinical problems (i.e., depression, anxiety) as well as documenting students' relationships with parents, teachers, and peers. The inclusion of clinical scales measuring sensation-seeking behaviors as well as social stress may result in important information for the development of intervention programs. In addition, the measurement of school functioning (i.e., School Maladjustment composite score) may be particularly relevant for school-based practitioners involved with classification or eligibility decisions. However, although the SRP assesses a number of relevant behavior domains, school-based practitioners may find that this measure does not assess a wide range of clinical disorders, such as attention problems or aggression. Therefore, this measure may be more suitable for a broad-band assessment of self-reported internalizing disorders and general school functioning.

Broad-Band Measure of Internalizing Disorders

The ISSC is the only broad-band self-report measure of internalizing disorders. This instrument addresses four clinical symptoms: anxiety, depression, social withdrawal, and somatic complaints. Two general composite scores can be computed: Negative Affect/General Distress, and Positive Affect. School-based practitioners will find that the ISSC affords a comprehensive assessment of a broad range of internalizing disorders. In addition, because the ISSC includes dimensions of positive and negative affect, these behavioral domains can be used when practitioners attempt to clinically differentiate anxiety from depression (Merrell, 1999). As delineated by the authors of the scale (Merrell & Walters, 1996), the ISSC was developed as a general screening measure for a wide range of internalizing disorders. Therefore, it is recommended that school-based practitioners use the ISSC for referral cases focusing on internalizing problem behaviors, such as depression or anxiety.

USING SELF-REPORT MEASURES TO ASSESS NARROW DOMAINS OF BEHAVIOR

Following the use of a broad-band measure, potential behavioral problems should be identified along the continuum of internalizing and externalizing disorders. Narrow-band measures should then be employed to further investigate specific dimensions of behavior that are of clinical significance. Using narrow-band self-report measures allows detailed information to be gathered regarding a student's perceived level of functioning (Eckert & DuPaul, 1996). As reviewed in our chapter on self-report measures (Eckert et al., 2000), a number of instruments have been developed for specific internalizing and externalizing disorders, such as anxiety, depression, peer relationships, self-

concept, attention problems, and conduct problems. Although it may appear that several self-report measures may be available for assessing similar domains of behavior (i.e., depression), the applicability of each measure may depend on the referring problem(s) as well as the scope of the measure. Thus, it is important that school-based practitioners be familiar with the general characteristics of narrow-band self-report measures. Because each measure may be useful for different purposes, we have provided an overview of these self-report measures across relevant domains (see Table 6.1). It is our intention that this will serve as a framework for comparing these measures and assisting in instrument selection. In the next sections, we illustrate how the general characteristics of narrow-band measures can be used in assessing specific aspects of students' emotional and behavioral functioning.

Narrow-Band Assessment of Anxiety and Related Disorders

The Multidimensional Anxiety Scale for Children (MASC; March, 1997) is one of the few narrow-band measures of anxiety and related disorders. In addition to containing clinical subscales in the area of Physical Symptoms and Harm Avoidance, the MASC also contains one subscale assessing social anxiety and a separate form (i.e., the MASC-10) that assesses general anxiety symptoms. Composite scores can be obtained for two major indexes, Anxiety Disorders and Inconsistency, as well as a total anxiety index. School-based practitioners may find that this scale provides relevant information regarding anxiety symptomatology. In addition, response patterns on the MASC may be useful in determining whether a generalized or specific anxiety disorder may be present (March, 1997). Furthermore, examination of individual items may assist school-based practitioners in selecting target behaviors for intervention.

Narrow-Band Assessment of Depression

Two narrow-band measures of depression can be used to assess students' functioning. First, the Children's Depression Inventory (CDI; Kovacs, 1981, 1992) assesses the severity of depressive symptoms in children and adolescents. Behavioral domains assessed by this scale include Total Depression Index, Anhedonia, Ineffectiveness, Interpersonal Problems, Negative Mood, and Negative Self-Esteem. Because the CDI is considered the most widely used measure of depression (Kamphaus & Frick, 1996), school-based practitioners may prefer to use this measure. However, it is important to note that the lack of a national normative sample has drawn criticism (Kavan, 1990; Knoff, 1990). Because of this limitation, it has been recommended that school-based practitioners adopt conservative guidelines for determining clinical cutoff scores (Merrell, 1999). In addition, there has been some dis-

cussion regarding whether the CDI may be a better indicator of distress, rather than depression (Cooper, 1990). Given that the CDI was not designed as a diagnostic measure of depression (Reynolds, 1992), it is recommended that school-based practitioners use this measure conservatively in the assessment process.

The RCDS and the Reynolds Adolescent Depression Scale (RADS; Reynolds, 1987) are also narrow-band measures of depression. Specifically, the RCDS measures symptoms associated with depression and includes the following clinical subscales: Anhedonia, Despondency–Worry, Dysphoric Mood, Generalized Demoralization–Despondency, and Somatic–Vegetative. The RADS measures five clinical subscales associated with depression, which include Anhedonia, Despondency and Worry, Generalized Demoralization, Self-Worth, and Somatic–Vegetative. To determine the severity of depressive symptoms, overall composite scores can be computed for both the RCDS and the RADS. In addition, 29 items have been found to relate to clinically defined symptoms of depression (Reynolds, 1992) and can be used for diagnostic purposes. Furthermore, a number of studies have documented the use of the RCDS and RADS as viable treatment outcome measures (Kahn, Kehle, Jenson, & Clark; 1990; Reynolds & Coats, 1986). Therefore, school-based practitioners may find the RCDS and RADS to be beneficial in screening, diagnosis, and treatment planning.

Narrow-Band Assessment of Peer Relationships and Social Skills

The Social Skills Rating System—Student Form (SSRS-S; Gresham & Elliott, 1990) is a multidomain self-report measure of social skills. The SSRS-S contains five subdomains of social skills: Assertion, Cooperation, Empathy, Interfering Behaviors, and Self-Control. One global composite, the Social Skills Index, is computed as an indicator of the student's assessment of his or her social skills. In addition, data are collected regarding the frequency and importance of social behaviors, which may assist school-based practitioners in selecting target behaviors for intervention and program planning (Eckert & DuPaul, 1996). The normative sample contains children with disabilities and may therefore be of particular relevance in assessing this population. School-based practitioners may find the SSRS-S useful in assessing students' perceptions of their social skills at school and at home.

The Assessment of Interpersonal Relations (AIR; Bracken & Kelly, 1993) is the only narrow-band self-report measure of interpersonal relations. Designed to assess the quality of students' interpersonal relationships with their peers, parents, and teachers, the AIR measures 15 relationship characteristics across five primary relationships (see Table 6.1). This multidimensional assessment results in five interpersonal relations subscales (i.e., Mother, Father, Male Peers, Female Peers, Teacher) and a total scale score (i.e., Total

Relationship Index). School-based practitioners may find the AIR to be a useful adjunct in the assessment of social skills and interpersonal relations, in that it can provide quantitative data regarding students' perceptions of primary relationships (Eckert & DuPaul, 1996).

Narrow-Band Assessment of Self-Concept

Two narrow-band measures of self-concept can be used to assess students' perceptions of their functioning: the Piers–Harris Children's Self-Concept Scale (PHCSCS; Piers, 1984) and the Multidimensional Self-Concept Scale (MSCS; Bracken, 1992). The PHCSCS assesses students' perceived self-esteem across six areas: Anxiety, Behavior, Happiness and Satisfaction, Intellectual and School Status, Physical Appearance and Attributes, and Popularity. Although the PHCSCS has been widely cited in research and clinical applications, the normative sample has been criticized as outdated (Eckert & DuPaul, 1996). School-based practitioners are strongly encouraged to use caution when interpreting scores from the PHCSCS for diagnostic purposes. The PHCSCS may be more appropriate for use as an adjunct to other measures of self-control or as a tool for examining patterns of behavioral clusters relative to the total scale score. Furthermore, because of empirical evidence suggesting that the PHCSCS is sensitive to treatment effects (Piers, 1984), school-based practitioners may find this measure useful for treatment planning and progress monitoring.

Using a multidimensional approach to the conceptualization of self-concept, the MSCS represents an important development in the assessment process. Because of its breadth, the MSCS assesses global self-concept and includes six subscales: Affect, Academic, Competence, Family, Physical, and Social. Unlike the PHCSCS, the MSCS possesses an adequate normative sample. Therefore, school-based practitioners can be confident in using scores obtained from the MSCS for various types of decision making. In addition, subscales can be administered and interpreted individually. Practitioners may find that the MSCS provides a more comprehensive assessment of self-concept.

Narrow-Band Assessment of Attention and Concentration Problems

The Adolescent Behavior Checklist (ABC; Adams, Kelley, & McCarthy, 1997) is one of the few self-report measures of attention problems. The measure was designed to assess the core symptoms of attention-deficit/hyperactivity disorder (ADHD) and associated problem areas. Accordingly, the ABC yields a total scale score as well as six clinical factors, which include Conduct Problems, Emotional Lability, Inattention, Impulsivity/Hyperactivity, Poor

Work Habits, and Social Problems. School-based practitioners may find this scale useful in obtaining information regarding adolescents' perceptions of their behavior and related problem areas.

Narrow-Band Assessment of Conduct Problems

There are few recent self-report measures of conduct disorder. The Self-Report Delinquency Scale (SRD; Elliott, Huizinga, & Ageton, 1985) is one measure that is widely used in longitudinal studies of conduct disorder and delinquency. Information obtained from the SRD indicates the frequency of conduct problems during the last year. These include criminal offenses, delinquent behaviors, and drug use. The SRD contains six summary subscales as well as a Total Self-Report Delinquency Score. The subscales of the SRD include hard drug use, illegal service crimes, predatory crimes against persons, predatory crimes against property, public disorder crimes, and status crimes. Although this scale is not recommended for diagnostic decision making, the SRD may assist school-based practitioners in measuring adolescents' reported frequency of conduct problems.

USING BROAD- AND NARROW-BAND SELF-REPORT MEASURES TO SCREEN FOR COMORBIDITY

An advantage of combining broad- and narrow-band measures is that this approach to assessment allows comorbid conditions to be examined along a continuum of internalizing and externalizing conditions. That is, broad-band measures of internalizing and externalizing disorders can be used to screen for potential behavior problems across broad domains of behavior, such as anxiety, depression, aggression, and attention problems. If multiple domains are identified, then school-based practitioners can enlist narrow-band measures to conduct a more detailed examination. This allows the assessment process to be guided by information gathered with the narrow-band measures. Therefore, based on the results of the broad-band measure, the assessment process will have to be adjusted.

To successfully assess comorbid conditions, it is important for school-based practitioners to be aware of the research examining and estimating the prevalence of such conditions. In our chapter discussing conceptual and theoretical issues associated with self-report measures, we identified a number of comorbid conditions likely to occur in the areas of anxiety, depression, attention and concentration problems, and conduct disorders (Eckert et al., 2000). For example, a number of empirical studies have documented the comorbidity of depression with other behavior disorders such as anxiety (Alessi & Magen, 1988; Finch, Lipovsky, & Casat, 1989; Strauss, Last, Hersen, & Kazdin,

1988), attention-deficit/hyperactivity disorder (Alessi & Magen, 1988; Anderson, Williams, McGee, & Silva, 1987; Jensen, Burke, & Garfinkel, 1988), conduct disorder (Alessi & Magen, 1988; Kovacs, Paulauskas, Gastonis, & Richards, 1988; Puig-Antich, 1982), eating disorders (Alessi, Krahn, Brehm, & Wittekindt, 1989), substance abuse (Akiskal et al., 1985; Kashini, Keller, Solomon, Reid, & Mazzola, 1985; Levy & Deykin, 1989), and suicidal behavior (Reynolds, 1994). Given that comorbidity occurs frequently with children and adolescents experiencing emotional and behavioral difficulties (Bird, Gould, & Staghezza, 1992), it is important for school-based practitioners to conduct a comprehensive assessment that addresses the referral problem as well as patterns of comorbidity relevant to the referral problem (Kamphaus & Frick, 1996). In Table 6.2, we have constructed a matrix illustrating the most common patterns of comorbidity along the continuum of internalizing and externalizing disorders. Practitioners may find this matrix helpful in evaluating possible comorbid conditions, as well as in planning the assessment process.

Decision-Making Framework for Combining Broad- and Narrow-Band Self-Report Measures

In addition to being aware of common patterns of comorbidity, it is important for practitioners to consider a framework for combining broad- and narrow-band self-report measures. The first step in this decision-making process is to review the referral information to determine whether broad-band measures that assess internalizing and externalizing behavior domains are warranted. For referral cases that present internalizing and externalizing problems, either the YSR or the SRP should be used. School-based practitioners

TABLE 6.2. A Matrix Illustrating the Comorbidity of Internalizing and Externalizing Behavior Disorders

	Internalizing behavior disorders			Externalizing behavior disorders		
	Anxiety	Depression	Eating disorders	Attention problems	Conduct disorder	Oppositional defiant disorder
Anxiety	—	Yes	No	Yes	Yes	No
Depression	Yes	—	Yes	Yes	Yes	No
Eating disorders	No	Yes	—	No	No	No
Attention problems	Yes	Yes	No	—	Yes	Yes
Conduct disorder	Yes	Yes	No	Yes	—	Yes
Oppositional defiant disorder	No	No	No	Yes	Yes	—

may consider selecting the ISSC for referral cases that focus predominately on internalizing problems. Following the administration of a broad-band self-report measure, behavior domains of clinical significance should be further examined with narrow-band self-report measures. Behavior domains that approach clinical significance should also be examined in further detail with corresponding self-report measures. Furthermore, given the questionable correspondence between children's and adolescents' self-report measures and informant reports, data obtained from parents or teachers should also be incorporated in the selection of narrow-band measures. Parent- or teacher-report data suggesting clinically significant behavior domains, particularly externalizing symptoms, should be explored in further detail.

The selection of appropriate narrow-band measures, based on clinically significant behavior domains, should focus on those that afford detailed examination. To assist practitioners in this decision making, we have developed frameworks for combining broad-band and narrow-band self-report measures. Figures 6.1, 6.2, and 6.3 illustrate these frameworks for combining the narrow-band measures reviewed in this chapter with the YSR, SRP, and ISSC, respectively. For example, in Figure 6.1, the broad behavior domains of the YSR are illustrated at the top. Solid arrows identify eight behavior domains measured by the YSR. If data obtained from the YSR in these behavior domains suggest clinical significance, further investigation is warranted. Dotted arrows identify corresponding narrow-band measures that school-based practitioners can select to obtain further information. That is, if the domain of Somatic Complaints reaches clinical significance on the YSR, either the MASC or MSCS may be administered.

Case Illustration of Combining Broad- and Narrow-Band Self-Report Measures

This final section presents a case illustration of how self-report measures can be used in school-based settings to assess students' perceived functioning in a number of domains. To illustrate combining broad- and narrow-band self-report measures within the context of a multimethod behavioral assessment, the case example describes the use of self-report measures with a young child experiencing externalizing and internalizing behavior problems. It is important to note that this illustration focuses on only one aspect of behavioral assessment, the use of self-report measures.

Tanner, an 11-year-old sixth-grade student, was referred for a psychological evaluation because of attention problems and withdrawn behaviors at home and in school. His parents contacted the school psychologist because they were concerned about his progress and adjustment in school. Tanner's parents reported that he had experienced difficulty concentrating for long periods of time since he was a young child. In addition, his parents reported

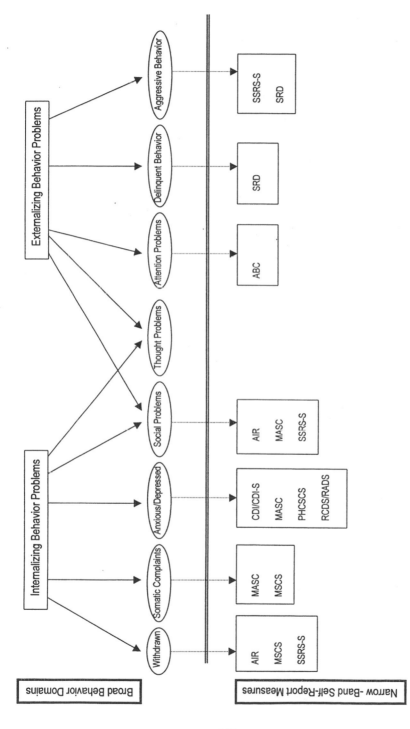

FIGURE 6.1. A decision-making framework for combining the Youth Self-Report with narrow-band self-report measures.

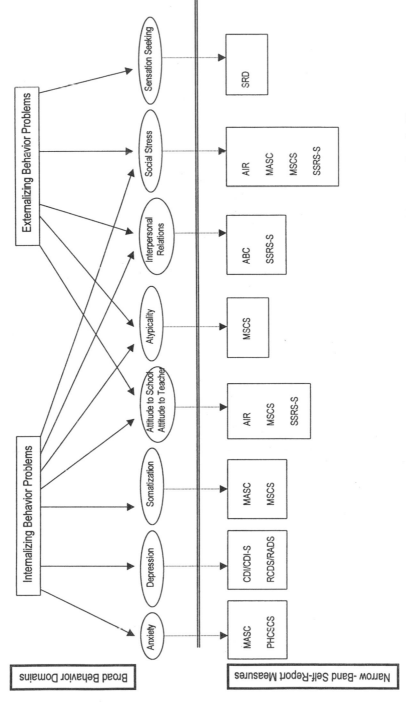

FIGURE 6.2. A decision-making framework for combining the Self-Report of Personality with narrow-band self-report measures.

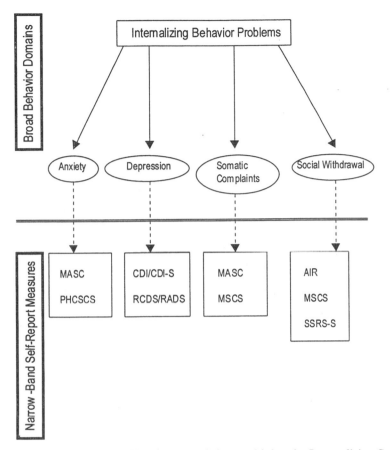

FIGURE 6.3. A decision-making framework for combining the Internalizing Symptoms Scale for Children with narrow-band self-report measures.

that Tanner had a history of impulsive and hyperactive behavior problems. Tanner's teachers reported that he was having problems with inattention and impulsivity in the classroom. Although Tanner demonstrated above average achievement in all content areas, his teachers reported that he continually expressed concern regarding his performance.

After reviewing the case, the school psychologist noted indicators of internalizing and externalizing behavior problems. Based on this review, the psychologist decided to administer the SRP of the BASC to serve as an initial screening of Tanner's emotional and behavioral functioning across a number of behavior domains. Tanner's ratings on the SRP revealed severe internalizing and externalizing problems. That is, significant clinical eleva-

tions were obtained for the Composite Scores of Clinical Maladjustment (98th percentile) and Emotional Symptoms Index (98th percentile). Further examination of subscale scores revealed clinical elevations in the areas of Anxiety (98th percentile), Depression (99th percentile), and Sense of Inadequacy (98th percentile). Ratings on the remaining subscales of the SRP did not reflect significant deviations in any other areas of functioning, such as Aggression, Conduct Problems, Somatization, Atypicality, or Social Skills.

Based on the results of the SRP, the school psychologist administered a number of narrow-band self-report measures to further examine the externalizing and internalizing symptoms and assist in diagnosis and treatment planning. To assess the anxiety symptomatology, Tanner was asked to complete the MASC. Results of this measure indicated clinically significant symptoms of anxiety on the MASC total score (T score $= 69$) and on the Anxiety Disorders Index (T score $= 70$). The school psychologist examined the scales of the MASC to determine whether all scales were elevated or whether there was a pattern of elevated scales. An examination revealed a pattern of elevated subscale scores for the Harm Avoidance Scale (T score $= 70$) and the Social Anxiety Scale (T score $= 69$). Further examination of subscale scores on these two scales suggested that Tanner was experiencing perfectionism symptoms and performance fear symptoms. To assess the depressive symptomatology, Tanner was asked to complete the RCDS. Results of this measure indicated severe self-perceptions of depression. His total scale score of 85 exceeded the clinical cutoff score. In addition, clinically elevated subscale scores were obtained for Generalized Demoralization (98th percentile), Despondency and Worry (97th percentile), and Dysphoric Mood (98th percentile). To assess the attention and concentration problems, Tanner was asked to complete the ABC. Total and subscale scores of the ABC revealed severe externalizing symptoms similar to those reported on the BASC. Clinically elevated scores were obtained for the Total Scale Score of the ABC as well as the Impulsivity/Hyperactivity and Inattention subscales.

The results of this case illustrate how self-report measures can be used as part of multimethod behavioral assessment. Although the information gathered in this case example assesses Tanner's perceived functioning in a number of domains, a number of important observations can be highlighted. First, Tanner's parents and teachers did not report anxiety or depression to be major concerns. Tanner was not viewed as a depressed or unduly anxious child at home or at school. The inclusion of a broad-band self-report measure allowed these two behavior domains to be assessed. Second, comorbid conditions may also have been present. Although the diagnosis of ADHD requires a history of ADHD characteristics, the present case illustrates how behaviors of this type can be screened with the use of self-report methodology.

SUMMARY

In this chapter we have reviewed the literature describing currently available child and adolescent self-report measures that may be useful within the context of a multimethod behavioral assessment. Specifically, we reviewed broad- and narrow-band self-report rating scales across a number of important measurement domains. In addition, we outlined a decision-making framework for combining broad- and narrow-band measures to assess the emotional and behavioral functioning of children and adolescents. It was our intent to illustrate how these two types of self-report measures can be combined to provide a comprehensive assessment of students' perceived functioning across a number of behavioral domains.

REFERENCES

Achenbach, T. M. (1991). *Manual for the Youth Self-Report and 1991 Profile.* Burlington: University of Vermont, Department of Psychiatry.

Achenbach, T. M., & McConaughy, S. H. (1992). Taxonomy of internalizing disorders of childhood and adolescence. In W. M. Reynolds (Ed.), *Internalizing disorders in children and adolescents* (pp. 19–60). New York: Wiley.

Adams, C. D., Kelley, M. L., & McCarthy, M. (1997). The Adolescent Behavior Checklist: Development and initial psychometric properties of a self-report measure for adolescents with ADHD. *Journal of Clinical Child Psychology, 26,* 77–86.

Akiskal, H. S., Downs, J., Jordan, P., Watson, S., Daugherty, D., & Pruitt, D. B. (1985). Affective disorders in referred children and younger siblings of manic-depressives: Mode of onset and prospective course. *Archives of General Psychiatry, 42,* 996–1003.

Alessi, N. E., Krahn, D., Brehm, D., & Wittekindt, J. (1989). Prepubertal anorexia nervosa and major depressive disorder. *Journal of the American Academy of Child and Adolescent Psychiatry, 28,* 380–384.

Alessi, N. E., & Magen, J. (1988). Comorbidity of other psychiatric disturbances in depressed psychiatrically hospitalized children. *American Journal of Psychiatry, 145,* 1582–1584.

Anderson, J. C., Williams, S., McGee, R., & Silva, P. A. (1987). DSM-III disorders in preadolescent children: Prevalence in a large sample from the general population. *Archives of General Psychiatry, 44,* 69–76.

Bird, H. R., Gould, M. S., & Stagheeza, B. (1992). Aggregating data from multiple informants in child psychiatry epidemiological research. *Journal of the American Academy of Child and Adolescent Psychiatry, 32,* 361–368.

Bracken, B. A. (1992). *Multidimensional Self-Concept Scale: Examiner's manual.* Austin, TX: PRO-ED.

Bracken, B. A., & Kelley, P. (1993). *Assessment of interpersonal relations.* Austin, TX: PRO-ED.

Breen, M., Eckert, T. L., & DuPaul, G. J. (1996). Interpreting child behavior questionnaires. In M. Breen & C. Fiedler (Eds.), *Behavioral approach to the assessment of emotionally disturbed youth: A handbook for school-based practitioners* (pp. 225–241). Austin, TX: PRO-ED.

Cone, J. D. (1978). The behavioral assessment grid (BAG): A conceptual framework and a taxonomy. *Behavior Therapy, 9,* 882–888.

Cooper, D. K. (1990). *Developmental trends in Children's Depression Inventory responses across age and gender.* Master's thesis, University of Georgia, Athens.

Eckert, T. L., Dunn, E. K., Guiney, K. M., & Codding, R. S. (2000). Self-reports: Theory and research in using rating scale measures. In E. S. Shapiro & T. R. Kratochwill (Eds.), *Behavioral assessment in schools (2nd ed.): Theory, research, and clinical foundations* (pp. 288–322). New York: Guilford Press.

Eckert, T. L., & DuPaul, G. J. (1996). Youth completed and narrow-band child behavior questionnaires. In M. Breen & C. Fiedler (Eds.), *Behavioral approach to the assessment of emotionally disturbed youth: A handbook for school-based practitioners* (pp. 289–357). Austin, TX: PRO-ED.

Elliott, D. S., Huizinga, D., & Ageton, S. S. (1985). *Explaining delinquency and drug use.* Beverly Hills, CA: Sage.

Elliott, S. N., Busse, R. T., & Gresham, F. M. (1993). Behavior rating scales: Issues of use and interpretation. *School Psychology Review, 22,* 313–321.

Finch, A. J., Lipovsky, J. A., & Casat, C. D. (1989). Anxiety and depression in children and adolescents: Negative affectivity or separate constructs? In P. C. Kendall & D. Watson (Eds.), *Anxiety and depression: Distinctive and overlapping features* (pp. 171–202). San Diego, CA: Academic Press.

Gresham, F. M., & Elliott, S. N. (1990). *The social skills rating system.* Circle Pines, MN: American Guidance.

Jensen, J. B., Burke, N., & Garfinkel, B. D. (1988). Depression and symptoms of attention deficit disorder with hyperactivity. *Journal of the American Academy of Child and Adolescent Psychiatry, 27,* 742–747.

Kahn, J. S., Kehle, T. J., Jenson, W. R., & Clark, E. (1990). Comparison of cognitive-behavioral, relaxation, and self-monitoring interventions for depression among middle-school students. *School Psychology Review, 19,* 196–211.

Kamphaus, R. W., & Frick, P. J. (1996). *Clinical assessment of child and adolescent personality and behavior.* Boston: Allyn and Bacon.

Kashini, J. H., Keller, M. B., Solmon, N., Reid, J. C., & Mazzola, D. (1985). Double depression in adolescent substance users. *Journal of Affective Disorders, 8,* 153–157.

Kavan, M. G. (1990). Review of the Children's Depression Inventory. In J. J. Kramer & J. C. Conoley (Eds.), *The supplement to the 10th Mental Measurements Yearbook* (pp. 46–48). Lincoln, NE: Buros Institute of Mental Measurements.

Knoff, H. M. (1990). Review of the Children's Depression Inventory. In J. J. Kramer & J. C. Conoley (Eds.), *The supplement to the 10th Mental Measurements Yearbook* (pp. 48–50). Lincoln, NE: Buros Institute of Mental Measurements.

Kovacs, M. (1981). Rating scales to assess depression in school-aged children. *Acta Paedopsychiatria, 46,* 305–315.

Kovacs, M. (1992). *Children's Depression Inventory.* Los Angeles: Multi-Health Systems.

Kovacs, M., Paulauskas, S. L., Gastonis, C., & Richards, C. (1988). Depressive disorders in childhood: III. A longitudinal study of comorbidity with and risk for conduct disorders. *Journal of Affective Disorders, 15,* 205–217.

Kratochwill, T. R., & Shapiro, E. S. (1988). Introduction: Conceptual foundations of behavioral assessment. In E. S. Shapiro & T. R. Kratochwill (Eds.), *Behavioral assessment in the schools* (pp. 384–454). New York: Guilford Press.

Levy, J. C., & Deykin, E. Y. (1989). Suicidality, depression, and substance abuse in adolescence. *American Journal of Psychiatry, 146,* 1462–1467.

March, J. S. (1997). *Multidimensional Anxiety Scale for Children: Technical manual.* New York: Multi-Health Systems.

Martens, B. K. (1993). Social labeling, precision of measurement, and problem solving: Key issues in the assessment of children's emotional problems. *School Psychology Review, 2,* 308–312.

McConaughy, S. H., & Ritter, D. R. (1995). Multidimensional assessment of emotional or behavioral disorders. In A. Thomas & J. Grimes (Eds.), *Best practices in school psychology–III* (pp. 865–878). Washington, DC: National Association of School Psychologists.

Merrell, K. W. (1999). *Behavioral, social, and emotional assessment of children.* Mahwah, NJ: Erlbaum.

Merrell, K. W., & Walters, A. S. (1996). *The Internalizing Symptoms Scale for Children: User's guide and technical manual.* Logan, UT: Utah State University, Department of Psychology.

Piers, E. V. (1984). *Revised manual for the Piers-Harris Children's Self-Concept Scale.* Los Angeles: Western Psychological Services.

Puig-Antich, J. (1982). Major depression and conduct disorder in prepuberty. *Journal of the American Academy of Child Psychiatry, 21,* 118–121.

Reynolds, C. R., & Kamphaus, R. W. (1992). *Behavior Assessment System for Children.* Circle Pines, MN: American Guidance Service.

Reynolds, W. M. (1987). *Professional manual for the Reynolds Adolescent Depression Scale.* Los Angeles: Western Psychological Services.

Reynolds, W. M. (1989). *Professional manual for the Reynolds Child Depression Scale.* Odessa, FL: Psychological Assessment Resources.

Reynolds, W. M. (1992). Depression in children and adolescents. In W. M. Reynolds (Ed.), *Internalizing disorders in children and adolescents* (pp. 149–254). New York: Wiley.

Reynolds, W. M. (1994). Assessment of depression in children and adolescents by self-report questionnaires. In W. M. Reynolds & H. F. Johnston (Eds.), *Handbook of depression in children and adolescents* (pp. 209–234). New York: Plenum Press.

Reynolds, W. M., & Coats, K. I. (1986). A comparison of cognitive-behavior therapy and relaxation training for the treatment of depression in adolescents. *Journal of Consulting and Clinical Psychology, 54,* 653–660.

Strauss, C. C., Last, C. G., Hersen, M., & Kazdin, A. E. (1988). Association between anxiety and depression in children and adolescents with anxiety disorders. *Journal of Abnormal Child Psychology, 16,* 57–68.

CHAPTER 7

♦♦♦

Self-Report:
Child Clinical Interviews

♦

STEPHANIE H. McCONAUGHY

To frame a discussion of child clinical interviews, it is important to distinguish between interviewing for assessment purposes and interviewing as a form of psychotherapy (Hughes & Baker, 1990; Sattler, 1998). Clinical assessment interviews are designed to obtain data on a child's functioning to diagnose problems and to make decisions about treatment. Psychotherapeutic interviews are designed to relieve emotional stress and to foster behavioral, cognitive, and affective change. Clinical assessment interviews usually cover specific content areas (e.g., presenting problems, relationships with friends and family, school performance, self perceptions), and are limited to one or two sessions. Psychotherapeutic interviews usually cover salient issues raised by the interviewee, use specific techniques (e.g., problem solving, recalling past experiences, experiencing affect), and include multiple sessions to achieve therapeutic goals. Clinical assessment interviews are also different from forensic interviews, which are designed to investigate specific issues for referral sources (e.g., child maltreatment), and survey interviews, which are designed to collect data on specific variables of interest to the researcher (e.g., epidemiological surveys).

Even when clinical assessment is the main purpose, different theoretical perspectives can shape the content and style of interviewing (Sattler, 1998). This chapter focuses on child interviews in the context of multimethod behavioral approaches to assessment. Accordingly, the following definition, adapted from Hughes and Baker (1990), guides the discussion:

> The child interview is a face-to-face interaction for the purpose of directly assessing a child's functioning in important life areas, as reported by the

child and observed by the interviewer, in order to identify current problems and competencies that have relevance for planning, implementing, or evaluating treatment.

After discussing the advantages of child interviews, subsequent sections present practical guidelines for semistructured interviewing. The Semistructured Clinical Interview for Children and Adolescents (SCICA; McConaughy & Achenbach, 1994) is then discussed as an example of an empirically based interview that dovetails with other measures in multimethod assessment. Final sections include case examples to illustrate how interview data can be integrated with data from other sources and how interview data contribute to intervention planning.

ADVANTAGES OF CHILD CLINICAL INTERVIEWS

Within the context of multimethod assessment, child interviews have several potential advantages. First, interviews provide opportunities for directly assessing children's own perceptions and subjective experiences of important events and people in their lives. We know from meta-analyses that agreement between reports from different informants is low to moderate at best, including agreement between children's self-reports and reports by parents, teachers, mental health workers, and peers (Achenbach, McConaughy, & Howell, 1987). Low agreement does not mean that one informant is wrong and the other right. Instead, it highlights the importance of obtaining information from multiple sources. Child interviews offer unique opportunities to assess children's own views of their problems and competencies and their beliefs and interpretations of experiences, social interactions, and environmental circumstances relevant to their problems.

A second advantage of child interviews is the opportunity to observe children's behavior and affect in a one-on-one interaction with an adult. Hughes and Baker (1990) outline several characteristics to observe in child interviews, including activity level, attention span, impulsivity, distractibility, reactions to frustration and praise, responsiveness to limit setting, communicative competence, nervous mannerisms, range of emotional expression, and logic of thought processes.

A third advantage of child interviews is the opportunity to establish rapport and trust with a child, which are necessary first steps for effective treatment. For many troubled children, the clinical interview may be their first experience of having an adult solicit their points of view on sensitive issues and discuss their problems in a nonjudgmental fashion. Even when assessment is the primary purpose of a child interview, effective communication between the interviewer and the child can foster an atmosphere of trust and provide a

model of caring adults who want to help children with their problems. In this respect, interviews, more than many other evaluation procedures, can serve as bridges between assessment and interventions.

Finally, child interviews have the advantage of flexibility, which may not be available in other assessment methods, such as rating scales, psychological tests, or direct observations in group settings. The degree of flexibility depends on whether a structured or semistructured format is used. Structured diagnostic interviews, such as the Diagnostic Interview Schedule for Children (DISC; Shaffer, 1992), have limited flexibility because they are usually designed to cover narrowly defined topics, such as reported symptoms and history related to symptoms. Semistructured interviews, in contrast, can cover a wide range of topics concerning children's functioning in different contexts, and they can be adapted to follow children's flow of conversation. Semistructured formats are also more compatible with behavioral assessment because they enable interviewers to question children about specific problems and probe for antecedents and consequences of the problems. For this reason, semistructured interviews are the main focus of this chapter. To advance effective interviewing, the next several sections present practical guidelines for arranging settings, explaining purposes and confidentiality, and formulating questions for semistructured interviews.

ARRANGING SETTINGS FOR CHILD INTERVIEWS

Child interviews should be conducted in relaxed, neutral settings that facilitate communication. For preschool children, Garbarino and Scott (1989) suggest using cushions or mats on the floor so that the interviewer can sit at the same level as the child. Interviews with children older than 5 can be conducted sitting in chairs at a table to facilitate note taking and drawing. The child should be provided with a suitably sized chair and allowed to leave the table occasionally. Having the interviewer sit at a diagonal to the right or left of the child, instead of on the opposite side of the table, can reduce the test-like aspect of the setting.

Before a child arrives for an interview, it is important to prepare the space so as to reduce distractions. For preschool children, clear desks and tables of extraneous or tempting materials and remove or relocate toys and games out of reach of the child. Such "childproofing" will help focus the child's attention on the task at hand. The removal of distractions is especially important in interviewing children with impulsive or disruptive behavior disorders. If the interview occurs in a private office, it is also a good idea to remove family pictures and personal mementos that may elicit questions or comments that focus on the interviewer's interests and relationships instead of the child's. Before interviewing adolescents, it may be helpful to remove toys, games, and other objects that suggest a child-like atmos-

phere, which may undermine adolescents' self-esteem or willingness to co-operate.

School psychologists and others with itinerant schedules may have limit-ed choices of settings for interviewing. However, it is helpful to stress to ad-ministrators the importance of having a familiar, neutral setting that assures the child of confidentiality and reduces anxiety. Interviews in schools should not be conducted in hallways or open spaces where the child can be seen or heard by other people. Interviewers should avoid using the principal's office or other rooms in the school that a child may associate with punishment, be-cause these settings may reduce communication and trust.

Young children, in particular, need time to become familiar with the in-terviewer and the setting. It is often helpful to let young children explore the space briefly before questioning begins. Having games available can also put children at ease. However, playing games before interviewing may produce resistance when the interviewer switches to questioning, which is usually not as much fun as games. If a child asks about playing games, the interviewer can explain that they are going to talk for a while first, but they can play a game at the end of the talk. Of course, if this strategy is used, the interview-er must allow time at the end to follow through on that commitment.

Young children, and even some adolescents, are not used to maintaining eye contact or carrying on lengthy conversations, especially with unfamiliar adults. Providing manipulatives, such as clay or drawing materials, can ease a child's discomfort while talking. Drawings can also be used as a supplement to direct questioning with 6- to12-year-old children and some adolescents. The kinetic family drawing (KFD; Burns, 1982) is often used to solicit infor-mation about family relationships, as explained later.

EXPLAINING PURPOSES AND CONFIDENTIALITY

At the beginning of any clinical interview, it is important to explain its pur-poses, why it was requested, and how the information will be used or shared with other people. It is usually helpful to begin by asking children why they think they are being seen. This allows the interviewer to identify any miscon-ceptions children may have and to explain the purpose, beginning with chil-dren's perspectives. For example, if a child was told that he or she will be playing games, the interviewer can explain when that may happen. Or if a child thinks the interview will be a test, the interviewer can explain that they will mostly be talking. Adolescents sometimes resist interviewing because they think it means they are crazy or stupid or in trouble for something. Initial ex-planations of purposes and confidentiality can alleviate such fears and im-prove cooperation.

In school settings, it is sometimes helpful to have a teacher or other trusted adult introduce the interviewer to the child. If the psychologist uses

"Doctor" as a title, then it is important to explain the difference between psychologists, or "talking doctors," and medical doctors so as to avoid misconceptions or fears associated with medical examinations. The following is an example of an introduction for an elementary child:

TEACHER: Linda, this is Dr. McConaughy. She's going to spend time talking with you this morning.

INTERVIEWER: Hello, Linda. I'm glad to meet you. Did you know you were going to see me today?

CHILD: Yeah, my mom told me.

INTERVIEWER (*walking down the hall with child*): What did your mom say we were going to do today?

CHILD: I dunno, play games and stuff.

INTERVIEWER (*in the room*): Well, let me tell what we'll be doing. I'm the school psychologist. I'm a talking doctor. I don't give shots or medicine. I talk to kids, get to know them, and help figure out their problems. So we are going to talk for a while, and later do some drawing while we are talking.

CHILD: Okay.

After a brief introduction, the interviewer should explain the guarantees and limits of confidentiality. This task can be done in the context of explaining purposes, the type of information sought, and the likely uses of the information. If the interviewer cannot guarantee confidentiality of some information, this issue should be made clear at the outset (e.g., reporting abuse or attempts to harm self or others). In most cases, interviewers can guarantee the confidentiality of children's direct statements and discuss the type of information that will go into reports at the end of the interview. For young children, introductory remarks should be phrased in language appropriate to their cognitive level and be kept as brief as possible. As an example, the SCICA has the following standard introduction:

"We are going to spend some time talking and doing things together, so that I can get to know you and learn about what you like and don't like. This is a private talk. I won't tell your parents or your teacher what you say unless you tell me it is okay. The only thing I might tell is if you said you were going to hurt yourself, hurt someone else, or if someone has hurt you." [If a taperecorder is used, the interviewer adds, "We are going to record our talk on this taperecorder to help remember our time together."]

For adolescents, more detailed introductions may be appropriate, especially if trust is an issue. Adolescents should also be told explicitly that a writ-

ten report will be one of the outcomes of the evaluation, if this is the case, as illustrated here:

INTERVIEWER (*in private room*): Hello, Danielle, I'm Dr. McConaughy. It's nice to meet you.

CHILD: Hello.

INTERVIEWER: Why do you think you are seeing me today?

CHILD: I don't know, probably because my teachers said to. Mr. Casey doesn't like me; I know that.

INTERVIEWER: Well, your teachers are concerned about you, so we can talk about that. But first, let me explain what will happen. I am the school psychologist. My job is to talk to kids about their problems and help them and their teachers figure out ways to deal with problems. This is a private talk. That means I won't tell your teachers or your parents what you say to me, unless you say it is okay. The things I do have to tell is if I think you are going to hurt yourself, hurt someone else, or someone has hurt you. The law says I have to report those things. I will be writing a report about what I learn about you, so at the end of our talk we can discuss what the report will cover. Do you understand?

CHILD: Yeah, I guess so.

INTERVIEWER: Well, first I would like to get to know you better. What do you like to do for fun—for instance, when you are not in school?

With all children, lengthy, technical introductions should be avoided. Too much adult talk at the beginning of the interview may be misunderstood. It may also create an impression that interviewers are more interested in their own agendas than in hearing children's viewpoints. Such initial perceptions can easily inhibit children's willingness to share their thoughts and feelings. After the introduction, interviewers can move quickly to questions on specific topics. In the preceding illustration, the interviewer chose not to begin discussion on the negative topic of Mr. Casey, so as to establish rapport on a more pleasant topic first. Later, when the interview moved to questions about school, the interviewer picked up on Danielle's opening statement: "When we first started talking, you said you thought Mr. Casey didn't like you. Tell me more about that."

SEMISTRUCTURED QUESTIONING STRATEGIES

Talking with an adult about feelings and personal issues may be a novel experience for most children (Bierman, 1983). When interviewing children, it is

important to be flexible and to adapt questioning strategies to their cognitive developmental level, language capabilities, and social interaction style. Semistructured formats are most amenable to these requirements, because they allow interviewers to use a variety of questioning strategies to promote communication and data gathering, as outlined in Table 7.1 (McConaughy, 1996; McConaughy & Achenbach, 1994).

Modifying Interviewer Talk

In many cultures, one of the first rules of polite conversation is that only one person should talk at a time. Interviewers can use this rule to their advantage by keeping interviewer talk at a minimum to encourage more child talk. Limiting the length of questions and interviewer comments creates more "conversation space" for child talk. Tailoring questions and vocabulary to a child's developmental level also helps to reduce stimulus complexity in an interview (Garbarino & Scott, 1989; Hughes & Baker, 1990; Witt, Cavell, Carey, & Martens, 1988). For example, interviewers should not ask a 6-year-old, "What sorts of activities or things are rewarding for you?" or "What kinds of

TABLE 7.1. Questioning Strategies for Semistructured Interviewing of Children and Adolescents

Do's	Don'ts
Limit length of questions and comments.	Avoid inserting embedded phrases or clauses.
Ask only one question at a time.	
Use the child's terms and phrases.	Avoid using psychological terms.
Use people's names instead of pronouns.	Avoid imposing the interviewer's agenda.
Follow the child's lead in conversation.	
Use open-ended questions along with probes.	Avoid too much direct questioning.
Solicit and restate feelings.	Avoid questions that can be answered "yes" or "no."
Use extenders to encourage more child talk.	Avoid "why" questions about motives.
Provide multiple-choice response options when probing abstract concepts.	Refrain from making judgmental comments.
Use direct requests to transition to new topics or tasks.	Avoid questions with obvious "right" answers.
Allow ample time for the child to respond and elaborate.	Don't follow every response with another question.
Rephrase or simplify questions when the child has misunderstood or not responded.	Avoid rhetorical questions.

Note. Adapted from McConaughy and Achenbach (1994, p. 68). Copyright 1994 by S. H. McConaughy and T. M. Achenbach. Adapted by permission.

activities are reinforcing for you?" Use of such psychological jargon will only be confusing. Instead, a more developmentally appropriate question may be, "What do you like to do for fun, like when you're not in school?" Using the child's terms and phrases in questions, as Garbarino and Scott (1989) suggest, is another good way to tailor language to the child's level. Examples of such terms are names for body parts, names of friends or family, and terms or phrases for rules at home or school. Using people's names instead of pronouns helps to reduce confusion, especially in discussing friends, teachers, and members of the family.

Asking only one question at a time and avoiding embedded phrases or clauses in questions also reduces stimulus complexity. For example, to elicit views and feelings about school, an interviewer can first ask, "What do you like best in school?" and then probe for elaboration, such as, "So, what do you like about gym?" Then, the interviewer can query for negative aspects of school by asking, "What do you like the least in school?" and follow up with probes. Sometimes it is helpful to add introductory remarks to create an open mind-set for sensitive issues or to give the child permission for negative responses. For example, after discussing likes and dislikes, the interviewer may probe for areas of difficulty by saying, "Most kids think some things in school are easy and other things are hard. What things are hard for you?"

Following the child's lead in conversation also helps to facilitate communication. Children usually remain interested and keep talking when they feel that they control the topics. They become less talkative when conversation is governed by the interviewer's agenda and feels more like a "test." However, the often meandering style of children's conversations can become confusing and irritating, especially if interviewers fear that key issues are being avoided. A protocol of topics and questions, like that provided by the SCICA (McConaughy & Achenbach, 1994), can help interviewers remember topics to be covered, while allowing freedom to follow children's conversations in the sequencing of topics.

Open-Ended Questions and Probes

Using open-ended questions and avoiding too much direct questioning go hand in hand as key interviewing strategies. Open-ended questions elicit more information than direct questioning and reduce the likelihood of leading the child to respond in only a certain way (Cox, Hopkinson, & Rutter, 1981; Witt, et al., 1988). Direct questions may also increase anxiety and generate resistance or denial in some children, especially if they perceive the questions as threatening or accusatory (Bierman, 1983). On the other hand, young children sometimes have difficulty responding to only open-ended questions without some direct questions and probes to clarify meaning. A good general strategy is to begin with easy questions that set the stage, and

then to intersperse open-ended questions with more direct questions that probe for elaboration or clarification of responses. As a general rule in this process, interviewers should ask only a few questions that can be answered with a simple "yes" or "no." For example, the following SCICA questions focus on relationships with friends:

> How many friends do you have?
> Do you think that is enough friends?
> Are your friends boys or girls?
> How old are your friends?

> What do you do with your friends?
> Do they come to your house?
> Do you go to their houses?
> How often?

> Tell me about someone you like.
> What do you like about _____?
> Tell me about someone you don't like.
> What don't you like about _____?

> Do you ever have problems getting along with other kids?
> What kinds of problems do you have?
> What do you try to do about _____?

Open-ended questions are especially good for eliciting children's feelings or reactions to events or other people's actions toward them. When children talk about sensitive issues, restating what they say shows that the interviewer accepts their feelings nonjudgmentally. Hughes and Baker (1990) also suggest that it may be necessary to explain that feelings do not make things happen and that many other children have the same kinds of feelings. To encourage children to share their feelings, they suggest telling them directly that their point of view is important, such as by saying: "No one else can tell me how you think or feel about things, so it is very important that I talk with you, and not just with your parents, or your teachers, or anyone else."

Avoiding "Why" Questions

Avoiding "why" questions about motives is the "don't" counterpart of the "do" for eliciting feelings. Young children often seem unaware of the motives behind their own actions or the actions of other people. Instead, they focus more on actions and events, or on "what happened" rather than "why it happened." The tendency for children to focus more on actions and events than on motives was illustrated by research on how people summarize short sto-

ries. McConaughy, Fitzhenry-Coor, and Howell (1983) asked fifth-grade children and college students to summarize the important parts of some short stories, each of which had a well-defined sequence of actions and events and clearly stated motives of the characters. Children emphasized the actions of characters and event sequences in the stories, using an "and-then" format for summarizing. College students summarized stories in terms of actions and events, but also described the characters' motives and feelings behind their actions.

Although older children may be more capable of focusing on motives than younger children, many adolescents still respond cautiously to "why" questions because they perceive them as accusations, threats, or tests of their knowledge. This can be especially true for adolescents with behavioral or emotional problems who have had many conflicts with adult authority figures. As an alternative to "why" questions, interviewers can use the reflective technique of restating children's reports of problems, and then soliciting their feelings, reactions, and potential solutions to the problems. For example, when children report being left out of games, instead of asking, "Why won't other kids play with you?" interviewers can say, "So other kids won't play with you. How does that make you feel?" and then ask later, "What do you do when they won't play with you?" Or when children describe fighting with peers or siblings, instead of asking, "Why did you get into that fight?" interviewers can ask, "What started the fight? What did you do then? How did that make you feel? What else could you do besides fighting when that happens?" Hughes and Baker (1990) also suggest turning "why" questions into "what" questions. For example, in a case in which a boy stole money from a teacher, they suggest asking, "What did you do with the money?" Asking, "Why did you take the money?" sets up a situation in which the boy is tempted to lie to protect himself and then is likely to be confronted by the interviewer, who already knows he did it. These alternatives to "why" questions can appear less threatening to children, as well as enable interviewers to evaluate children's range of affect, understanding of behavioral causes and effects, and their ability to generate solutions to problems.

Refraining from Judgmental Comments

Refraining from judgmental comments is another key strategy. Judgmental comments can be positive (e.g., "That's nice"; "What a good drawing.") or negative (e.g., "That's too bad"; "I wonder what your teacher would say about that."). Because children naturally look to adults for approval or disapproval, judgmental comments can easily shape their responses. Too many positive comments or too much praise can encourage children to modify their responses to fit what they believe an adult wants to hear. Negative judgmental comments can produce resistance or refusal to talk if children fear reprimands

or disapproval. An alternative is to use what Hughes and Baker (1990) call "extenders" (e.g., "Uh huh, umm"; "Okay"; "Tell me more about that") to encourage children to reveal feelings and opinions more freely. If children have trouble expressing feelings or seem reluctant to say anything negative, interviewers can use structured probes that include several different response options. For example, when a child reports hating reading, the interviewer may say, "Some kids don't like reading because the words are too hard, or it's boring, or it's no fun. What is it about reading that you don't like?"

Presenting multiple choice options is one way to reduce response complexity, especially when children have trouble answering open-ended questions about abstract concepts like feelings (Hughes & Baker, 1990; Witt et al., 1988). Multiple choices can also be used to probe sensitive issues and topics on which the interviewer has prior knowledge from referral sources. For example, in a case in which a mother reports that her child fears being attacked by a bully at school, the interviewer can broach the topic as follows: "A lot of kids I know are afraid of things, like being in the dark, or going to school, or that a big kid on the playground will hurt them. What are you afraid of?"

Minimizing Resistance

Several strategies listed toward the bottom of Table 7.1 alert interviewers to pitfalls that can lead to resistance or inhibit spontaneous talk from a child. For example, interviewers should avoid asking questions with obvious "right" answers (Hughes & Baker, 1990). Questions of this kind create a test-like atmosphere that can stifle communication. Similarly, interviewers should avoid following every response from the child with another question. This tactic can also create the feeling of being tested. In school-based assessments, interviewers have to be particularly sensitive not to create test-like atmospheres, because children may initially equate interviewers with teachers.

"Rhetorical questions" are forms of polite conversation in which adults use question formats when they really intend to give commands. Interview examples include asking children, "Would you like to draw me a picture of your family?" "Would you like to talk about your family?" "Would you like to tell me about school?" A classic example is a parent's asking, "Would you like to straighten up your room?" Young children often misinterpret such rhetorical questions as presenting real "yes" or "no" options, whereas adults really want only positive responses or compliance. When children logically answer "no" to such questions, the scene is set for resistance if adults try to enforce compliance. As an alternative, interviewers can state direct requests or polite commands to initiate transitions to new topics or activities. For example, they may say, "Draw me a picture of your family"; "Now let's talk about your family. Who are the people in your family? Who lives in your home?" "Tell me about school. What do you like best in school?"

Because many children are not accustomed to prolonged conversations with adults, they may need time to think about their responses or to elaborate on responses. This issue is especially true for children with expressive language problems or learning disabilities, and inhibited, shy children. For these types of children, interviewers should allow ample time for them to collect their thoughts before asking another question or probing for responses. Interviewers should resist the natural urge to fill silent spaces in conversation with more interviewer talk. As cautioned earlier, too much interviewer talk can cause children to "shut down." If a child does not respond after a brief pause, or if the child seems to have misunderstood the question, the interviewer can rephrase or simplify the original question or give multiple-choice response options. Sometimes it is helpful to ask the child to repeat or rephrase questions. However, this strategy should not be used very often, because it, too, can create a test-like atmosphere, especially for children who have receptive and expressive language problems.

Interspersing Nonverbal Activities

Interspersing nonverbal activities with questioning is a key strategy for interviewing preschool and elementary children. For many children, and even some adolescents, interviewers can request a kinetic family drawing (KFD; Burns, 1982). To do this, the interviewer provides paper and pencil and tells the child, "Draw a picture of your family doing something together." After the drawing is completed, the interviewer asks the child to describe the drawing and family members depicted. The following are examples of SCICA questions about the family drawing:

What are they doing?
What kind of a person is _____? Tell me three words to describe _____.
How does _____feel in that picture?
What is _____thinking?
Whom do you get along with best/least?
What is going to happen next in your picture?

The KFD and related questions are used to solicit children's perceptions of each family member and to describe their relationships with them. The content of the drawing can also be informative in terms of the positioning of family members and who has been included and who has been left out. Burns (1982) also provides rules for scoring the KFD as a projective test, but this is not necessary for clinical interviewing.

Hughes and Baker (1990) and Witt et al. (1988) suggest several other nonverbal techniques that can be incorporated into interviews with young children or children who are reluctant to engage in conversation. For exam-

ple, interviewers can present pictures of happy, sad, mad, or scared faces and ask children to point to a picture that depicts how they felt in certain situations. When exploring options for reward systems, interviewers may present a list of different choices and ask children to select favorites or to rate each on a scale of 1 to 10 (Jensen, Rhode, & Reavis, 1994). Encouraging children to enact a situation with or without props (e.g., "Show me") can be another good alternative to verbal description. Using puppets as props for asking and answering questions can also be more effective than asking direct questions with some young children.

For young children, play materials should be available for use at the interviewer's discretion. These generally include wooden blocks, small doll family figures, dollhouse furniture, and perhaps a dollhouse. Play sessions provide opportunities for interviewers to observe children's behavior and themes depicted in play. During play, interviewers can judiciously interject comments and questions to assess whether the play actually depicts events and relationships in the child's family so as to avoid invalid inferences about meaning of the play. For example, if a 6-year-old boy's play depicts family violence, the interviewer can describe the dolls' actions as the boy plays and then comment, "There is a lot of fighting in that family. Is that what happens in your house?" Interviewers can also use doll figures as concrete referents for depicting specific events, such as family members in a divorce situation (Hughes & Baker, 1990). For more detailed descriptions of play interviews, see Garbarino and Scott (1989), Hughes and Baker (1990), and Witt et al. (1988). These authors also discuss other nonverbal techniques, including sentence completion tasks, feeling scales, thought bubbles, and vignettes depicting social problem solving.

Dealing with Lying or Cheating

On the Child Behavior Checklist/4–18 (CBCL; Achenbach, 1991a) 18% to 31% of parents of children in the normative sample reported that their child had lied or cheated in the past 6 months. For children referred for mental health services, 54% to 66% of parents reported lying or cheating. Analyses of CBCL item scores revealed significantly higher scores for lying and cheating among boys than girls and among older than younger referred children. On the Teacher's Report Form (TRF; Achenbach, 1991b), 30% to 40% of teachers reported lying or cheating by children referred for mental health or special education services. These findings demonstrate the high frequency of lying or cheating among children, especially those with problems severe enough to warrant clinical referral.

Children lie or cheat for a variety of reasons, including attempts to deny feelings, avoid failure, gain a desired outcome or advantage, maintain self-esteem, or avoid reprimand or punishment (Hughes & Baker, 1990). In clini-

cal interviews children may be tempted to lie because they are anxious about talking with a strange adult, they want to please or impress the interviewer, or they are afraid they will get in trouble. To ensure the validity of children's self-reports, interviewers must avoid creating situations that may inadvertently induce children to lie or "stretch the truth." One strategy is to avoid "did you" or "why" questions about misbehavior that tempt children to deny a problem, especially when the interviewer has already received the answer from other sources (e.g., "Did you take the money?" "Did you hit that kid?" "Why did you hit him?").

Young children may also appear to lie because they have difficulty distinguishing fantasy from reality or feelings from actual behavior, or they have difficulty expressing such distinctions in words. Interviewers can deal with these situations by verbalizing these distinctions for the child. For example, when a child exaggerates or describes something that obviously could not have happened, the interviewer can say, "Sounds as though you really wished it could happen that way." Or the interviewer can restate the child's feelings and then ask about reality versus fantasy. For example, after a 7-year-old boy told an exaggerated tale of single-handedly rescuing his father from a motorcycle accident, the interviewer replied, "Sounds as if that was really scary, and you wanted to save your father. Was that what really happened or something you wish had happened?" Given this option, the boy was able to identify the rescue as his wish. He then talked freely about his reactions to the accident, which had indeed occurred, and expressed his lingering fears about separation and injury to his parents and himself.

CLOSING THE INTERVIEW

Comprehensive child assessment interviews often take 60 to 90 minutes, depending on the breadth of topics covered and the child's verbal style. At the end of the session, the interviewer should readdress issues of confidentiality. This task can be done by briefly summarizing the content of the interview and asking the child's permission to discuss certain issues with other adults, such as parents and teachers. Interviewers should also inform children when a follow-up meeting is planned with parents and/or teachers. For older children, interviewers should briefly summarize the general content of what will be included in any written reports. The following example illustrates closing an interview with a 7-year-old girl who reported frequent fighting with her sister and trouble completing schoolwork:

INTERVIEWER: Well, that was a pretty long talk about a lot of different things—school, your friends, your family, what makes you happy, sad, and mad, and things that are problems for you. I really appreciate the way you

shared your feelings with me. Do you remember what I said about this being a private talk?

CHILD: Yeah, you said you wouldn't tell my mom.

INTERVIEWER: That's right. Now, one important thing I learned was about all that fighting with your sister and how you feel you always get blamed. I think that would be important to talk about with your mom, so we can figure out better ways to deal with it. Is that okay with you?

CHILD: Yeah, okay . . . but don't tell Mom I called Cindy a jerk.

INTERVIEWER: No, I won't tell Mom about the "jerk" part. I'll just tell her about the fighting and how you get blamed.

CHILD: Okay.

INTERVIEWER: I'm also going to talk to your mom and your teachers about your problems in finishing your work in school and how you would like some extra help.

CHILD: Okay. Can I go now?

Usually, brief wrap-ups are sufficient to reassure children about confidentiality and to inform them about reports of interview findings. If a child is particularly concerned about confidentiality even after such closing remarks, the interviewer can usually tailor subsequent reports to parents and teachers in the form of observations, clinical impressions, and data regarding referral complaints and related issues. To further protect confidentiality in written reports, interviewers should refrain from quoting children's exact words during interviews, except as required for reporting abuse, danger to self, or danger to others.

SEMISTRUCTURED CLINICAL INTERVIEW FOR CHILDREN AND ADOLESCENTS (SCICA)

The SCICA is an example of a standardized semistructured interview appropriate for ages 6 to 18. It can be administered in approximately 60 to 90 minutes, depending on whether optional sections are included. The SCICA Protocol Form outlines topics, open-ended questions and probes, and tasks to be covered in nine broad areas of functioning: (1) activities, school, job; (2) friends; (3) family relations; (4) fantasies; (5) self-perception, feelings; (6) parent/teacher reported problems; (7) achievement tests (optional); (8) screen for fine and gross motor abnormalities (for ages 6 to 12, optional); and (9) somatic complaints, alcohol, drugs, trouble with the law (for ages 13 to 18). Interviewers should follow the standard procedures for administering the

SCICA, but are free to tailor questions and probes to fit the child's character-istics and developmental level. For adolescents, more structured questions are included to cover somatic complaints, alcohol and substance use, and trouble with the law. In addition to outlining questions and tasks, the SCICA Proto-col Form provides space for recording the interviewer's observations of the child's behavior, affect, and interaction style, as well as the child's self-reports of problems.

SCICA Observation and Self-Report Forms

After the SCICA is completed, the interviewer scores the child on the SCICA Observation and Self-Report Forms. The Observation Form con-tains 120 problem items to be scored for ages 6 to 18, plus an open-ended item for recording up to three additional problems observed during the inter-view. The Self-Report Form contains 114 problem items to be scored for ages 6 to 18, plus an open-ended item for recording up to three additional prob-lems reported by the child during the interview. Eleven additional self-report items for ages 13 to 18 cover specific somatic complaints, substance use, and trouble with the law.

Items on the SCICA Observation Form describe aspects of the child's behavior, affect, and interaction style observed during the interview. Inter-viewers are instructed to score only the item that most specifically describes a particular observation during the interview, using the following 4-point scale: "For each item that describes the subject's behavior during the interview, cir-cle: 0 if there was no occurrence, 1 if there was a very slight or ambiguous occurrence, 2 if there was a definite occurrence with mild to moderate inten-sity and less than 3 minutes' duration, and 3 if there was a definite occur-rence with severe intensity or 3 or more minutes' duration."

SCICA self-report items describe problems a child may report during an interview. The self-report items are scored on the same 4-point scale as observation items, except that the 0 to 3 scores are intended to reflect the du-ration or intensity of the child's discussion of the problems.

SCICA Profile

To provide a quantitative picture of children's functioning during child inter-views, McConaughy and Achenbach (1994) developed a SCICA scoring pro-file for ages 6 to 12, modeled on scoring profiles for the CBCL, TRF, and Youth Self-Report (YSR; Achenbach, 1991c). The SCICA profile consists of eight syndrome scales and two broad groupings of Internalizing and Exter-nalizing problems derived from ratings of 168 clinically referred subjects. In-terviews were videotaped for each subject and rated by an observer of the videotape as well as by the interviewer. Averaged interviewer–observer scores

for each item were submitted to principal components analyses to derive sets of items that co-occurred to form syndromes. Five syndrome scales were derived from observation items: Anxious, Attention Problems, Resistant, Strange, and Withdrawn. Three syndromes were derived from self-report items: Aggressive Behavior, Anxious/Depressed, and Family Problems. Principal factor analyses of the correlations among the syndrome scales identified Internalizing and Externalizing groupings of syndromes.

To develop the SCICA scoring profile, normalized T scores were assigned to raw scores obtained for 237 clinically referred children for each syndrome scale, Internalizing, Externalizing, Total Observations, and Total Self-Reports. Scoring an individual child on the SCICA profile provides a visual representation of high and low scores for problems, as compared with the reference sample of 237 clinically referred children aged 6 to 12. Raw scores and T scores of individual children can also be compared to means and standard deviations for demographically matched samples of 53 clinically referred children and 53 nonreferred children aged 6 to 12. Mean score comparisons provide measures of deviance for individual children as compared with the SCICA clinically referred and nonreferred samples. However, there are no clinical cutpoints for the SCICA scales that demarcate clinical versus normal ranges of scores, as there are for the CBCL, TRF, and YSR (Achenbach, 1991a; 1991b; 1991c). The reason for this difference is that the SCICA T scores are based on a *clinically referred sample* rather than the normative samples used to derive T scores for the CBCL, TRF, and YSR.

Reliability and Validity

The SCICA *Manual* (McConaughy & Achenbach, 1994) reports data on the reliability and validity of the SCICA profile for ages 6 to 12. For 168 children, interrater reliabilities were obtained between interviewers and videotape observers. Reliabilities were moderate for Total Observations and Total Self-Reports (.52 and .58, respectively), but higher for Internalizing (.64) and Externalizing (.72). For the SCICA syndromes, the Resistant scale showed the highest reliability (.80) and the Anxious scale showed the lowest reliability (.45). Interrater reliabilities for the remaining syndromes ranged from .57 to .76. Test–retest reliabilities on a sample of 20 children were .69 for Internalizing, .84 for Externalizing, .89 for total observations, and .73 for total self-reports. Significant test–retest correlations for the syndromes ranged from .54 for Anxious/Depressed to .75 for Anxious, demonstrating the degree of consistency in observations and self-reports during the child interview. However, a nonsignificant correlation of .30 for Withdrawn suggested that children varied considerably from one time to the next on this particular dimension. The SCICA showed good discriminative validity for differentiating referred versus nonreferred children (McConaughy & Achenbach, 1994) and differ-

entiating children classified as having emotional/behavioral disabilities (EBD) versus learning disabilities (LD), according to special education criteria (McConaughy & Achenbach, 1996).

INTERVIEWS IN THE CONTEXT OF MULTIMETHOD ASSESSMENT

As indicated earlier, agreement among different types of informants is far from perfect (Achenbach et al., 1987). This can be true even under the best of circumstances. Accordingly, no one data source, including child interviews, can substitute for all other sources. Child interviews can be especially useful in assessing children's own views and understanding of their problems and observing their behavior, interaction styles, and coping strategies during the interview. Information obtained from child interviews must then be integrated with data from other sources, such as parent and teacher reports, cognitive and personality assessment, developmental and educational records, medical examinations, and so on. Integration of multiple kinds of data can guide practitioners in evaluating children's problems and competencies and selecting appropriate interventions. To facilitate this process, Achenbach and McConaughy (1997) have described a model of multiaxial assessment, outlined in Table 7.2, which integrates parent reports, teacher reports, cognitive assessment, physical assessment, and direct assessment of the child.

The five axes in Table 7.2 represent major areas of child assessment, with an emphasis on standardized empirically based measures. Not all axes

TABLE 7.2. Data Sources for Multiaxial Assessment

I. Parent reports	II. Teacher reports	III. Cognitive tests	IV. Physical assessment	V. Direct assessment of the child
Parent interview	Teacher interview	Cognitive ability	Medical examinations	Child interview
Standardized parent rating scales	Standardized teacher rating scales	Achievement	Neurological examinations	Standardized self-reports
Background questionnaires/ forms	School records	Perceptual–motor skills	Relevant illnesses or disabilities	Direct observations
	Background questionnaires/ forms	Speech and language	Medications	Personality tests

Note. Based on Achenbach and McConaughy (1997).

may be relevant to all cases, and for certain cases additional axes may also be appropriate, such as in assessing family functioning for forensic cases. For most school-age children, Axes I and II will be relevant, inasmuch as parents and teachers are major referral sources and are among the most knowledge-able informants on children's functioning. Axes I and II include standardized parent and teacher rating scales, such as the CBCL and TRF, along with par-ent and teacher interviews, developmental history, and school records. Axis III includes standardized procedures for assessing ability, achievement, lan-guage, and perceptual–motor functioning, as done by school psychologists and other practitioners. Axis IV covers physical characteristics, medical and neurological examinations, and medical history and medications. Axis V in-cludes procedures for direct assessment of children, excluding cognitive as-sessment. This is where child clinical interviews, such as the SCICA, fit into multiaxial assessment, along with standardized self-reports like the YSR and direct observations, such as obtained on the Direct Observation Form (DOF; Achenbach, 1986; McConaughy, Achenbach, & Gent, 1988), and standard-ized personality assessment.

    This chapter has focused specifically on the SCICA as an example of a standardized child interview because it was designed to mesh with other em-pirically based measures in the multiaxial model. To facilitate cross-infor-mant comparisons, many SCICA observation and self-report items were drawn from similar items scored by parents on the CBCL and teachers on the TRF. In addition, SCICA broad scales and syndrome scales were derived from statistical analyses similar to those used to derive the CBCL, TRF, and YSR scales. The pattern of high and low scores obtained on the SCICA scoring profile can thus be easily compared with scores on similar scales of the CBCL, TRF, and YSR. For children aged 5 to 14, practitioners can also compare SCICA scores to similar scores on the DOF, used for rating obser-vations of children in group settings, such as in classrooms and at recess. Such comparisons across measures can highlight similarities and differences in the types of problems exhibited during the child clinical interview and problems reported by other informants or observed in other settings. In the next section, two case examples illustrate how interview data can be integrat-ed with other information in multimethod assessment. For both cases, the as-sessment process included parent and teacher interviews, the CBCL and TRF, individual cognitive and achievement testing, and physical assessment, as well as direct interviewing of the child. For the purpose of this chapter, the information obtained through the child interview, the SCICA, is highlighted.

Case Example: Linda, Age 8

Linda, an 8-year-old, was referred for evaluation to the school psychologist because of her slow progress in school, despite having repeated a grade. Her

parents and teacher wondered whether she had attention-deficit/hyperactivity disorder (ADHD). They complained that she seemed very disorganized and "spacey," and did not appear to understand her schoolwork. It was a constant battle to get her to do homework. Half the time, Linda forgot to bring home school papers and books. Other times, even when she had the necessary materials, Linda seemed "clueless" about what the teacher wanted her to do. Linda's parents tried to help her with homework, but their attempts usually ended in heated arguments and their sending her to her room.

School staff reported that Linda had been retained in first grade because of social immaturity and difficulty learning to read. Linda's current second grade teacher described her as somewhat shy, moody, and still socially immature. She said that Linda had very few friends in school and often stayed on the fringe of activities at recess. When she tried to join into games, other children rejected her because she argued and was too "bossy." Many days, Linda arrived at school looking sad or grumpy. She complained frequently to her teacher about arguments with her parents. Linda also argued about assignments and failed to finish her work, which resulted in staying in for recess. Linda's teacher agreed that she seemed confused about her schoolwork and demanded a lot of attention. However, the teacher felt that Linda was capable of doing the work.

Interview with Linda

When Linda arrived for the SCICA with the school psychologist, she seemed shy and somewhat sullen, but she warmed up after a few minutes of conversation. She was restless in her seat throughout the interview and sometimes fidgeted with her hair and clothing. Linda also tested the limits, for example, by putting her feet up on the table and grabbing objects from the interviewer's desk. Each time she misbehaved, she peeked at the interviewer for a reaction. When discussing family issues, Linda sometimes reverted to a babyish voice. Her mood fluctuated from being happy when talking about her toys and activities to being sad, sullen, or angry when discussing her family and the rules and punishments at home.

Linda seemed eager to have an adult listen to her opinions and feelings. When asked about school, Linda said she liked reading and math, but sometimes the work was too hard. She admitted not completing homework because it was "boring," or she didn't know what she was supposed to do. Linda liked having a teacher help her with her schoolwork, which often happened when she stayed in during recess to make up missing assignments. Linda said she didn't care whether she missed recess, because the other kids didn't like her and wouldn't play with her. However, she seemed to be unaware of what she did to annoy other kids or what she could do differently to win more friends.

Much of Linda's conversation during the SCICA focused on conflicts with her parents. When the psychologist suggested doing a kinetic family drawing, Linda refused. Eventually, she drew a large picture of her father's head. She erased many times and often commented that she couldn't draw or that the drawing didn't look right. She complained that her father always worked, didn't pay enough attention to her, and was mean and grumpy. Linda expressed ambivalent feelings about her mother, first saying she was nice because she bought her things, then later stating that she hated her mother. She said she liked her younger brother best, but that he was a "pest." Then Linda decided that she hated everyone in her family, and liked herself best.

Linda reported being punished frequently at home, including being spanked hard, but she could not identify specific behaviors that led to the punishments. When queried further, Linda explained that her parents gave her points on a chart that she could cash in for money to buy things. Linda liked earning points, but she was angry about not being able to choose what to buy with her money. She was also clearly aware of disagreements between her parents about how to deal with her behavior, and she seemed to play one parent against the other. Linda's perspective on conflicts with her parents is illustrated in the following excerpt from the SCICA:

INTERVIEWER: We were talking about the people in your family. You said your mom was nice. What else about her?

LINDA: She's nice most of the time. I like her a lot. She has candy. And whenever Dad disagrees with something I've done, she always wins and gets me something. That's nice, and she doesn't make me pay for it. She pays for it with her own money. Because I'm saving up for this dumb old puzzle! (*Changes her expression, looks disgusted and angry.*)

INTERVIEWER: You're saving up for a puzzle?

LINDA: Dad said I had to.

INTERVIEWER: Oh . . . so Dad said you had to save up for the dumb old puzzle, huh?

LINDA: Yeah. He said that when I got my ears pierced, I had to save up for it because I was gonna pay for the earrings. But I said I didn't want to. And then he said you have to save up for a puzzle that costs hundreds of dollars. And Mom said I can only save up $5, and she'll save the rest.

INTERVIEWER: Do you want the puzzle?

LINDA: No! (*Looks angry.*) I want this big soft thing (*rubs her face*) that you can squeeze. It's a giant panda about that tall. (*Shows how tall from the floor.*) But Dad says I can't get it, and he says it probably costs $200. He says, "If you

want it, I'm not helping you, because I don't want you to have it!" (*Imitates her father's voice in a singsong way.*)

INTERVIEWER: Oh, I see. Well, I still don't get whose idea it was to get the puzzle, then.

LINDA: *Dad's!* (*Looks angry again.*)

INTERVIEWER: And it's your money that you're saving for earning points?

LINDA: Yeah. I should get what *I* want. (*Voice gets louder, angrier.*)

INTERVIEWER: Yeah. I see what you mean. You earned the points and you want to buy what you want.

LINDA: Yeah. It's not fair!

On the SCICA profile, shown in Figure 7.1, Linda's T score for observed problems (OB T = 58) was at the 82nd percentile and her score for self-reported problems (SR T = 63) was at the 90th percentile, as compared with scores for the SCICA clinical sample. Her Externalizing score was above the 82nd percentile and her Internalizing score was near the 50th percentile. The SCICA profile showed peaks on the Family Problems and Resistant syndromes, with scores above the 93rd percentile. On the Family Problems syndrome, the interviewer scored Linda's reports of being harmed by a parent (spanked very hard); punished a lot; treated unfairly at home; hating her parent(s); lacking attention from parents; not getting along with parents; and screaming. On the Resistant syndrome, the interviewer scored 16 of 26 observed problems, such as argues; complains of tasks being too hard; impatient; resistant or refuses to comply; shows off, clowns, or acts silly; sudden changes in mood or feelings; temper tantrums, hot temper or seems angry; and wants to quit or does quit. Linda's score on the Attention Problems syndrome was above the 50th percentile for the clinical sample for problems such as acts too young for age; contradicts or reverses own statements; doesn't sit still, restless, or hyperactive; fidgets; gross motor difficulty or clumsy; needs repetition of questions or instructions; and out of seat.

Linda's Total Problem and Externalizing scores on the SCICA were more than one standard deviation above mean scores for the SCICA clinical sample, indicating many problems as compared with other children referred to mental health practitioners. Her scores on the Family Problems and Resistant syndromes were also more than one standard deviation above the mean, and all other SCICA scores were similar to the mean scores for the clinical sample. Linda's scores on all of the SCICA scales were more than one standard deviation above mean scores for the nonreferred SCICA sample, indicating that she was showing more problems during the interview than typical

Internalizing   Externalizing   T_Score

T_Score		Metadata
-95	ID# Linda	
-90	Girl Age: 8	
	DATE FILLED:	
-85	INTERVR:	
-80	OBSERVR:	
	AGENCY: 36	
-75		
-70		
-65	# ITEMS	71
-60	TOT OB	60
	OB T	58
-55	TOT SR	54
	SR T	63
	INTERNAL	17
-50	INT T	52
	EXTERNAL	47
-45	EXT T	61
-40		
-38		

Clin %ile (left axis): 93, 84, 69, 50, 31, 16, 11

Scale	Raw score ladder (top → bottom)
1-SR ANXIOUS/DEPRESSED	63, 60, 57, 53, 51, 47, 44, 41, 38, 34, 33, 28, 27, 22, 21, 17, ##, 12, 11, 9, 8, 6, 4
2-OB ANXIOUS	35, 31, 29, 28, 26, 24, 22, 21, 19, 18, 14, 12, 11, 9, 8, 6, 5, ##, 2
3-SR FAMILY PROBLEMS	32, 30, 29, 25, 23, 22, 20, 19, ##, 13, 12, 10, 9, 6, 3, 2, 1
4-OB WITHDRAWN	61, 58, 56, 53, 51, 48, 46, 43, 41, 38, 36, 33, 31, 27, 21, 16, ##, 10, 8, 5, 4, 2
5-SR AGGRESSIVE BEHAVIOR	43, 40, 39, 36, 34, 31, 29, 27, 25, 22, 20, 18, 16, 13, 12, ##, 6, 5, 3, 2, 1
6-OB ATTENTION PROBLEMS	41, 39, 38, 34, 32, 31, 29, 28, 24, 22, 21, 19, 16, 14, ##, 10, 8, 7, 6, 5, 4
7-OB STRANGE	51, 48, 45, 42, 39, 36, 33, 30, 27, 24, 21, 18, 15, 12, 11, 9, ##, 5, 3, 1, 0
8-OB RESISTANT	74, 70, 66, 61, 58, 53, 50, 45, 42, 37, 34, 29, ##, 21, 19, 16, 14, 11, 9, 6, 4, 3, 2

Scale scores (bottom axis): 0-3, 0-1, 0, 0-1, 0, 0-2, 0, 0-1

0 128.Confused	0 23.Confused	1 135.HarmdPar	0 5.Apathetic	1 122.Mean	1 4.ActYoung	0 1.OverConfid	1 6.Argues
0 134.Lonely	0 29.Difficlt	2 136.Punished	0 9.AvoidsEye	2 130.DisobHom	0 22.Concrete	0 3.Giggles	0 7.AskFeedback
0 137.SelfConsc	Directns	3 142.Unfair	0 56.NoConver	0 131.DisobSch	1 24.Reverses	1 15.Brags	1 10.Irresponsible
0 141.Fearful	0 44.Difficlt	Home	0 57.NoFantsy	0 132.Impulsiv	0 31.Doesnt	0 16.BurpFart	0 14.BlameInterv
0 144.Concentr	Express	0 143.Unfair	2 63.NeedCoax	0 140.Suspics	Concentr	2 17.MindOff	2 21.ComplainHard
0 146.Underact	1 46.Doesnt	School	0 72.WontTalk	0 145.SitStill	3 32.Doesnt	0 18.ChewsClth	1 27.Defiant
1 147.Sad	Remember	0 151.TooNeat	2 73.WTFeeling	0 155.Destroys	SitStill	0 26.Daydreams	1 28.DemandsMet
0 157.Directns	0 50.Fears	3 177.HatesPar	2 74.WontGues	OwnThngs	1 33.Distract	1 30.Disjoint	1 36.Explosive
2 158.Learning	Mistakes	2 181.NoAttent	2 77.DontKnow	0 156.Destroys	2 38.Fidgets	Conversat	0 40.OffTask
0 160.FrMistake	2 52.Confidnc	3 186.NotGet	0 79.Secretiv	Others	2 42.Clumsy	0 35.Exaggerat	0 43.Guesses
1 162.Fears	0 65.Nervous	AlongPar	0 80.Overtird	2 173.Fights	0 45.Understnd	0 41.LongRespns	2 48.Impatient
1 164.Guilty	0 68.AnxPleas	1 196.Screams	1 82.NoHumor	0 175.BadComp	0 53.Lapses	0 51.Jokes	0 49.Impulsive
0 168.OutToGet	1 83.SelfCons	0 229.Headache	0 85.Shy	0 178.HateTchr	1 64.NdRepeat	0 55.Leave	0 59.OddNoises
0 169.Overtired	0 102.TooNeat	0 234.Stomache	0 86.SlowVerb	0 182.NoGuilt	0 66.Twitches	Toilet	1 60.MessyWork
0 171.Worthless	0 103.Fearful	15 TOTAL	0 87.SlowWarm	0 188.Attacks	1 67.OutOfSeat	0 71.PlaySexPrt	1 61.Misbehaves
1 174.Teased	0 104.Tremors	73 CLIN T	0 89.Stares	2 205.Temper	0 88.SpeechPrb	0 75.RepeatActs	2 76.Resistant
1 179.Nightmare	4 TOTAL		1 93.Stubborn	0 207.Threaten	12 TOTAL	0 91.Strange	0 78.Screams
0 185.NotLiked	49 CLIN T		0 106.Underact	7 TOTAL	55 CLIN T	Behavior	1 84.ShowsOff
2 192.NGetAlong			2 107.Sad	57 CLIN T		0 92.Strange	1 95.MoodChange
0 193.NoFriends			0 111.Quiet			Ideas	0 97.Suspicious
3 194.SchoolWork			0 114.Withdrawn			2 98.Swears	0 99.TalksSelf
1 214.Worries			12 TOTAL			0 100.TalkMuch	2 101.TemperAngry
13 TOTAL			57 CLIN T			6 TOTAL	2 105.Manipulates
56 CLIN T						55 CLIN T	0 110.Loud
							2 112.Quits
							1 115.Careless
							22 TOTAL
							66 CLIN T

FIGURE 7.1. SCICA profile for Linda, age 8.

for other children her age (see McConaughy & Achenbach, 1994, for details on scoring the SCICA).

Summary of Findings for Linda

Linda's case illustrates the contributions of the child interview in assessing attention problems and externalizing behavior reported by parents and teachers. On the CBCL and TRF, Linda's parents and teacher scored her in the borderline clinical range above the 95th percentile on the Aggressive Behavior and Attention Problems scales. Linda's teacher also scored her in the clinical range on the TRF Attention Problems and Social Problems scales. These results indicated that Linda's parents and teachers were reporting more problems than typically reported for girls her age. During the SCICA, the school psychologist had ample opportunity to observe similar problems, particularly Linda's resistance to adult requests and attempts to control situations, as well as her attention problems. The combined evidence from the multiaxial assessment supported diagnoses of oppositional defiant disorder (ODD) and attention-deficit/hyperactivity disorder (ADHD)-combined type, according to the *Diagnostic and Statistical Manual of Mental Disorders,* fourth edition (DSM-IV; American Psychiatric Association, 1994).[1]

Linda's own perspective on her problems was especially revealing regarding conflicts with her parents and her reactions to discipline procedures at home. Linda's parents corroborated her reports about a home-based point system and their control of the reward system. Linda's parents also acknowledged use of physical punishments (spanking), but expressed frustration about the lack of effectiveness of their discipline efforts. Linda's perspective on schoolwork was also enlightening, especially her comments suggesting that she enjoyed the extra attention from her teachers when she stayed in for recess to complete her work. Such data from the child interview added important information for designing interventions, as discussed in the next section.

Interventions for Linda

When the school psychologist met with Linda's parents and teacher, she used the scored CBCL, TRF, and SCICA profiles to illustrate the patterns of problems identified from each data source. Linda's parents and teacher saw that there was evidence to support their original suspicion of ADHD. However, the CBCL, TRF, and SCICA profiles also revealed severe aggressive, oppositional behavior and social problems that were not the main focus of the original referral complaints. Given these results, the school psychologist advised Linda's parents to seek mental health services to improve their behavior management strategies at home. She referred them to a local clinic

that used Barkley's (1997) parent training program for children with ODD. Without violating confidentiality, she explained how the child interview revealed Linda's feelings about unfair rules and reward systems at home. She stressed the importance of giving Linda some control over the reward choices in order to motivate better compliance. She also encouraged Linda's parents, especially her father, to provide more attention when Linda was behaving appropriately, such as praising and rewarding her for completing chores or homework.

At school, the school psychologist consulted with Linda's teachers to develop an incentive plan for completing assignments. A school–home note system was also established to improve communication about homework (Kelly, 1990). Because Linda had expressed such a positive attitude about earning points on a behavior chart at home, a similar system was developed at school that rewarded her for independent effort and work completion. Linda earned points each day for meeting behavioral targets and then cashed in her points according to a menu of rewards. Linda still stayed in for recess when she failed to complete homework, but her teacher refused to give her any special attention during this time. The teacher also instituted other classroom accommodations to address Linda's attention problems, such as reducing the amount of work given at any one time. After several weeks Linda's productivity in class began to improve and she missed fewer recesses. Eventually, she began saving points on her chart for more "costly" rewards at the end of the week instead of immediate, daily rewards.

To address her social problems, Linda was joined with five other children in the *Tough Kids Social Skills Program* (Sheridan, 1997), conducted by the school psychologist. Linda's teacher provided additional opportunities in class for Linda to practice specific skills that she had learned each week.

Case Example: Charlie, Age 9

From first grade on, Charlie had received special education services for a learning disability in math. He also received remedial reading instruction in first grade, but by fourth grade he had become a proficient reader. From first to fourth grade, Charlie continued to struggle in math, even with special education. When he entered the middle grades, Charlie's teachers began to worry about his emotional sensitivity regarding his learning problems and his reluctance to participate in cooperative learning groups. Charlie's parents were also concerned about his emotional outbursts over homework. When the time came for Charlie's triennial special education evaluation, his teachers and parents agreed to an evaluation of his emotional functioning along with the usual cognitive and academic assessment for learning disabilities.

On the CBCL, Charlie's mother and father both scored him in the borderline clinical range on the Social Problems scale, and his mother scored

him in the clinical range on the Internalizing and Anxious/Depressed scales. On the TRF, Charlie's special education and fourth grade teachers scored him in the borderline to clinical range on the Internalizing, Anxious/Depressed, and Withdrawn scales.

Interview with Charlie

During the SCICA, Charlie was anxious and tense much of the time. He sat rigidly in his chair and fidgeted with his clothes. He spoke in a halting monotone and often paused for long periods to choose his words. He initially avoided eye contact and seemed quite self-conscious. Attempts at humor fell flat, although Charlie eventually warmed up as he described his interests and activities. He said that he enjoyed watching sports on TV, and he wanted to try out for the school baseball team. He liked playing catch with his dad, although this happened infrequently because his dad worked late and many weekends. Charlie liked caring for his many pets at home and enjoyed family outings to the park, where he could go off by himself to observe birds and animals. He wanted to be a field biologist when he grew up.

Charlie reported having one very close friend, whom he saw about once a week. This friend shared his interests in animals and was easy to talk to. Charlie said other kids teased him at school and left him out of their activities. When asked about schoolwork, Charlie said he liked science and social studies because he felt he was good in those subjects. He readily admitted having problems in math, but liked getting special help outside of the classroom. He especially liked working with one girl in his class who was good in math. He was glad that his teachers allowed him to use a calculator, because he had trouble with multiplication and division and could not remember math facts. When he became a field biologist, Charlie said, he would have an assistant help him with "the number stuff." Charlie desperately wanted good grades and hated disappointing his parents with a poor report card. He felt that he was capable of B's and C's in most subjects, except math. However, he thought that his dad wanted him to get all A's.

Charlie's drawing of his family during the SCICA was notable for his very slow and meticulous approach. He checked with the interviewer several times about details and expectations for the drawing. He drew with his head close to the table and afterward complained that his hand hurt from the pressure. His picture depicted his entire family going off in the car to the park. Charlie admitted that he argued a lot with his sister, who deliberately tried to embarrass him. He seemed at a loss for ways to cope with his sister's tactics, even though she was several years younger than Charlie. He reported getting angry when his sister messed up things in his room, particularly his toy animal collection and science paraphernalia. Charlie also reported being upset by arguments between his parents, which sometimes concerned his home-

work but often had nothing to do with him. He had recently begun hiding homework to avoid confrontations with his parents.

Charlie's SCICA profile, displayed in Figure 7.2, showed peaks for self-reported problems on the Anxious/Depressed syndrome and for observed problems on the Anxious syndrome. On both SCICA scales, Charlie scored at or above the 90th percentile as compared with the SCICA clinical sample of 6- to 12-year-olds. Charlie also scored above the 50th percentile on the SCICA Family Problems, Withdrawn, and Attention Problems scales. His scores on the remaining syndromes were much lower and closer to the mean for the SCICA sample of nonreferred children.

Summary of Findings for Charlie

Charlie's case illustrates the contribution of the child interview for assessing internalizing problems in a boy with a long-standing learning disability. The SCICA enabled the school psychologist to directly observe Charlie's anxiousness and social awkwardness and hear his views of his learning and social problems. High scores on the SCICA Anxious/Depressed and Anxious syndromes corroborated parent and teacher reports of anxiety, depressed affect, and social problems. Such findings are consistent with research showing significant internalizing problems among children with LD as compared with nonreferred samples (McConaughy & Achenbach, 1996; McConaughy, Mattison, & Peterson, 1994) and among individuals with nonverbal LD, in particular (Rourke, 1988). During the SCICA, Charlie exhibited several of the behaviors found to be associated with nonverbal LD, including social anxiety, difficulty assessing cause and effect in social interactions, failure to appreciate humor, and a halting manner of speaking (Rourke & Fuerst, 1992). These findings, combined with other evidence, underscored the importance of addressing Charlie's emotional and social needs, as well as his learning problems, in home and school interventions.

Interventions and Outcomes for Charlie

High Internalizing scores on his mother's CBCL, the two TRFs, and the SCICA convinced Charlie's parents that his level of anxiety was not typical for boys his age. They agreed to seek mental health services with a local psychologist who specialized in cognitive behavioral therapy techniques for children with anxiety disorders (Kendall & Panichelli-Mindel, 1995). The psychologist also provided family therapy to develop strategies for reducing conflicts between Charlie and his parents and Charlie and his younger sister.

In school, Charlie continued to have an individualized education program (IEP) for special education services in math. Hands-on projects, practical activities, and computer games were used to demonstrate new mathemat-

T Score

-95 ID# CHARLIE
-90 Boy Age: 9
-85 DATE FILLED:
INTERVR:
-80 RATER:
AGENCY: 36

Internalizing   Externalizing

	1-SR ANXIOUS/ DEPRESSED	2-OB ANXIOUS	3-SR FAMILY PROBLEMS	4-OB WITHDRAWN	5-SR AGGRESSIVE BEHAVIOR	6-OB ATTENTION PROBLEMS	7-OB STRANGE	8-OB RESISTANT	T Score
	63	35	32	61	43	41	51	74	
	60	31	30	58	40	39	48	70	
	57	29	29	56	39	38	45	66	
	53	28	25	53	36		42	61	# ITEMS 60
	51	26	23	51	34	34	39	58	TOT OB 53
	47	24	22	48	31	32	36	53	OB T 55
	44	22	20	46	29	31	33	50	TOT SR 36
	41	21	19	43	27	29	30	45	SR T 54
	38			41	25	28	27	42	INTERNAL 39
	34			38	22		24	37	INT T 69
Clin	33	18		36	20	24	21	34	EXTERNAL 14
%ile	28	14	15	33	18	22	18	29	EXT T 42
	27	12	13	31	16	21	15	26	
93	22	11	12	27	13	19	12	21	
	##		10	21	12		11	19	
	17	9	9	16		16		16	
84	16	8		##	8	14	9	14	
	12	6	6	10	6	12	6	11	
69	11	5		8	5		5	9	
	9			5		8		6	
50	8	4	2	4	3	7		4	
					2	6	1	3	
31	6	2	1	2		5			
	4					4			
16									
11	0-3	0-1	0	0-1	1	0-2	0	0-1	

SCICA profile for Charlie, age 9.

0 128.Confused	0 23.Confused	0 135.HarmdPar	0 5.Apathetic	0 122.Mean	0 4.ActYoung	0 1.OverConfid	0 6.Argues
1 134.Lonely	0 29.Difficlt	0 136.Punished	0 9.AvoidsEye	0 130.DisobHom	0 22.Concrete	0 3.Giggles	1 7.AskFeedback
2 137.SelfConsc	Directns	1 142.Unfair	1 56.NoConver	0 131.DisobSch	1 24.Reverses	0 15.Brags	0 10.Irresponsible
Directns	3 44.Difficlt	Home	1 57.NoFantsy	0 132.Impulsiv	0 31.Doesnt	0 16.BurpFart	0 14.BlameInterv
1 141.Fearful	Home	0 143.Unfair	0 63.NeedCoax	0 140.Suspics	Concentr	1 17.MindOff	0 21.ComplainHard
2 144.Concentr	0 46.Doesnt	School	0 72.WontTalk	0 145.SitStill	1 32.Doesnt	0 18.ChewsClth	0 27.Defiant
0 146.Underact	Remember	1 151.TooNeat	1 73.WTFeeling	0 155.Destroys	SitStill	0 26.Daydreams	0 28.DemandsMet
0 147.Sad	1 50.Fears	0 177.HatesPar	0 74.WontGues	OwnThngs	1 33.Distract	1 30.Disjoint	0 36.Explosive
0 157.Directns	Mistakes	1 181.NoAttent	0 77.DontKnow	0 156.Destroys	2 38.Fidgets	Conversat	0 40.OffTask
3 158.Learning	2 52.Confidnc	0 186.NotGet	0 79.Secretiv	Others	1 42.Clumsy	0 35.Exaggerat	0 43.Guesses
0 160.FrMistake	3 65.Nervous	AlongW	0 80.Overtird	0 173.Fights	0 45.Understnd	0 41.LongRespns	0 48.Impatient
2 162.Fears	1 68.AnxPleas	0 196.Screams	1 82.NoHumor	0 175.BadComp	0 53.Lapses	0 51.Jokes	0 49.Impulsive
0 164.Guilty	3 83.SelfCons	2 229.Headache	2 85.Shy	0 178.HateTchr	1 64.NdRepeat	0 55.Leave	0 59.OddNoises
0 168.OutToGet	3 102.TooNeat	0 234.Stomache	1 86.SlowVerb	0 182.NoGuilt	1 66.Twitches	Toilet	0 60.MessyWork
0 169.Overtired	1 103.Fearful	3 TOTAL	1 87.SlowWarm	0 188.Attacks	1 67.OutOfSeat	0 71.PlaySexPrt	0 61.Misbehaves
1 171.Worthless	0 104.Tremors	54 CLIN T	0 89.Stares	0 205.Temper	1 88.SpeechPrb	0 75.RepeatActs	0 76.Resistant
2 174.Teased	19 TOTAL		0 93.Stubborn	0 207.Threaten	10 TOTAL	0 91.Strange	0 78.Screams
0 179.Nightmare	75 CLIN T		0 106.Underact	0 TOTAL	53 CLIN T	Behavior	0 84.ShowsOff
0 185.NotLiked			0 107.Sad	38 CLIN T		0 92.Strange	0 95.MoodChange
0 192.NGetAlong			1 111.Quiet			Ideas	0 97.Suspicious
0 193.NoFriends			0 114.Withdrawn			0 98.Swears	1 99.TalksSelf
3 194.SchoolWork			11 TOTAL			0 100.TalkMuch	0 101.TemperAngry
3 214.Worries			56 CLIN T			2 TOTAL	0 105.Manipulates
20 TOTAL						46 CLIN T	0 110.Loud
63 CLIN T							0 112.Quits
							0 115.Careless
							2 TOTAL
							41 CLIN T

FIGURE 7.2. SCICA profile for Charlie, age 9.

ical concepts and train computational skills. Charlie continued to use a calculator for math, although his father had reservations about this practice. The girl Charlie identified in the SCICA agreed to serve as a peer tutor in math. Charlie's parents also agreed to collaborate with his teachers on a school–home note system for monitoring and planning homework (Kelly, 1990).

To capitalize on Charlie's interests in science and animals, his teachers arranged a special science project for him and two other students, depicting animal habitats for the Spring science fair. To improve his self-esteem and capitalize on his good reading skills, the school psychologist recommended novels and biographies about people who had successfully coped with LD and social problems. He also recommended reading material on LD and child development to Charlie's parents. To expand Charlie's social interactions, the school psychologist supported his efforts to join the school baseball team and science club. SCICA findings also persuaded Charlie's parents to allow him to participate in a school-based social skills group.

At the end of the school year Charlie received passing grades in all subjects and was promoted to fifth grade. However, he continued to score below average on standardized mathematics tests. Because he was a special education student, Charlie's math grades were adapted to his individual level of achievement in place of grade-level comparisons. On a follow-up TRF from Charlie's fourth grade teacher and a CBCL from his mother, Charlie's Internalizing scores dropped into the normal range, indicating considerable improvement since the beginning of the school year.

SUMMARY

This chapter described child clinical interviews for obtaining children's self-reports of their competencies and problems. Child interviews also provide opportunities for directly observing children's behavior and emotional functioning in a one-on-one situation. Semistructured interview formats were emphasized because of their flexibility and compatibility with children's different developmental levels and conversational styles and their compatibility with behavioral assessment. Practical guidelines were offered on questioning strategies for semistructured interviews.

Although they are often considered central to clinical assessment, interviews are only one of several data sources for evaluating children's functioning. Because agreement across data sources is limited, it is important to compare information obtained from child interviews with information from parents, teachers, and other data sources. The SCICA (McConaughy & Achenbach, 1994) was described as an example of a semistructured interview designed to dovetail with other empirically based measures, including

standardized parent and teacher rating scales. When combined with other methods of assessment as done in these cases, child interviews can contribute important and unique information for evaluating children's emotional and behavioral functioning.

NOTE

1. Other assessment procedures from those listed in Table 7.1 are also necessary for making valid DSM-IV diagnoses, such as ADHD and ODD. Because the focus of this chapter is on child clinical interviews, data from other assessment procedures are not discussed in case examples.

REFERENCES

Achenbach, T. M. (1986). *Direct Observation Form.* Burlington: University of Vermont, Department of Psychiatry.

Achenbach, T. M. (1991a). *Manual for the Child Behavior Checklist/4–18 and 1991 Profile.* Burlington: University of Vermont, Department of Psychiatry.

Achenbach, T. M. (1991b). *Manual for the Teacher's Report Form and 1991 Profile.* Burlington: University of Vermont, Department of Psychiatry.

Achenbach, T. M. (1991c). *Manual for the Youth Self-Report and 1991 Profile.* Burlington: University of Vermont, Department of Psychiatry.

Achenbach, T. M., & McConaughy, S. H. (1997). *Empirically based assessment of child and adolescent psychopathology: Practical applications.* Thousand Oaks, CA: Sage.

Achenbach, T. M., McConaughy, S. H., & Howell, C. T. (1987). Child/adolescent behavioral and emotional problems: Implications of cross-informant correlations for situational specificity. *Psychological Bulletin, 101,* 213–232.

American Psychiatric Association. (1994). *Diagnostic and statistical manual of mental disorders* (4th ed.). Washington, DC: Author.

Barkley, R. A. (1997). *Defiant children (2nd ed.): A clinician's manual for assessment and parent training.* New York: Guilford Press.

Bierman, K. L. (1983). Cognitive development and clinical interviews with children. In B. B. Lahey & A. E. Kazdin (Eds.), *Advances in clinical child psychology* (Vol. 6, pp. 217–250). New York: Plenum Press.

Burns, R. C. (1982). *Self-growth in families: Kinetic family drawings (K-F-D) research and application.* New York: Brunner/Mazel.

Cox, A., Hopkinson, K., & Rutter, M. (1981). Psychiatric interviewing techniques II. Naturalistic study: Eliciting factual information. *British Journal of Psychiatry, 138,* 283–291.

Garbarino, J., & Scott, F. M. (1989). *What children can tell us.* San Francisco: Jossey-Bass.

Hughes, J. N., & Baker, D. B. (1990). *The clinical child interview.* New York: Guilford Press.

Jenson, W. R., Rhode, G., & Reavis, H. K. (1994). *The Tough Kid Tool Box*. Longmont, CO: Sopris West.

Kelly, M. L. (1990). *School–home notes: Promoting children's classroom success*. New York: Guilford Press.

Kendall, P. C., & Panichelli-Mindel, S. M. (1995). Cognitive-behavioral treatments. *Journal of Abnormal Child Psychology, 23*, 107–124.

McConaughy, S. H. (1996). The interview process. In M. Breen & C. Fiedler (Eds.), *Behavioral approach to the assessment of youth with emotional/behavioral disorders: A handbook for school-based practitioners* (pp. 181–223). Austin. TX: PRO-ED.

McConaughy, S. H., & Achenbach, T. M. (1994). *Manual for the Semistructured Clinical Interview for Children and Adolescents*. Burlington: University of Vermont, Department of Psychiatry.

McConaughy, S. H., & Achenbach, T. M. (1996). Contributions of a child interview to multimethod assessment of children with EBD and LD. *School Psychology Review, 25*, 24–39.

McConaughy, S. H., Achenbach, T. M., & Gent, C. L. (1988). Multiaxial empirically based assessment: Parent, teacher, observational, cognitive, and personality correlates of Child Behavior Profiles for 6–11-year-old boys. *Journal of Abnormal Child Psychology, 16*, 485–509.

McConaughy, S. H., Fitzhenry-Coor, I., & Howell, D. C. (1983). Developmental differences in story schemata. In K. E. Nelson (Ed.), *Children's language* (Vol. 4, pp. 385–421). Hillsdale, NJ: Erlbaum.

McConaughy, S. H., Mattison, R. E., & Peterson, R. L. (1994). Behavioral/emotional problems of children with serious emotional disturbance and learning disabilities. *School Psychology Review, 23*, 81–98.

Rourke, B. P. (1988). Socioemotional disturbances of learning disabled children. *Journal of Consulting and Clinical Psychology, 56*, 801–810.

Rourke, B. P., & Fuerst, D. R. (1992). Psychosocial dimensions of learning disability subtypes: Neuropsychological studies in the Windsor laboratory. *School Psychology Review, 21*, 361–374.

Sattler, J. M. (1998). *Clinical and forensic interviewing of children and families*. San Diego, CA: Author.

Shaffer, D. (1992). *NIMH Diagnostic Interview Schedule for Children, Version 2. 3*. New York: Columbia University, Division of Child and Adolescent Psychiatry.

Sheridan, S. M. (1997). *The tough kid social skills book*. Longmont, CO: Sopris West.

Witt, J. C., Cavell, T. A., Carey, M. P., & Martens, B. (1988). Child self-report: Interviewing techniques and rating scales. In E. S. Shapiro & R. R. Kratochwill (Eds.), *Behavioral assessment in schools: Conceptual foundations and practical applications* (pp. 384–454). New York: Guilford Press.

CHAPTER 8

◆◆◆

Informant Report:
Rating Scale Measures

◆

KENNETH W. MERRELL

During the last two decades of the 20th century, the use of behavior rating scales emerged as one of the most popular forms of child behavior assessment (Wilson & Reschly, 1996). Today school and clinical child psychologists routinely utilize child behavior rating scales as either primary components of multisource assessment designs or as key means of obtaining behavioral information prior to, during, and following interventions. Although rating scale measures were eschewed by many behaviorally oriented practitioners and researchers during the 1960s and 1970s as unreliable and not ecologically valid, important advances in research and development in rating scale technology during the 1970s and 1980s strengthened the position and acceptability of this form of assessment (Elliott, Busse, & Gresham, 1993; Merrell, 1999). In fact, behavior rating scale informant reports are now considered to be an important component of a functional assessment of child and adolescent behavior in school settings (Alberto & Troutman, 1996). Clearly, the transformation of behavior rating scale measures as clinical assessment tools for children, within a relatively short time, from their formerly marginal position to the widespread acceptance they now enjoy has been truly remarkable.

The purpose of this chapter is to give an overview of some of the theoretical, technical, and practical aspects of using rating scale measures, and to analyze this assessment method in terms of its clinical use in assessing behavioral, social, and emotional problems of children and adolescents within school settings. First, a brief discussion regarding the characteristics of rating scales and the advantages and problems they present is offered. Next, some of

the technical and measurement issues involving rating scales are discussed. A number of the child behavior rating scales that are most widely used in school settings in the United States are discussed briefly, along with their major features. Finally, some recommended best practices for using child behavior rating scales in school settings are presented.

CHARACTERISTICS OF RATING SCALE MEASURES

Rating scale measures provide a standardized format for an informant's summary judgments regarding a child or adolescent's behavioral characteristics. A broad range of informants may potentially complete a rating scale, although parents and teachers are the respondents most commonly involved. Because the focus of this volume is on school-based behavioral assessment, the examples regarding rating scale informants are limited primarily to teachers. However, the concepts, discussion, and issues concerning behavior rating scales are identical for all informants.

Behavior rating scales have been considered a less direct assessment method than either direct behavioral observation or structured behavioral interviewing (McMahon, 1984), because they tend to measure *perceptions* of behavior rather than providing a firsthand measure of the existence of a behavior. However, rating scales are clearly an objective assessment method. Martin (1988) described four characteristics necessary for a measurement tool to be considered objective: (1) individual differences in responses to stimuli, which are relatively consistent across times, items, and situations; (2) comparison of responses of one person to those of other persons; (3) the use of norms for comparison purposes; and (4) responses are shown to be related to other stimuli in some meaningful way. Behavior rating scales, almost without exception, meet these criteria of objectivity.

Because of their objectivity, rating scale measures have been found to yield behavioral assessment data that are more reliable than the data typically obtained through unstructured interviewing or projective–expressive techniques (Martin, Hooper, & Snow, 1986; Merrell, 1999). In addition, because systematic and direct observations of child behavior may require several observations over a period of time to yield reliable data, particularly when younger children are being observed (Doll & Elliott, 1994), rating scale measures appear to offer several advantages for reliability over direct observation, even though the two methods tap somewhat differing constructs. Direct behavioral observation provides a measure of clearly specified behaviors that occur within a specific environmental context and within a given time constraint. Behavior rating scales, on the other hand, provide summative judgments of general types of behavioral characteristics that may have occurred in a variety of settings and over a long period of time. Both methods

of behavioral assessment are important in the overall clinical analysis of behavior.

It is important to differentiate rating scale measures from behavior checklists, a historical precursor to rating scales as they are currently used. Behavior checklists provide several behavioral descriptors, and if the informant perceives the symptom to be present, he or she simply checks the item. After the checklist is completed, checked items are typically summed into a total score, most often by simply totaling the number of symptoms or characteristics that have been checked by the informant. Therefore, behavior checklists are considered to be *additive* tools (Merrell, 1999). Rating scales, as they are now commonly used, not only allow the informant a means of indicating whether a specific symptom is present, but also provide a way of estimating *to what degree* symptoms may be present. For example, a commonly used 3-point rating scale allows the informant to rate a specific behavior descriptor from 0 to 2, with 0 indicating the symptom is "never" present, 1 indicating the symptom is "sometimes" present, and 2 indicating the symptom is "frequently" present. Because rating scales allow the informant to differentially weight particular behavioral characteristics, and because each weighting selected corresponds with a specific numerical value and frequency or intensity description, rating scales are said to be *algebraic* in nature, because they involve symbolic numeric representation of specific levels or intensities of behavioral characteristics (Merrell, 1999). The algebraic format provided by rating scales is generally preferred to the additive format of checklists because it allows for more precise measurement of behavioral frequency or intensity. Although the checklist format for evaluating child behavior is still used, it has been largely abandoned among today's behavior assessment instruments in favor of the more sophisticated rating scale format.

ADVANTAGES AND PROBLEMS

It is not surprising that rating scales have enjoyed such widespread popularity and use in recent years. The truth is that this method of assessment offers several unique advantages in comparison with other methods. Six of the primary advantages or strengths, which have been previously noted by this author (e.g., Merrell, 1999), are as follows:

1. In comparison with direct observation of behavior, rating scales require less professional time and training for effective use.
2. Behavior rating scales may provide information on low-frequency but potentially important behaviors that might not be identified in time-limited direct observation sessions. For example, violent and assaultive behaviors by a particular student may not occur on a constant or consistent sched-

ule. Therefore, these behaviors would likely be missed within the constraints of conducting two or three brief direct observations. However, these are critically important behaviors, and an examiner cannot afford to miss them in the course of an assessment.

3. Behavior rating scales tend to provide assessment data that are considerably more reliable than data provided through unstructured interviews or projective–expressive techniques.

4. Behavior rating scales offer one of the few assessment methods useful for providing information on students who cannot readily provide self-report information. For example, a child with limited verbal ability because of a significant developmental delay would typically not be able to provide useful self-report information regarding his or her behavior, nor would an adolescent who is temporarily not accessible to school personnel because of having been suspended from school. In both cases, rating scale measures may provide some highly useful behavioral information.

5. Rating scales capitalize on observations over a period of time in a child or adolescent's "natural" environment (i.e., school or home setting).

6. Rating scales may effectively exploit the judgments and observations, over time, of persons who are very familiar with the student's behavior, such as classroom teachers, who may thus be considered "expert" informants.

These distinct advantages of rating scales clearly illustrate some of the reasons they have become so widely used. In short, they are quite capable of capturing essential behavioral information in a short amount of time, at moderate cost, and with a great deal of technical precision and practical utility.

Although rating scale measures may offer some distinct advantages, they are also beset with certain problems or disadvantages that must be considered. In considering these inherent problems, it is worth noting that rating scales are not alone in having limitations. In fact, each of the several methods of behavioral assessment contains inherent limiting factors that present challenges for effectively conducting assessments. Therefore, the current preferred professional practice for overcoming the limitations presented by a particular assessment method is to conduct a multimethod, multisource, multisetting assessment, wherein the strengths of several methods in combination may be helpful in counteracting the limitations of any one method (Merrell, 1999).

The basic measurement problems inherent in behavior rating scales were formally articulated by Saal, Downey, and Lahey (1980) and later discussed in terms more specific to school and clinical child psychology by Martin et al. (1986). These problems are generally divided into two classes of measurement bias or error: *bias of response* and *error variance*. Bias of response refers to the error in measurement produced by the way that informants who

complete rating scales use the scales. There are three specific types of response bias. A *halo effect* refers to rating a student in a decidedly positive or negative way just because that student possesses positive or negative characteristics, which can be unrelated to the rating scale task, that somehow influence the rater. *Leniency or severity* refers to the tendency of some raters to have an overgenerous or overcritical response set in general and whose ratings may be consistently higher or lower than warranted. *Central tendency effects* refer to the inclination of some raters to consistently select midpoint ratings, thus avoiding end points of the scale.

In contrast to response bias, error variance has less to do with the way a particular rater approaches the task of completing the rating scale measure, and more to do with a general representation of some of the problems encountered because of the very nature of this assessment method. Four particular types of error variance relevant to rating scale measures were listed by Martin et al. (1986), consistent with the earlier work of Saal et al. (1980). *Source variance* refers to the subjectivity or unique evaluative characteristics of the rater, including any idiosyncratic ways in which they may complete the rating scales. Source variance is therefore closely related to response bias. *Setting variance*, on the other hand, is an entirely different type of error than source variance. Setting variance is a result of the fact that individuals behave somewhat differently in each setting in which they must respond, assumably because of the differing stimulus/antecedent conditions and reinforcing or punishing properties specific to those settings. Kazdin (1979) has articulated this issue in terms of situational specificity of behavior. Although situational specificity may be accurately thought of as a form of variance, it does not necessarily involve error but may accurately reflect the fact that behavior varies from place to place because of differing conditions. *Temporal variance* refers to the tendency of behavior ratings to be only moderately consistent over time. Perhaps partly because of actual changes in behavior over time and partly because of changes or inconsistency in a rater's approach to the measurement task over time, it is likely that behavior rating scales will yield test–retest coefficients that are not nearly as strong as those that would be found with ability or achievement measures. Thus, this type of variance may be related to both the construct being measured as well as source variance. In addition, *instrument variance* is a phenomenon that reflects the fact that various rating scales, even those purported to measure similar constructs, may actually measure slightly differing hypothetical constructs because of differences in item content, item wording, or rating scale format. For example, the Teacher Report Form (TRF) and the Behavior Assessment System for Children (BASC) teacher form (which are both discussed later in this chapter), are purported to measure essentially the same constructs, with some minor differences. However, the demonstrated correlations among these measures, although strong, reflect enough unaccounted variance to allow the

assumption that there is only a moderate degree of variance shared between the two instruments and the constructs they measure. Another reason for instrument variance is the necessary fact that each rating scale utilizes unique normative samples. If the norm samples are not randomly selected and entirely representative of the population as a whole, then variance among instruments may be normally expected because of these sampling differences.

A final potential problem to consider in regard to rating scale measures is the actual nature of the rating task. Rating scales seem to measure an informant's *perceptions* of a particular behavior or characteristics. Although this is an objective form of measurement, it is important to recognize that objective perceptions may be different from objective reality. Therefore, rating scales do not actually provide direct measures of behavior as it occurs in a given setting, but provide a summary judgment of specific behavioral characteristics, based on the experience of the rater that provides a basis for his or her perception. Although these problems associated with rating scales are important to consider, it must also be considered that each form of measurement presents unique problems and that no method is without error. Specific suggestions for overcoming some of the measurement problems with rating scales are offered later in this chapter.

OTHER TECHNICAL CONSIDERATIONS

In addition to rater bias and error variance, there are other important technical issues to consider in selecting and using behavior rating scales. Some of the more commonly identified of these technical issues are considered in this section. Because the major focus of this text is practical considerations for assessment, a comprehensive discussion of technical and theoretical issues is beyond the scope of this chapter. Thus, readers are referred to other sources (e.g., Martin et al., 1986; Merrell, 1999, 2000; Saal et al., 1980) for a more detailed treatment of these topics.

One of the most basic measurement variables that may affect the technical or psychometric properties of a rating scale is the actual *rating format* of the scale and how it is constructed. The two rating formats that appear to be the most common for child behavior rating scales are 3-point and 5-point scales. Each numerical value in the rating format is keyed or anchored to a descriptor (for example, 0 = never, 1 = sometimes, 2 = frequently). As a general rule, more accurate ratings are obtained when there is a concrete definition for each possible level. In other words, descriptors such as "sometimes" and "frequently" may be more effective if the rating scale provides examples for these categories. Although 3-point and 5-point rating formats appear to be the most widely used in construction of child behavior rating scales, there has actually been very little discussion of how many rating points or levels are

appropriate. Worthen, Borg, and White (1993) suggested that a common error in scale construction is the use of too many levels. The assumption here is that a higher level of inference is needed in making ratings when more possible rating points are involved, which increases the difficulty in reliably discriminating among the various rating levels. In general, a good heuristic is for scale developers to use the fewest rating levels needed to make an appropriate rating discrimination, and to avoid scales that require an excessive amount of inference in making discriminations among rating points. It is also important to ensure that rating levels and anchor points of a measure are meaningful and easy to understand.

A technical characteristic of rating scales that may potentially introduce variance into the ratings is the *time element* to be considered in making the rating. According to Worthen et al. (1993), there is a general tendency for recent events and behaviors to be given disproportionate consideration as an informant completes a rating scale. For example, it seems to be easier to remember a child's behavioral characteristics observed during the previous 2-week period than those observed during the previous 3-month period. Rating scales clearly differ in regard to the time period on which the ratings are supposed to be based. The most common time periods that child behavior rating scales appear to be based on range from about 1 month to about 6 months.

Although there are no empirical data to support this assertion, it seems likely that as the time element or rating period for the scale increases, the ratings of behavior become less specific and objective, and increasingly holistic and general. Although such holistic and general ratings may be reliable and valid for many purposes, they are likely to be measuring a somewhat different construct than would be measured if the rating format of a scale were anchored to a short and recent time frame. It seems likely that behavior rating scales that are anchored to very brief and discrete time periods are more likely to measure specific occurrences or estimates of behavior, whereas rating scales anchored to a longer time period are measuring general perceptions of behavioral characteristics over time and across settings. It is unclear how the time element in a rating format will actually affect the data that are yielded from the scale, but this is an issue that should at least be considered by users of rating scales. The issue may be particularly important in school-based assessment in the early stages of an academic year, when a teacher who may be asked to complete a rating has not had an opportunity to interact with the student or observe that student's behavior for more than a few weeks.

Another technical issue to consider in regard to rating scale measures is that it may be easier for raters to remember or recall *unusual or novel behaviors* than it is to remember ordinary or typical behaviors (Worthen et al., 1993). If this is the case, then typical uneventful behaviors may be assigned less proportional weight during the rating than novel, unusual, or highly distinctive behaviors. Again, there is little empirical evidence to support this idea (other

than general findings from the field of memory regarding recall of novel versus ordinary events), but it is worth considering. Intuitively, many psychologists and special education consultants understand the idea that a regular classroom teacher may be likely to pay less attention to the times that a particular student is behaving like the other students than to the occasions when he or she is engaging in disruptive or unusual behavior.

Of additional concern regarding the technical characteristics of rating scale measures are the *directions for use* provided with the instrument. Some scales include highly detailed and specific instructions for completing the ratings, whereas other scales may provide a minimum of directions and clarifications. It is recommended that users of rating scale measures select instruments that provide clear and concrete directions, as well as decision rules for dealing with unclear distinctions in rating student characteristics (Gronlund & Linn, 1990). This recommendation simply reflects a commonsense way of increasing the objectivity and reliability of the task of completing child behavior rating scales.

In sum, some of the same technical characteristics that make behavior rating scales an appealing method of measurement may also have potential to negatively affect the reliability and validity of the ratings that are ultimately obtained with these measures. As with any type of measurement and evaluation system, users of behavior rating scales are advised to evaluate a potential instrument based on the important technical characteristics it includes or lacks, and to make decisions that will lead to increased reliability and validity of the overall assessment.

OVERVIEW OF SELECTED BEHAVIOR RATING SCALES FOR USE IN SCHOOL SETTINGS

Because this volume is intended to be a practical guide for child behavior assessment in school settings, a major focus of this chapter is to provide descriptive information and summary comments about some of the more recent, technically sound, and widely used rating scale measures designed for use in school settings. The characteristics and potential uses of some of the best of the latest generation of school-based behavior rating scales, which readers may find useful for specific purposes, are discussed in this section. Readers who desire detailed evaluations or critiques of these or similar measures should refer to more comprehensive sources, such as a recent volume by this author (Merrell,1999) or the most recent edition of the thoroughly exhaustive *Mental Measurements Yearbook* (Impara & Plake, 1998). It is sufficient to state that the instruments discussed herein have all been deemed, in my opinion, to meet or exceed minimum standards for technical adequacy and usefulness.

The behavior rating scales discussed in this section are divided into two major groups: general-purpose problem behavior rating scales and specific-purpose behavior rating scales. The general-purpose problem behavior rating scales include four of the most widely used instruments designed for global screening of child behavior problems in school settings. The specific-purpose behavior rating scales are divided into two categories: rating scales designed for screening and assessment of attention-deficit/hyperactivity disorder (ADHD) and social behavior rating scales. Of course, there are many other technically sound and useful instruments available for these purposes besides those discussed in this chapter, and there are certainly some additional specialized types of behavior rating scales other than social behavior or ADHD measures. The instruments included in this chapter are a sampling of some of the best of an ever increasing array of widely available behavior rating scales.

General-Purpose Problem Behavior Rating Scales

For our purposes, a general purpose problem behavior rating scale is one that is designed for screening and assessment of a broad rather than narrow range of child behavior problems. Four of the most widely available and used general purpose problem behavior scales designed for assessment in school settings are reviewed in this section: The Behavior Assessment System for Children, Devereux Behavior Rating Scale—School Form, Revised Behavior Problem Checklist, and Teacher Report Form. Of course, there are a large number of general purpose problem behavior rating scales that have acceptable technical properties and should prove useful for school-based behavior assessment, but space limitations of this chapter preclude a review of all but a few. The four instruments reviewed in this section, as well as a sampling of other school-based instruments that are available, are summarized in Table 8.1.

Behavior Assessment System for Children

The Behavior Assessment System for Children (BASC; Reynolds & Kamphaus, 1992) includes a variety of rating scales, self-report forms, and a direct observation and interview form. This overview focuses only on the teacher rating scales of the BASC. These measures, including a preschool-age version (ages 4 to 5), a child version (ages 6 to 11), and an adolescent version (ages 12 to 18), are separately normed and somewhat unique from each other, but still share many similarities. The BASC teacher rating scales are comprehensive, designed to assess a variety of problem behaviors, school difficulties, and adaptive skills, and include between 126 and 148 items. The items are rated using an N = "never," S = "sometimes," O = "often," and A = "al-

TABLE 8.1. A Sampling of General-Purpose Child Behavior Rating Scales for Use in School Settings

Instrument	Publisher	Purpose	Norm sample	Items and subscales
Behavior Assessment System for Children— TRS-C	American Guidance Service 4201 Woodland Rd. Circle Pines, MN 55014-1796 800-328-2560	Comprehensive assessment of child and adolescent behavioral, emotional, and adaptive problems and competencies; parent and self-report versions are also available.	Teacher ratings of more than 2,000 students ages 6–18	126 to 148 items, 20 scales and subscales
Behavior Evaluation Scale, 2nd edition	Hawthorne Educational Services 800 Gray Oak Dr. Columbia, MO 65201 800-542-1673	Evaluation of students with behavior problems for eligibility, placement, and programming; based on IDEA definition of behavior disorders/ emotional disturbance; a home version is also available.	Parent and teacher ratings of 2,272 students ages 5–18	76 items, 5 subscales
Behavior Rating Profile, 2nd edition, Teacher Rating Scale	PRO-ED 8700 Shoal Creek Blvd. Austin, TX 78757–6869 800-897-3202	Evaluation of problem behaviors, adaptive skills, and interpersonal relationships; parent, student, and peer report forms are also available.	Teacher ratings of 1,452 students ages 6–18	30 items, no subscales
Devereux Behavior Rating Scale—school form	The Psychological Corporation	Evaluation of behavioral characteristics that may indicate	Teacher ratings of more than 3,000	40 items, 4 subscales

Name	Contact	Description	Sample	Items/Subscales
	555 Academic Court San Antonio, TX 78204–2498 800-211-8378	...severe emotional disturbances in children and adolescents.	students ages 5–18	
Preschool and Kindergarten behavior scales	PRO-ED 8700 Shoal Creek Blvd. Austin, TX 78757–6869 800-897-3202	Evaluation of social skills and emotional–behavioral problems of young children (ages 3–6), for child find screening, assessment, and determining program/service eligibility.	2,855 parent and teacher ratings of children ages 3–6	34 social skills items with 3 subscales; 42 problem behavior items with 5 subscales
Revised Behavior Problem Checklist	Psychological Assessment Resources P.O. Box 998 Odessa, FL 33556 800-331-8378	Evaluation of behavioral and emotional problems in children and adolescents; may be used by teachers or parents.	Teacher ratings of 869 students ages 5–18	89 items, 6 subscales
Teacher Report Form	University Associates in Psychiatry 1 S. Prospect St. Burlington, VT 05401-3456 802-656-8313	Evaluation of behavioral and emotional problems in children and adolescents; a parent-report version (Child Behavior Checklist) is also available.	Teacher ratings of 1,391 students ages 4–18	120 problem behavior items with 8 subscales

most always" format. The BASC rating form is easy to use. After the rating is completed, the examiner tears off the top perforated edge and separates the forms, which reveals an item scoring page and a summary page with Clinical and Adaptive Profiles. Norm tables in the test manual are consulted for appropriate raw score conversions by rating form, and by age and gender of the child. Raw scores on BASC rating scales are converted to T scores and five possible classification levels (e.g., ranging from "very low" to "clinically significant"). The BASC rating scales also include a validity scale designed to detect excessively negative responses made by a teacher.

The complex empirically derived structure of the BASC rating scale consists of composite and scale scores. The Externalizing Problems composite includes Aggression, Hyperactivity, and Conduct Problems scales. The Internalizing Problems composite includes Anxiety, Depression, and Somatization scales. The School Problems composite includes Attention Problems and Learning Problems scales. There are two other problem scales, namely, Atypicality and Withdrawal, that do not belong in either the Externalizing or the Internalizing composite. The Adaptive Skills composite includes the scales of Adaptability (for the child version only), Leadership, Social Skills, and Study Skills. The Behavioral Symptoms Index, sort of a composite problem behavior total score, includes Aggression, Hyperactivity, Anxiety, Depression, Attention Problems, and Atypicality scale scores.

The child and adolescent versions of the BASC were developed with the use of well-stratified samples from a large number of testing sites in the United States and Canada. The normative group for the BASC teacher rating scales includes 1,259 respondents for the child form, and 809 respondents for the adolescent form. Internal consistency reliability estimates for the teacher rating versions of the BASC are high, with most scale values in the .80 to .90 range. Short-term test–retest coefficients (ranging from 2 to 8 weeks) for the various forms have median values spanning the .70s to .80s range. Long-term stability (7 months) of the child version of the teacher rating scale (TRS-C) was investigated, with coefficients ranging from .27 (Atypicality) to .90 (Study Skills). Interrater reliability studies across pairs of teachers conducted with the TRS-C yielded coefficients ranging from .44 (Depression) to .93 (Learning Problems). Numerous types of validity evidence are also presented in the BASC technical manual. Studies showing correlations between these teacher rating scales and several other teacher rating scales provide evidence of convergent and discriminant construct validity. BASC profiles of various clinical groups (children with conduct disorder, behavior disorder, depression, emotional disturbance, ADHD, learning disability, mental retardation, autism), when compared with the normative mean scores, provide strong evidence of the construct validity of the teacher rating scales through demonstrating sensitivity and discriminating power to theory-based group differences.

Overall, the BASC, including the teacher rating scales discussed herein, is impressive. These general-purpose problem behavior rating scales were developed using state-of-the-art standards and methods, have an impressive empirical research base, and are easy to use. One of the few drawbacks of the BASC teacher rating scales may be that their extensive length may make them difficult to use for routine screening work, and certainly for frequent progress monitoring. However, as a thorough and comprehensive system of behavior rating scales, the BASC is representative of the best of what is currently available.

Devereux Behavior Rating Scale—School Form

The Devereux Behavior Rating Scale—School Form (Naglieri, LeBuffe, & Pfeiffer, 1993) is designed for use by school personnel in assessing emotional–behavioral disturbance in children and adolescents. A separately normed parent version of the scale is also available. The school form includes two versions, one designed for use with children ages 5 through 12 years, and the other for youth ages 13 through 18 years. These are relatively brief scales, with each form containing 40 items. The items are rated with the use of a 5-point scale (ranging from "never" to "very frequently") indicating how often the child engages in specific behaviors. For each form there are four subscales, which address the individual areas identified in the federal definition of Emotional Disturbance in the Individuals with Disabilities Education Act, including Interpersonal Problems, Inappropriate Behaviors/Feelings, Depression, and Physical Symptoms/Fears. A total score, which is the sum of all items on the form, is also included. The subscale raw scores are converted to standard scores based on a mean of 10 and a standard deviation (SD) of 3, whereas the converted total score is based on a mean of 100 and an SD of 15. Specific problem behaviors can also be identified from the rating sheet, which signifies scores for individual items that are equal to or exceed 1 SD above the mean.

The Devereux Behavior Rating Scale was standardized on a national sample of 2,042 children and 1,111 adolescents who attended regular education classes. The national standardization sample was representative of the larger U.S. population in terms of gender, community size, race, and ethnicity as indexed by 1990 and 1991 U.S. Census data. Separate norms are provided for each age group and are further subdivided by gender and rater. These scales have been shown to have high total scale internal consistency, with coefficients ranging from .92 to .97, and subscale score coefficients ranging from .70 to .94. One-week retest correlation coefficients for the total score ranged between .69 (adolescent) and .85 (children) in a regular education setting sample. Clinical sample correlation coefficients ranged between .75 for a 24-hour retest interval and .52 for a 4-week retest interval. Two in-

terrater reliability studies presented in the test manual indicate a total scale reliability of .40 and .53, and subscale coefficients ranging from .36 to .60. Criterion-related validity was assessed by determining the extent to which ratings discriminated between normal clinically diagnosed groups and is substantiated by six studies presented in the manual.

In sum, the Devereux Scale—School Form is a useful tool for assessing the presence of moderate to severe emotional disturbance in children and adolescents. It also appears to be a useful tool for identifying specific problem areas and for evaluating the appropriateness of special education placement. Furthermore, because it is relatively brief, the Devereux Behavior Rating Scale—School Form appears to be a potentially useful tool for the planning and progress monitoring of these individual students following specialized placement or during interventions.

Revised Behavior Problem Checklist

The Revised Behavior Problem Checklist (RBPC; Quay & Peterson, 1987, 1996), is a well-researched and widely used problem behavior rating scale. The 1987/1996 version of the RBPC is a revision of Quay's original Behavior Problem Checklist, developed in the 1960s, one of the pioneering efforts in the modern advancement of child behavior rating scales. It includes 89 problem behavior items that are rated using a 3-point scale (0 = "not a problem" to 2 = "severe problem"). The scale may be completed by anyone who is familiar with the child's behavior and is appropriate for use by either parents or teachers (the setting components of the behavior descriptors are generic). It is designed to be used with children and adolescents ages 5 through 16. Completion of the RBPC typically takes about 10 minutes. The scale includes six empirically derived factor or subscale scores (Conduct Disorder, Socialized Aggression, Attention Problems–Immaturity, Anxiety–Withdrawal, Psychotic Behavior, and Motor Excess), which are converted to T scores using tables in the manual for differing types of normative groups based on grade-level ranges and gender. Supplemental norms for a variety of comparison groups (i.e., youth in specific settings or with specific types of identified competencies or problems) are also provided in the RBPC. The general raw score to T score conversion tables are based on teacher ratings of a sample of 869 cases of nonreferred public school children in South Carolina, New Jersey, and Iowa.

Technical data presented in the RBPC manual, and in more than 80 published studies to date, indicate that the instrument has adequate to excellent psychometric properties. Several types of reliability data on the RBPC have been demonstrated. Internal consistency coefficients range from .70 to .95 for the six scales across various subsamples. Interrater reliability coefficients from a small number of teachers range from .52 to .85 for the six

scales, whereas agreement between mothers and fathers on this instrument has been shown to range from .55 to .93. Test–retest reliability of the RBPC, using teacher ratings at 2-month intervals, has been shown to range from .49 to .83. The RBPC has been demonstrated to differentiate effectively between clinical or special education groups and typical youth, thus providing evidence of construct validity. Strong convergent validity has been shown to exist between the RBPC and other assessment instruments. In addition, RBPC ratings have been shown to have strong predictive validity for later conduct and substance abuse problems, and to have strong convergence with peer sociometric nominations and ratings.

Although it is a general-purpose problem behavior rating scale, the RBPC appears to be particularly relevant in assessing conduct disorders and general antisocial behavior. In fact, numerous studies with incarcerated, delinquent, antisocial, and conduct disordered youth have provided strong evidence of validity for this use of the RBPC. Although the standardization samples for the RBPC are not as extensive or geographically stratified as those for several rating scales that have been developed more recently, its strong psychometric properties and extensive research base provide a foundation for confidence in its continued use.

Teacher Report Form

Part of Achenbach's comprehensive cross-informant rating system (which includes teacher, parent, and self-report forms), the Teacher Report Form (TRF; Achenbach, 1991a) is a sophisticated and widely researched global problem behavior rating scale designed for use by teachers. Similar in structure to the Child Behavior Checklist (Achenbach, 1991b), its parent-report counterpart, the TRF includes 120 problem behavior items that are rated on a 0 = "not true" to 2 = "very true or often true" format. This scale is designed for use with students ages 5 to 18. In addition to problem behavior items, the TRF also includes several items designed to measure adaptive school-related skills. The TRF national standardization sample is based on a well-stratified sample of 1,391 cases, with supplemental normative groups also included for students from specific situations, such as special education participation. The TRF can be scored with the use of several means, including hand-scoring profiles and templates, as well as a computer-assisted scoring program and machine-readable forms for mail-in scanning and scoring. Raw scores are converted to T scores and percentile ranks. The *broad-band* scores include a total problems score, an internalizing problems score, and an externalizing problems score. Eight empirically derived *narrow-band* (subscale) scores are also produced: Aggressive Behavior, Anxious/Depressed, Attention Problems, Delinquent Behavior, Social Problems, Somatic Complaints, Thought Problems, and Withdrawn.

Extensive evidence of reliability and validity for the TRF is presented in the technical manual and in more than 60 published studies to date. The TRF scales have been shown to have high internal consistency reliability (.80s to .90s) and strong stability at various retest intervals, including median reliability coefficients of .90 at 7 days, .84 at 15 days, .74 at 2 months, and .68 at 4 months. Interrater or cross-informant reliability of the TRF between teacher and classroom aides has been reported to range from .42 to .72, whereas cross-informant reliability of the TRF and other child behavior checklist instruments has shown average coefficients of approximately .30. Extensive evidence supports the validity of the TRF as a measure of child psychopathology. Several studies have demonstrated its sensitivity to group differences (e.g., students with behavioral–emotional disorders in comparison with regular education students), as well as significant correlations with other behavior rating scales. The subscale structure of the TRF and its companion instruments has been found to replicate quite well across various subsamples and specific standardization groups.

In sum, the TRF is a sophisticated teacher rating scale designed to screen for psychopathology in children and youth. It is particularly useful with students who may exhibit serious behavioral and emotional problems, which is the specific focus of its items. On the other hand, the highly clinical nature of many of the TRF items (for example, descriptions of psychotic-like behaviors, sexual self-stimulation and deviancy, and abnormal behavior involving bowel and bladder functions) may make it less pertinent for screening routine social behaviors. Overall, however, the TRF has numerous advantages as well as excellent empirical support.

Specific-Purpose Behavior Rating Scales: ADHD

In recent years, attention-deficit/hyperactivity disorder (ADHD) has become a widely recognized and discussed psychological disorder among both children and adults, but particularly among children. Although the disability classification categories of the Individuals with Disabilities Act of 1997 (IDEA) do not consider ADHD as a separate disability category for special education services, it is clear that many students with learning disabilities also have ADHD or many ADHD characteristics, and it is also true that many students who receive special education services under the federal law because of emotional or behavioral disorders (i.e., emotionally disturbed) have ADHD either as a component of other conduct or affect problems, or as their primary presenting problem. Other than the original Conners rating scales, few behavior rating scales were initially designed primarily for assessment of ADHD. However, in recent years, this situation has changed substantially. Because of the frequent misdiagnosis and classification of ADHD, as well as the increased emphasis on this disorder in general, several behavior rating scales designed specifically for assessment of ADHD have been devel-

oped since the late 1980s. Four of these measures are discussed in this section: the ADHD Rating Scale—IV, the ADHD Symptoms Rating Scale, the Attention Deficit Disorders Evaluation Scale, and the Conners Rating Scales—Revised. These four instruments, as well as a sampling of additional ADHD rating scales, are summarized in Table 8.2.

ADHD Rating Scale—IV

The brief (18-item) ADHD Rating Scale—IV (ADHD-IV; DuPaul, Power, Anastopoulos, & Reid, 1998) is designed for use by parents and teachers for diagnosing ADHD symptoms and assessing treatment response in children ages 5 to 18. The 18 items are linked specifically to the 18 symptom descriptors of the *Diagnostic and Statistical Manual of Mental Disorders,* fourth edition (DSM-IV; American Psychiatric Association, 1994), and are thus based on the classification system's organization of ADHD symptoms into the Inattention and Hyperactivity–Impulsivity domains (9 items each). This two-domain structure of the ADHD-IV is also empirically validated on the basis of factor analytic research. To prevent rater bias in responding to the two types of symptoms, individual items across the two domains are alternated in the list of 18 items. The items are rated using a 4-point scale ("never or rarely" to "very often"). The two domain scores and a total score are converted to percentile ranks based on separate gender and age (5 to 7, 8 to 10, 11 to 13, 14 to 18) groupings. These score conversion tables are based on national norms, with approximately 2,000 well-stratified cases for both the parent and teacher norms represented in the national standardization sample.

Reliability and validity evidence is presented in the ADHD-IV manual and in separate published studies (e.g., DuPaul, 1991; DuPaul et al., 1997; DuPaul, Anastopoulos, et al., 1998). This scale has been shown to have strong internal consistency reliability (.86 to .96), and strong test–retest reliability (.78 to .90) at 4-week intervals. Interrater agreement between parents and teachers has been shown to range from .40 to .45, which is the expected range for cross-informant reliability across settings. Evidence of convergent and discriminant construct validity for the ADHD-IV includes correlational comparisons with other behavior rating scales, and comparisons with direct observations of student behavior in classroom settings. In addition, the scale has been shown to discriminate effectively between children with and without ADHD.

The ADHD-IV offers many advantages, is easy to use, and is psychometrically sound. The brief 18-item format might be considered a disadvantage (in that it does not provide as much evaluation depth as scales with larger item pools, but it is clearly advantageous in other ways. The brief format of this scale makes it ideal for tracking treatment progress and for conducting initial screening when a more in-depth assessment is not possible at the time.

TABLE 8.2. A Sampling of Specific-Purpose Child Behavior Rating Scales: School-Based Measures for ADHD

Instrument	Publisher	Purpose	Norm sample	Items and subscales
ADD-H Comprehensive Teacher's Rating Scale, 2nd Edition	Metritech Inc. 4106 Fieldstone Rd. Champaign, IL 61821 217-398-4868	Evaluation of ADHD symptoms in children and early adolescents.	Teacher ratings of more than 4,000 students in grades K-8	24 items, 4 factors
ADHD Rating Scale—IV	Guilford Publications 72 Spring St. New York, NY 10012 800-365-7006	Diagnosis of ADHD and measuring treatment response in children and adolescents; may be completed by parents or teachers.	Parent and teacher ratings of more than 2,000 children and youth ages 5–18.	18 items, 2 subscales
ADHD Symptoms Rating Scale	Wide Range Inc. 15 Ashley Place, Suite 1A Wilmington, DE 1904 800-221-WRAT	Evaluation of ADHD symptoms in children and adolescents; parent report version is also available.	Teacher ratings of more than 1,000 students ages 5–18	56 items, 2 subscales
Attention Deficit Disorders Evaluation Scales—School Version, 2nd Edition	Hawthorne Educational Services 800 Gray Oak Dr. Columbia, MO 65201 800-542-1673	Evaluation and diagnosis of ADHD in children and youth; home version is also available.	Teacher ratings of more than 5,000 students, ages 4–18	56 items, 2 subscales
Attention Deficit/ Hyperactivity Disorder Test	PRO-ED 8700 Shoal Creek Blvd. Austin, TX 78757-6869 800-897-3202	Evaluation of ADHD in children, adolescents, and young adults.	Parent and teacher ratings of more than 1,200 individuals ages 3–23	36 items, 3 subscales
Conners Rating Scales— Revised, Teacher Versions	Multi-Health Systems 908 Niagra Falls Blvd. North Tonowanda, NY 14120-2060 800-456-3003	Assessment of ADHD symptoms and related problem behaviors; parent and self-report forms are also available.	Teacher ratings of approximately 2,000 children and adolescents ages 3–17	28–item version with 4 subscales; 59-item version with 8 subscales

ADHD Symptoms Rating Scale

The ADHD Symptoms Rating Scale (ADHD-SRS; Holland, Gimpel, & Merrell, in press), is a 56-item behavior rating scale designed to assist in evaluating ADHD characteristics of school-age children (grades K–12). This scale may be completed by either teachers or parents; separate norms are available for each group. The 56 items were developed specifically based on the assessment criteria for ADHD from the DSM-IV. In the development of the ADHD-SRS, several possible items for each of the 18 DSM-IV symptom descriptors for ADHD were generated, and after field testing and evaluation of possible items, an average of about three items for each of these descriptors was retained. The items are rated using a 4-point scale based on the estimated frequency of observed behavior (e.g., "behavior does not occur" to "behavior occurs one to several times an hour"). The empirically derived subscale structure of the ADHD-SRS for both the teacher and parent norms is very consistent with the two domains of ADHD symptoms from DSM-IV, and thus are labeled Inattention and Hyperactive-Impulsive. The standardization sample for this instrument is derived from a nationwide sample and includes more than 1,000 cases for both the parent and teacher norms.

Research evidence (Holland, Gimpel, & Merrell, 1998) indicates that the ADHD-SRS has adequate to excellent technical and psychometric properties. Internal consistency reliability of the total score has been shown to be in the .98 to .99 range. Test–retest reliability of teacher ratings at a 2-week interval was .95 to .97. Cross-informant correspondence across settings and between parents and teachers was shown to be in the expected range of about .30. To date, the validity of the ADHD-SRS has been demonstrated through the finding of strong score correlations with other ADHD measures (including the Conners scales, the ADHD-IV, and the Attention Deficit Disorders Evaluation Scale [ADDES]) and through the finding of significant differences between the scores of typical children and children who have been diagnosed as having ADHD.

The ADHD-SRS is practical and easy to use and balances its relatively brief length with the advantage of providing an average of about three characteristic rating items for each of the DSM-IV symptom descriptors. The division of the two subscales into the Inattentive and Hyperactive–Impulsive domains, consistent with the DSM-IV, and the addition of a total score make this instrument potentially useful for initial assessment and classification purposes, as well as for tracking intervention progress.

Attention Deficit Disorders Evaluation Scale

The Attention Deficit Disorders Evaluation Scale (ADDES; McCarney, 1995) is a 56-item rating scale designed for use by teachers in assessing ADHD characteristics in school-age children. A 50-item version of this in-

strument for use by parents is also available. Like the ADHD-SRS and the ADHD-IV, this instrument was designed to reflect the symptom content found in the DSM-IV diagnostic criteria for ADHD, and it also includes subscales reflecting inattentiveness and hyperactivity–impulsivity. The items are rated using a 5-point rating scale that is anchored to frequency of observed behaviors (0 = "does not engage in the behavior" to 4 = "one to several times per hour") rather than a traditional Likert scale format. The teacher rating version of this scale was standardized using a large national normative sample of ratings of 5,795 students provided by 2,414 teachers.

Based on evidence presented in the technical manual, the stability of ADDES scores internally, across raters and across time, appears to be solid. Internal consistency coefficients are reported in the .90s range, the average correlation among pairs of teacher raters is reported at .85, and test–retest reliability ranges from .88 to .97. Convergent construct validity evidence for this scale is demonstrated through strong score correlations with other behavior rating scales, including the Conners Rating Scales.

In sum, the ADDES offers several advantages and appears to be technically adequate. It may prove to be a useful assessment tool for screening ADHD symptoms, making classification and treatment decisions, and tracking intervention progress.

Conners Rating Scales—Revised

The Conners Rating Scales are among the best known and most widely used of all child behavior rating scales. The most recent revision of these scales, the Conners Rating Scales—Revised (CRS-R; Conners, 1997), designed for use with children ages 3 to 17, is discussed in this section. Unlike the other ADHD rating scales discussed herein, the Conners scales come in a variety of forms of varying length and content (with separate forms and norms for parents and teachers), and in some cases (the longer versions), the item content is not focused exclusively on ADHD symptoms. In some respects, the longer versions of the Conners scales might be best considered as general-purpose problem behavior rating scales. However, according to its author, the primary focus of this rating scale system has been, and continues to be, assessment of children who exhibit ADHD symptoms (Conners, 1997, p. 5). Therefore, these scales are included in the discussion of specific-purpose behavior rating scales.

The longest form of the teacher version CRS-R includes 59 items, and a shorter form includes 28 items. In addition, a 27-item teacher rating scale based on the 18 core DSM-IV characteristics for ADHD and the inattentive/hyperactive–impulsive domain breakdown is available. This latter version is referred to as the Conners ADHD/DSM-IV Scales. However, the items representing the 18 core DSM-IV symptoms are similar across the

three teacher rating scale versions. Therefore, the longer version provides a more comprehensive screen for behavior problems, whereas the shorter versions provide a more narrowly focused screen for ADHD problems. All versions of the CRS-R utilize a common 4-point rating scale (ranging from 0 = "not at all" to 3 = "pretty much"). The standardization sample for the CRS-R is large (more than 2,000 cases) and well stratified across both the United States and Canada.

The technical manual for the CRS-R is comprehensive and includes extensive evidence regarding the development, use, and psychometric properties of the scales. Internal consistency of the CRS-R has been shown to range from the .70s to .90s, depending on the specific version and subscale involved. Test–retest reliability at 6- to 8-week intervals is reported to range from .47 to .88. The subscale/factorial structures of the scales are empirically derived and robust. The technical manual includes a large array of validity evidence, such as strong correlations with other rating scales, and significant discriminating power between various groups of children who would be theoretically expected to have different levels of ratings, based on their clinical status.

The CRS-R offers the advantage of several forms of varying length and content, each with a common normative sample and core of 18 ADHD symptom indicators. This system also offers the advantage of a thoroughly detailed technical manual with extensive empirical support. Although the focus of this rating system is clearly ADHD symptoms, the longer versions of the scales may be useful in evaluating comorbid behavioral concerns, such as conduct problems, antisocial behavior, passivity, and social withdrawal.

Specific-Purpose Behavior Rating Scales: Social Skills/Social Behavior

Another behavioral domain in which specific-purpose behavior rating scales have emerged is the area of social skills or social behavior. In recent years the importance of adequate social–behavioral development has been the focus of increased attention. This greater emphasis is perhaps partly the result of research findings showing that social behavior problems in early childhood may be linked to long-term negative outcomes, and perhaps partly due to the tremendous cost to society of the significant problems of antisocial behavior among youth (Merrell & Gimpel, 1998). The first nationally standardized and psychometrically sound social behavior rating scales began to emerge in the 1980s, and there are currently several good choices available in this area. Three of these instruments are discussed here, including the School Social Behavior Scales, the Social Skills Rating System, and the Walker–McConnell Scales of Social Competence and School Adjustment. These three instruments are also summarized in Table 8.3.

TABLE 8.3. A Sampling of Specific-Purpose Child Behavior Rating Scales: School-Based Measures for Social Skills

Instrument	Publisher	Purpose	Norm sample	Items and subscales
School Social Behavior Scales	PRO-ED 8700 Shoal Creek Blvd. Austin, TX 78757-6869 800-897-3202	Assessment of social competence and antisocial behavior; a parent report form is under development.	1,858 students ages 5–18	32 social competence items with 3 subscales; 33 antisocial behavior items with 3 subscales.
Social Skills Rating System	American Guidance Service 4201 Woodland Rd. Circle Pines, MN 55014-1796 800-328-2560	Assessment of social skills and academic competence, with a brief problem behavior screen; parent and self-report forms are also available.	Varies, based on specific form; more than 4,000 students for all versions combined	Number of items varies slightly, depending on form and age range; elementary teacher rating form includes 57 items with 6 subscales.
Walker–McConnell Scales of Social Competence and School Adjustment	Singular Publishing Group 4101 West "A" St., Suite 325 San Diego, CA 92101-7904 800-521-8545	Assessment of teacher- and peer-preferred social competencies.	Approximately 2,000 students ages 5–18	43-item elementary-age version includes 3 subscales; 53-item adolescent version includes 4 subscales.

School Social Behavior Scales

Designed specifically for use in educational settings, the School Social Behavior Scales (SSBS; Merrell, 1993) is a teacher rating scale aimed at evaluating social behaviors of K–12 students. The SSBS includes 65 items on two separate conormed scales: Scale A: Social Competence (32 items) and Scale B: Antisocial Behavior (33 items). All items are rated using a 5-point scale (1 = never to 5 = frequently). The empirically derived structure for each scale includes three subscales. Scale A includes the Interpersonal Skills, Self-Management Skills, and Academic Skills subscales, as well as a total score. Scale B includes the Hostile–Irritable, Antisocial–Aggressive, and Demanding–Disruptive subscales, as well as a total score. All subscale and total scores are converted to Social Functioning Levels, which serve as general indicators of the normative range of skill deficits or problem excesses. In addition, the total scores for each scale are converted to standard scores and percentile ranks. Scoring of the SSBS items and scales is accomplished using a very simple scoring key that is printed on the rating form. Both scales of the SSBS were standardized with a sample of 1,855 K–12 students from several U.S. states.

Internal consistency reliability of the SSBS total scores and subscales has been shown to range from .91 to .98. Test–retest reliability at 3-week intervals is reported at .76 to .83 for the Social Competence scores and at .60 to .73 for the Antisocial Behavior scores. Interrater reliability between resource room teachers and paraprofessional aides ranges from .72 to .83 for the Social Competence scores and from .53 to .71 for the Antisocial Behavior scores. Validity of the SSBS has been supported through research documented in the manual, and through several published studies. Convergent and discriminant construct validity of the SSBS has been demonstrated through correlation studies with several other behavior rating scales. Extensive research documenting the discriminating power and sensitivity to group differences with various educational groups has been published, including special education students, gifted students, regular education students, and at-risk students without identified disabilities. Moreover, the subscale structure of the SSBS has been supported through additional confirmatory factor analyses, which strengthen the theoretical foundation for the scale design.

The SSBS has the advantage of being focused exclusively on *social behavior* and providing a comprehensive screen of both social competence and antisocial behavior of students in school settings. It is also very easy to administer and score, relatively brief, and addresses routine social competencies and problems of youth, rather than low-rate clinical behaviors. Because the SSBS is focused exclusively on social behavior, it should be supplemented with problem-specific assessment tools if problems such as ADHD or depression are a major concern. A version of the SSBS for use by parents and other community-based informants is currently under development (Merrell &

Caldarella, 1999; Robbins & Merrell, in press), and should be available within a year of publication of this book.

Social Skills Rating System

The Social Skills Rating System (SSRS; Gresham & Elliott, 1990) is a multicomponent social skills rating system aimed at behaviors that affect parent–child relations, teacher–student relations, and peer acceptance. The entire system includes separate rating scales for teachers and parents, as well as a self-report form for students. The teacher rating form of the SSRS, the specific focus of this overview, includes separate forms for ages 3 to 5, grades K to 6, and grades 7 to 12. The three forms are similar in organization, but some of the content differs according to developmental considerations of the particular age range. The elementary-level version includes 57 items divided into three scales: Social Skills (30 items), Problem Behaviors (18 items), and Academic Competence (9 items). For Social Skills and Problem Behaviors items, teachers respond to descriptions using a 3-point response format based on how often a given behavior occurs (0 = never, 1 = sometimes, and 2 = very often). For the Social Skills items, teachers are also asked to rate (on a 3-point scale) how important a skill is to success in the classroom. The importance rating is not used to calculate ratings for each scale but is used for planning interventions. On the Academic Competence scale, teachers rate students as compared with other students on a 5-point scale. All raw scores are converted to standard scores ($M = 100$, $SD = 15$). The combined SSRS forms were standardized using a nationwide sample of more than 4,000 cases. The specific standardization groups for each of the three teacher rating forms are considered to be adequate to good.

For the teacher forms of the SSRS, reliability was measured using internal consistency, (i.e., alpha coefficients ranged from .74 to .95), interrater, and test–retest (i.e., .75 to .93 correlations across the three scales) procedures. Criterion-related and construct validity of these scales has been demonstrated through the finding of significant correlations between the SSRS and other rating scales. The empirically derived subscales for Social Competence (Cooperation, Assertion, and Self-Control) and Problem Behavior (Internalizing Problems, Externalizing Problems, Hyperactivity) are based on sound analytic procedures. The external research base for the SSRS is growing, and additional validity evidence continues to accrue.

The primary advantage of the SSRS is that it is an integrated, multicomponent system of instruments for use by teachers, parents, and students, one of the few social skills rating scales that includes a comprehensive parent report version. The manual is very well written, and the rating instruments are easy to understand and use. Because the Problem Behavior scale items are few in number, this scale should be considered as a brief screen, and if

possible problems are detected, a more thorough assessment using comprehensive problem behavior assessment tools is advised.

Walker–McConnell Scales of Social Competence and School Adjustment

Like the SSBS, the Walker–McConnell Scales of Social Competence and School Adjustment (SSCSA; Walker & McConnell, 1995a, 1995b) are social behavior rating scales designed specifically for teachers and other school-based professionals. However, the SSCSA focuses exclusively on the domain of social competence and does not include an antisocial behavior screen. Two versions of the scale are available—an elementary version for use with students in grades K to 6 and an adolescent version for use with students in grades 7 to 12. The elementary version contains 43 positively worded items that reflect adaptive social–behavioral competencies within the school environment and includes three empirically derived subscales (Teacher-Preferred Social Behavior, Peer-Preferred Social Behavior, and School Adjustment Behavior). The adolescent version, which includes the same three subscales, includes the 43 items included in the elementary version (although 9 are reworded to reflect adolescent-specific concerns), plus 10 additional items that constitute a fourth subscale and are designed to measure self-related social adjustment and empathy. The items are rated using a 5-point scale ranging from 1 ("never occurs") to 5 ("frequently occurs"). The scale yields standard scores on three subscales ($M = 10$, $SD = 3$), as well as a total score ($M = 100$, $SD = 15$), which is a composite of the three subscales. The scales were standardized with ratings of approximately 2,000 students representing all four U.S. geographical regions.

Studies undertaken during the development of the SSCSA, which are cited in the technical manuals, indicate adequate to excellent psychometric properties. Reliability of the scales was established using test–retest (e.g., .88 to .92 correlations over a 3-week period with 323 subjects), internal consistency (e.g., alpha coefficients ranging from .95 to .97), and interrater (e.g., a .53 correlation between teachers' and aides' ratings on the total score in a day treatment facility) procedures. Validity of the scales was evaluated using a variety of procedures. Sensitivity of the scales to theory-based group differences was indicated in studies that found the scales to differentiate between groups of students who would be expected to differ behaviorally (behavior disordered and normal, antisocial and normal, behaviorally at risk and normal, and those with and without learning problems). Criterion-related validity was demonstrated by the finding of significant correlations between the scales and various criterion variables, such as other rating scales, sociometric ratings, academic achievement measures, and a systematic behavioral screening procedure. Construct validity of the scales has been demonstrated by

strong correlations between evaluative comments on students from their peers and teacher ratings on the scales, and by finding low social skills ratings to be strongly associated with the emergence of antisocial behavior in a longitudinal study of at-risk boys. The factor structure of the two scales has been shown to be robust.

Both versions of the SSCSA are brief, easy to use, and contain items that are highly relevant for assessing social skills in educational settings. The research base underlying the scales is exemplary. Because neither version of the SSCSA was designed to measure problem behaviors, these instruments should be supplemented with an appropriate problem behavior assessment if warranted by the referral issues.

RECOMMENDATIONS FOR BEST PRACTICE

Effective use of behavior rating scales requires more than an understanding of their characteristics and the availability of good tools. It is true that there have been numerous advances and improvements in rating scale technology in recent years, and these advances have led to a general improvement in the way they are used in school settings. However, there is still a need to identify the specific ways in which these measures can be most effectively used to assess conduct problems and related behavioral concerns in school settings. The following list of "best practice" suggestions has been derived from my own and colleagues' research and clinical experience in using rating scale measures, as well as from the experiences of other writers. It reflects an attempt to develop a conservative framework for effective use of behavior rating scale measures that may be generalized into practical applications across school settings. These suggestions should not be considered absolute. It is quite possible that within another two decades the field will have advanced to the point where more specific suggestions for improved use of behavior rating scales can be identified

1. *Use only rating scales with adequate technical properties.* One of the problems that hindered the widespread acceptance of rating scale measures prior to the 1980s was the poor technical and psychometric properties of many of the instruments in use at that time. Fortunately, there are now numerous technically adequate behavior rating scales available for a wide variety of purposes. The instruments reviewed in detail in this chapter all meet or exceed, in my estimation, minimum standards for technical adequacy. The list of instruments is certainly not exhaustive. However, there are still instruments in use, some of which may be in widespread use, that have not been demonstrated to have such sound technical properties. Of course, it is important to recognize that an instrument that is untested or unproven (i.e., with-

out sufficient technical and research documentation) may actually have acceptable or even excellent technical properties. However, such a presumption of adequacy should *not* be made if the test developer(s) have not made an effort to document the technical properties sufficiently. The final burden of determining whether a particular rating scale has acceptable technical properties, and may thus be used with confidence for specific purposes, falls on the end user of the instrument, who should carefully consult the available evidence (such as the technical manual and published research and reviews) before making a decision. In evaluating the merits of a particular rating scale measure, the minimum standards discussed in the jointly produced *Standards for Educational and Psychological Testing* (1985) may be helpful. However, these standards are general and are not developed to be specific to any particular method of assessment. It is important to consider that rating scale measures comprise a unique assessment methodology and, as such, have different advantages and problem areas than other assessment methods. At a minimum, selection of a rating scale measure should be contingent upon evidence that (1) the construct(s) purported to be measured by the rating scale are indeed measured by it, (2) the standardization sample adequately reflects the population among which the instrument will be used, (3) the instrument is acceptably consistent or reliable, and (4) there is evidence that the instrument is valid for the specific purposes for which it is intended to be used. In considering these minimum criteria, it is important to keep in mind that behavior rating scale measures should, because of their unique nature, be judged from a somewhat different perspective than academic achievement or cognitive ability measures. For example, cognitive ability has been shown to be quite stable over time, and it may be expected that a valid measure of intelligence will yield test–retest reliabilities in the .80 to .90 range over time, even when relatively long time intervals are considered. Because social and emotional behavior is considerably more variable over time than cognitive ability, such strong consistency should not be expected with behavior rating scales. Reliability or consistency of rating scale scores across various raters may be modest because of the situational specificity of child behavior (Achenbach, McConaughy, & Howell, 1987). However, strong internal consistency coefficients should be expected in rating scale measures, as should strong convergent validity coefficients, a theoretically sound subscale structure, and the demonstrated ability to differentiate among clinical and general populations.

2. *Use rating scales routinely for early screening.* Effective screening practices involve the systematic identification, with a high degree of accuracy, of children who may be in the early stages of developing behavioral, social, or emotional problems. Those children identified as "good suspects" are then evaluated more thoroughly to determine whether their problems warrant special program eligibility and/or intervention services. The purpose of screening for social–emotional problems is usually for *secondary prevention,*

which is prevention of the existing problem from becoming worse (Kauffman, 1997). Screening for early intervention is one of the best uses of behavior rating scales, given that they cover a wide variety of important behaviors and take very little time to administer and score. For general screening purposes, it is recommended that children or youth whose rating scale scores are *one or more standard deviations* above instrument normative means, in terms of problem behavior excesses or social competence deficits, be evaluated in more detail. This practice will narrow the screening pool to approximately 16% of the overall population, and the selected group can then be evaluated more comprehensively. This screening criterion will typically result in some false-positive errors or identification of some students who do not require further evaluation or services, but such errors should be easy to detect upon further evaluation and consideration. Moreover, a one-standard-deviation screening criterion will seldom result in false-negative errors, or failure to identify children who are truly at risk. For screening purposes, false-positive error is generally more acceptable than false-negative error (Merrell, 1999).

3. *Use the "aggregation principle."* This principle involves obtaining ratings from a variety of sources and using a variety of measures (Martin et al., 1986; Merrell, 1999). Because of source and setting variance, each set of ratings will present a slightly different picture. In using rating scales for purposes other than routine screening (in which one rating may be sufficient), obtaining rating scale data that is aggregated in this manner is recommended as a way of identifying the particular behavioral excesses or deficits that are most consistent and troublesome across settings and from the perspectives of various informants. In other words, we should expect some differences in how various teachers rate the same student, even if they are using the same assessment tool for their ratings. However, in cases where there are significant behavioral problems or deficits, it is likely that they will be consistent across settings, sources, and measures. In other cases, where a behavioral concern is truly situation-specific, the use of an aggregated assessment design may be of great help in determining which behaviors may be most problematic under specific conditions.

4. *Design interventions to match specific problems.* A best practice in providing interventions for students with challenging behaviors is to specifically match the intervention to the most critical problem excesses or skill deficits (Merrell, 1999; Merrell & Gimpel, 1998; Peacock Hill Working Group, 1991). This matching process is the opposite of a "one size fits all" mentality in designing interventions, whereby any student who is identified as having significant behavioral concerns is recommended to receive a generic behavioral intervention of some kind. Such a global (if not vague) approach to intervention will typically fail to target the most important problems in a sufficiently specific manner, and the result will typically be weak or inconsistent

intervention gains. A simple and potentially effective way to link rating scale data to intervention is to carefully review the completed rating scales and list items or clusters of items that are rated as the most significant concerns. If any of these items are rated consistently problematic across raters and settings, it is particularly important to specify them in designing the intervention. Once a narrowed list of key behaviors has been identified and targeted, specific intervention techniques that precisely match those behaviors can be selected. This particular method is quite consistent with the Keystone Behavior Strategy that has been touted as a promising way to effectively link assessment data to intervention planning (Nelson & Hayes, 1986; Shapiro, 1996).

5. *Use rating scales to assess progress during and following intervention.* Continuous assessment and monitoring of student progress following the initial assessment and during treatment has been shown to be important in the successful implementation of behavioral interventions (Kerr & Nelson, 1989). One might easily evaluate progress toward behavioral intervention goals by obtaining weekly or biweekly ratings, and such continuous measurement may be helpful in modifying the intervention if it proves not to produce the desired effect (Merrell & Gimpel, 1998). In reality, full-length rating scale measures may be too long and time-consuming for frequent and repeated use. In such circumstances, it is easy and reasonable, following the initial assessment, to select from the rating scales a few critical behavioral items that were targeted for intervention and use these few items as a brief informal measure of intervention progress. An additional comprehensive assessment *following* the intervention can also be a useful tool. The primary reasons for conducting a follow-up assessment is to determine how well the intervention effects have been maintained over time (e.g., after 3 months) and how well the behavioral changes have generalized to other settings (e.g., other classrooms). Information gathered from a follow-up assessment may help determine whether additional interventions or "booster sessions" are needed.

CONCLUSIONS

As this chapter has indicated, rating scale measures have proven to be among the most popular assessment technologies in recent years for assessing behavioral, social, and emotional problems and competencies of children and youth. Although the behavior rating scales available prior to about 1980 often were of poor technical quality and were not enthusiastically accepted by researchers, the situation changed drastically during the latter two decades of the 20th century. In general, the technical adequacy of rating scale measures for assessing behavior of children and youth is now substantially improved, and the availability of such measures seems to be increasing dramatically. In

fact, practitioners who need to select a behavior rating scale for use in particular circumstances now often find themselves with an almost bewildering array of potentially good choices of instruments. The several general- and specific-purpose behavior rating scales discussed in this chapter are examples of the most recent and most technically advanced rating scale measures currently available.

Despite the many advances in this arena, it is simply naive to think that the problems inherent in using behavior rating scales are no longer at issue, or that there is no more room for advancement in the field. On the contrary, there are still numerous challenges in using behavior rating scales that should be considered by practitioners and researchers within the context of multimethod, multisource, multisetting assessment designs. Perhaps the most substantial and elusive challenge at present is to learn how behavior rating scales may best be linked to effective and practical delivery of behavioral interventions.

REFERENCES

Achenbach, T. M. (1991a). *Manual for the Teacher's Report Form and 1991 profile*. Burlington: University of Vermont, Department of Psychiatry.

Achenbach, T. M. (1991b). *Manual for the Child Behavior Checklist and 1991 profile*. Burlington: University of Vermont, Department of Psychiatry.

Achenbach, T. M., McConaughy, S. H., & Howell, C. T. (1987). Child/adolescent behavioral and emotional problems: Implications of cross-informant correlations for situational specificity. *Psychological Bulletin, 101*, 213–232.

Alberto, P. A., & Troutman, A. C. (1996). *Applied behavior analysis for teachers* (4th ed.). Columbus, OH: Merrill.

American Psychiatric Association. (1994). *Diagnostic and statistical manual of mental disorders* (4th ed.). Washington, DC: Author.

Conners, C. K.(1997). *Conners rating scales—revised technical manual*. Toronto: Multi-Health Systems.

Doll, B., & Elliott, S. N. (1994). Representativeness of observed preschool social behaviors: How many data are enough? *Journal of Early Intervention, 18*, 227–238.

DuPaul, G. J. (1991). Parent and teacher ratings of AD/HD symptoms: Psychometric properties in a community-based sample. *Journal of Clinical Child Psychology, 20*, 245–253.

DuPaul, G. J., Anastopoulos, A. D., Power, T. J., Reid, R., Ikeda, M., & McGoey, K. (1998). Parent ratings of attention-deficit/hyperactivity disorder symptoms: Factor structure and normative data. *Journal of Psychopathology and Behavioral Assessment, 20*, 83–102.

DuPaul, G. J., Power, T. J., Anastopoulos, A. D., & Reid, R. (1998). *ADHD Rating Scale–IV: Checklists, norms, and clinical interpretation*. New York: Guilford Press.

DuPaul, G. J., Power, T. J., Anastopoulos, A. D., Reid, R., McGoey, K., & Ikeda, M.

(1997). Teacher ratings of attention-deficit/hyperactivity disorder: Factor structure and normative data. *Psychological Assessment, 9,* 436–444.

Elliott, S. N., Busse, R. T., & Gresham, F. M. (1993). Behavior rating scales: Issues of use and development. *School Psychology Review, 22,* 313–321.

Gresham, F. M., & Elliott, S. N. (1990). *The social skills rating system.* Circle Pines, MN: American Guidance.

Gronlund, N. E., & Linn, R. L. (1990). *Measurement and evaluation in teaching* (6th ed.). New York: Macmillan.

Holland, M. L., Gimpel, G. A., & Merrell, K. W. (1998). Innovations in assessing ADHD: Development, psychometric properties, and factor structure of the ADHD Symptoms Rating Scale. *Journal of Psychopathology and Behavioral Assessment, 20,* 307–332.

Holland, M. L., Gimpel, G. A., & Merrell, K. W. (in press). *ADHD Symptoms Rating Scale.* Wilmington, DE: Wide Range.

Impara, J. C., & Plake, B. S. (Eds.) (1998). *The thirteenth mental measurements yearbook.* Lincoln: Buros Institute of Mental Measurements, University of Nebraska.

Kauffman, J. M. (1997). *Characteristics of behavior disorders of children and youth* (6th ed.). Upper Saddle River, NJ: Prentice-Hall.

Kazdin, A. E. (1979). Situational specificity: The two-edged sword of behavioral assessment. *Behavioral Assessment, 1,* 57–75.

Kerr, M. M., & Nelson, C. M. (1989). *Strategies for managing behavior problems in the classroom* (2nd ed.). Columbus, OH: Merrill.

Martin, R. P. (1988). *Assessment of personality and behavior problems: Infancy through adolescence.* New York: Guilford Press.

Martin, R. P., Hooper, S., & Snow, J. (1986). Behavior rating scale approaches to personality assessment in children and adolescents. In H. Knoff (Ed.), *The assessment of child and adolescent personality* (pp. 309–351). New York: Guilford Press.

McCarney, S. B. (1995). *Attention Deficit Disorders Evaluation scale—school version.* Columbia, MO: Hawthorne Educational Services.

McMahon, R. J. (1984). Behavioral checklists and rating scales. In T. H. Ollendick & M. Herson (Eds.), *Child behavioral assessment: Principles and practices* (pp. 80–105). New York: Pergamon Press.

Merrell, K. W. (1993). *School Social Behavior Scales* Austin, TX: PRO-ED.

Merrell, K. W. (1999). *Behavioral, social, and emotional assessment of children and adolescents.* Mahwah, NJ: Erlbaum.

Merrell, K. W. (2000). Informant reports: Theory and research in using child behavior rating scales in school settings. In E. S. Shapiro & T. R. Kratochwill (Eds.), *Behavioral assessment in schools* (2nd ed.): *Theory, research, and clinical foundations* (pp. 233–256). New York: Guilford Press.

Merrell, K. W., & Caldarella, P. (1999). Social-behavioral assessment of at-risk early adolescent students: Psychometric characteristics and validity of a parent report form of the School Social Behavior Scales. *Journal of Psychoeducational Assessment, 17,* 36–49.

Merrell, K. W., & Gimpel, G. A. (1998). *Social skills of children and adolescents: Conceptualization, assessment, treatment.* Mahwah, NJ: Erlbaum.

Naglieri, J. A., LeBuffe, P.A., & Pfeiffer, S. I. (1993). *Devereux Behavior Rating Scale—school form.* San Antonio, TX: Psychological Corporation.

Nelson, R. O., & Hayes, S. C. (Eds.). (1986). *Conceptual foundations of behavioral assessment*. New York: Guilford Press.

Peacock Hill Working Group. (1991). Problems and promises in special education and related services for children and youth with emotional or behavioral disorders. *Behavioral Disorders, 16*, 299–313.

Quay, H. C., & Peterson, D. R. (1987). *Manual for the Revised Behavior Problem Checklist*. Coral Gables, FL: Author.

Quay, H. C., & Peterson, D. R. (1996). *Manual for the Revised Behavior Problem Checklist— PAR version*. Odessa, FL: Psychological Assessment Resources.

Reynolds, C. R., & Kamphaus, R. W. (1992). *Behavior assessment system for children*. Circle Pines, MN: American Guidance Service.

Robbins, R., & Merrell, K. W. (in press). Cross-information comparisons of the Home and Community Social Behavior Scales and the School Social Behavior Scales. *Diagnostique*.

Saal, F. E., Downey, R. G., & Lahey, M. A. (1980). Rating the ratings: Assessing the psychometric quality of rating data. *Psychological Bulletin, 88*, 413–428.

Shapiro, E. S. (1996). *Academic skills problems: Direct assessment and intervention* (2nd ed.). New York: Guilford Press.

Standards for educational and psychological testing (1985). Washington, DC: American Psychological Association.

Walker, H. M., & McConnell, S. R. (1995a). *Walker–McConnell Scale of Social Competence and School Adjustment: Elementary version*. San Diego, CA: Singular Publishing Group.

Walker, H. M., & McConnell, S. R. (1995b). *Walker–McConnell Scale of Social Competence and School Adjustment: Adolescent version*. San Diego, CA: Singular Publishing Group.

Wilson, M. S., & Reschly, D. J. (1996). Assessment in school psychology training and practice. *School Psychology Review, 25*, 9–23.

Worthen, B. R., Borg, W. R, & White, K. R. (1993). *Measurement and evaluation in the schools: A practical guide*. White Plains, NY: Addison-Wesley/Longman.

CHAPTER 9

♦♦♦

Informant Report:
Parent and Teacher Interviews

♦

R. T. BUSSE
BARBARA RYBSKI BEAVER

Interviewing is a hallmark of assessment processes and perhaps the most common method used to obtain information to evaluate individuals. Indeed, whether seeking employment, applying to graduate school, or engaging in psychotherapy, most of us have been or will be the subject of an interview at some time in our lives. At a basic level, interviews involve questions and responses based on a particular focus for evaluation, such as determining suitability for employment or admission to a program of study. In psychological and psychoeducational settings, the focus of an interview varies with the purpose of the assessment. For example, interviews may be conducted to aid in diagnostic formulations or to facilitate problem-solving interventions. Within school-based settings, interviews are conducted to facilitate decisions regarding placement in special education programs and to aid in planning and implementing interventions.

The interviewing of parents and teachers, in addition to the children themselves, has long been a standard component in assessing the behavior problems of children and adolescents. In the 1950s and 1960s, assessments of children primarily relied on interviews with parents and other informants (Groth-Marnat, 1997). These interviews were often unstructured, their content depending on the interest and aim of the individual interviewer and informants. Early research comparing informant interviews with self-reports found that parents and children contributed information on different aspects of the children's behavior. For example, mothers were more likely to report overt behavior problems, particularly those that posed a problem for the

adults in the child's life. In contrast, children were more likely to report covert concerns, such as symptoms of anxiety and depression (Lapouse & Monk, 1964).

The utilization of parent reports continued in the 1970s as the focus of school-based assessment shifted toward a behavioral analysis model. Concurrently, as researchers and clinicians became more interested in obtaining detailed and specific reports of behaviors, there was increased concern about the reliability and validity of unstructured interview formats. Historically, interviews regarding children's problems focused on either loosely structured diagnostic or descriptive information (Edelbrock & Costello, 1990). With the publication of the third edition of the *Diagnostic and Statistical Manual of Mental Disorders* (DSM-III; American Psychiatric Association, 1980), which provided more explicit and operationalized criteria for childhood disorders, came an increased call for standardized diagnostic interviews with children and parents. Not all researchers and clinicians, however, were or are concerned with reaching a specific categorical diagnosis. For these interviewers, describing children's behaviors and understanding the functional relationships of behavior became paramount. Thus, regardless of whether a specific diagnostic classification is needed, the goal of assessment is increasingly conceptualized to include the ability to obtain a thorough functional assessment of problem behaviors. To that end, the major purpose of this chapter is to present a problem-solving focus for school-based interviewing of parents and teachers within a functional assessment approach. We begin with a brief overview of interview methods and the use of interviews within a functional assessment, follow with a discussion of general interviewing processes and guidelines, and conclude with a case illustration of a functional assessment interview.

INTERVIEW METHODS

As noted earlier, interview methods vary widely in style and format, ranging from rather didactic question-and-answer sessions, often influenced by the medical model, to more open-ended psychodynamically influenced styles and highly structured and standardized diagnostic formats. The method used depends on the theoretical framework (e.g., psychodynamic, behavioral) from which the interviewer works and on the purpose(s) of the interview. There are three general interview formats: structured, unstructured, and semistructured. Structured psychological interviews provide a standardized method for asking questions and are most often based on diagnostic systems such as outlined in the *Diagnostic and Statistical Manual of Mental Disorders* (DSM). Examples of structured interviews that include parent versions (cited in Sattler, 1998) are the Child and Adolescent Psychiatric Assessment (CAPA; Angold, Cox, Rutter, & Siminoff, 1996), the Child Assessment Schedule (CAS;

Hodges, 1997), the Diagnostic Interview for Children and Adolescents—Revised (DICA-R; Reich, 1996), and the Diagnostic Interview Schedule for Children (DISC-IV; Shaffer, 1996). Structured interviews have the advantages of maximizing reliability and validity and minimizing interviewer biases and inferences (Sattler, 1998). The major disadvantages of structured interviews are that they focus on diagnosis rather than intervention, they face obsolescence when the diagnostic system from which they are derived is revised, and, because they focus on psychiatric diagnosis, they are currently of limited use in school settings.

The second general format is the *unstructured* interview. As the name implies, unstructured interviews do not follow a standard format; rather, the interviewer "goes with the flow" to obtain information within a highly flexible framework. In contrast to a structured interview, the greatest advantage of an unstructured interview lies in its flexibility. It allows the interviewer to tailor the interview to the individual situation. With this format the interviewer is free to follow the concerns of the parent or teacher rather than being limited to standard, and possibly irrelevant, questions. Given that unstructured interviews are typically guided toward some clinical focus, they are not completely without structure. The obvious disadvantage to this format is that the minimal level of structure leads to problems with the psychometric properties of the interview. It can also be difficult to compare information obtained from unstructured interviews with that of different informants, because very different topics may have been covered.

The third interview format, the *semistructured* interview, is a standard format that allows for a certain flexibility in questioning and responding to an interviewee. Typically, a semistructured interview provides the interviewer with a framework and specific questions, still allowing the interviewer to follow up as needed. The Schedule for Affective Disorders and Schizophrenia for School-Age Children—Epidemiological Version 5 (K-SADS-E5; Orvaschel, 1995) has been regarded as a semistructured diagnostic interview format. There are also several school-based examples that can be categorized as semistructured interviews. One example that is useful for assessing academic problems is the Teacher Interview Form for Academic Problems (Shapiro, 1996). For descriptive information regarding a child's history, a useful method that can be employed in either an interview or self-completed format is provided by the parent Structured Developmental History of the Behavior Assessment System for Children (BASC; Reynolds & Kamphaus, 1992). An example that applies to both parents and teachers is the behavioral consultation interview system of Bergan and Kratochwill (Bergan & Kratochwill, 1990; Kratochwill & Bergan, 1990), which provides a standard format for conducting behavioral interviews. The major advantage of semistructured interviews is their flexibility in gathering information while maintaining a standard format. The major disadvantages of such interviews are

that they tend to be relatively weak in regard to established reliability and validity and that the interviewer must be well trained in the clinical aspects of
interviewing.

All three of the interview formats may also be conceptualized in terms
of the level of information the interview is designed to obtain. Each type of
interview may be used to garner detailed and specific information or more
general descriptions of a problem or situation. With regard to content, *omnibus* formats are designed for gathering a wide range of information, such as
data obtained in developmental history interviews and multiple-disorder-
related interviews (e.g., Child Assessment Schedule). The main advantage of
omnibus formats is that the interviewer can gather information on a variety
of issues and behaviors that can be used to aid in generating hypotheses regarding diagnosis and potential interventions. The greatest disadvantages of
omnibus interviews are that they may be time-consuming and may not provide sufficient specification for designing interventions.

Behavior-specific interviews are more narrow in scope and focus on the assessment of one or a limited number of specific problems. Behavior-specific
formats are useful when the presenting problem is identified in general and
the purpose of the assessment is to focus on a specific behavior. For example,
the Teacher Interview Form for Academic Problems is a semistructured format that focuses on academic difficulties and provides an efficient method for
gathering information that is directly pertinent to behavior of concern. The
major disadvantage of behavior-specific interviews is that the initial referral
issue may have been misidentified and, if so, the interviewer may have to
switch to a different interview format.

Finally, *problem-solving* interviews are open to presenting concerns, with
the focus of the interview driven by the presenting problem and directed toward intervention. For example, behavioral consultation interviewing provides a problem-solving format for identifying and specifying behavior priorities within the interview, thereby allowing flexibility regarding problem focus. Problem-solving interviews differ from behavior-specific interviews in
that the initial focus is more exploratory and includes defining the problem
situation rather than simply assessing specific behaviors. In practice, it is likely that problem-solving interviews will include behavior-specific interviewing
as a component of the interview process.

The selections of interview format and content level are driven by the
purpose of the interview. Within the context of assessment, an interviewer
may wish to obtain a thorough description of problem behaviors in order to
reach a diagnosis, and thus the interviewer may combine interview formats
to best suit the process of the assessment. Combining interview formats—
such as beginning with an open-ended interview and moving toward a more
structured format—may be useful if parents appear anxious or resistant during an assessment. In deciding on the format for the interview, the interview-

er also must take into account the specific goals of the assessment. For example, omnibus diagnostic interviews entail obtaining information specific to determining a diagnosis, such as family and developmental history, psychiatric history, history of substance abuse, and symptom information (e.g., onset, duration, frequency) and may therefore take a more historical approach. In contrast, problem-solving interviews are less concerned with diagnosis and, instead, focus on understanding problem behaviors and current situations and linking assessment with intervention. With this overview of interview methods in mind, we turn to a discussion of the use of interviews within a functional assessment of behavior.

PARENT AND TEACHER INTERVIEWS AS PART OF A FUNCTIONAL ASSESSMENT

Functional assessment is a process that involves gathering data regarding antecedent and consequent conditions surrounding a behavior to generate hypotheses about the function(s) of the behavior. Lewis and Sugai (1996) summarized three basic functions of problem behavior: (1) to increase access to social attention, (2) to avoid aversive tasks or situations, and (3) self-reinforcement. Thus, the focus of a functional assessment of behavior (FAB) is on the environmental (e.g., punishment, setting events) and individual organismic (e.g., motivation) variables that are functionally related to behavioral occurrences.

Informant interviews play a clear role in any functional assessment. Best practices call for assessment that uses multiple methods (e.g., interview, observation, rating scales) with multiple individuals (e.g., child, parent, teacher) in multiple settings (e.g., home, school, community) to generate data. Thus, a functional assessment interview is an integral component in providing convergent evidence toward generating hypotheses about the function of behavior and potential interventions (Lentz & Wehmann, 1995). Informant interviews have obvious importance in understanding the environmental stimuli affecting a child's behavior, and in understanding the reciprocal impact of behavior on the child's environment. For example, through interviewing a parent, it may be learned that a child's behavior is "not a problem" at home because of modifications the parents have made in their standards and home environment.

Parental informants can provide a variety of information about the child, including family history and demographics, a description of the problem and the parents' usual responses to problem behaviors, levels of familial distress over the problem, and information regarding environmental stimuli related to the problem. Parents may also discuss their impressions of their child's strengths and weaknesses. Interviewing parent informants also pro-

vides for an assessment of the parents' abilities to act as mediators of the child's behavior. For example, what level of insight do they have into the causal and maintaining factors of the problem, including their own role in the problem? As part of the assessment process, the interviewer may also note how parents relate to their child and, if more than one parent is interviewed, how they relate to each other.

Although parents are likely to be the informants who best know the child, teachers provide invaluable information regarding behavior in school settings. In general, teachers may provide information about the functional aspects of social behaviors, peer relationships, and academic skills of which parents may be unaware. Certainly, teachers, much more than parents, have experience with and have observed the child in school-based academic and social situations. Furthermore, teachers typically have contact with a wider range of children and can therefore provide information based on normative comparisons. Just as interviewers can assess parents as participants in the intervention process, they can engage teacher informants to determine their willingness to have a role in the assessment and intervention.

Whereas parents and teachers are typically the informants of first choice, situations arise wherein other informants may best serve as the primary sources. Among these alternative informants are parent surrogates such as foster parents and grandparents or other relatives, case workers, and support staff such as aides or caretakers. The selection of informants depends on which of the them are most familiar with the child and which can provide information on behaviors of concern in the environments that are targeted for change.

Selection of Interview Format

Prior to conducting the interview, several decisions must be made: determining which informants to interview, deciding what types of information must be obtained, and selecting an interview format. Among the various structured informant interview frameworks and methods, most (e.g., DICA-R, DISC) are designed for diagnostic purposes and, as such, have limited use in a functional assessment. Behavioral interviewing, however, is well suited to functional assessment because it is based on the behavioral principles around which a functional assessment of behavior is designed. Indeed, functional assessment, although relatively new as a specific topic in school-based assessment, has long been an integral component of behavioral assessment models.

Whereas many practitioners work from a behavioral interviewing model, they may use an unstructured format that can lead to difficulties with the validity of the assessment. In contrast, a semistructured format, by definition, provides the structure within which behavioral variables can be assessed, while allowing flexibility in using clinical problem-solving skills in determin-

ing which variables should be the focus of the interview. From a functional behavior standpoint, there is no single identifying variable that can help us understand an individual's behavior—that is, behavior is best understood and remediated through an idiographic, individualized assessment. Thus, from this perspective, a problem-solving interview format provides the flexibility necessary for a functional assessment.

A behavioral interviewing method that is both semistructured and problem-solving oriented is found in the behavioral consultation model fostered by Bergan (1977) and expanded by Bergan and Kratochwill (Bergan & Kratochwill, 1990; Kratochwill & Bergan, 1990). Within this model, three interviews are conducted to identify a problem (Problem Identification Interview, PII), to analyze the problem and develop a plan (Problem Analysis Interview, PAI), and to evaluate treatment outcomes (Treatment Evaluation Interview, TEI). The interviews are designed to provide a standardized framework for problem solving in regard to children's difficulties that draws on the foundations and principles of behavioral assessment and therapy. Behavioral consultation interviews have been shown to evidence high levels of reliability (e.g., Bergan & Tombari, 1975, 1976; Kratochwill, Elliott, & Busse, 1995) and to possess adequate content and criterion-related validity (Beaver & Busse, 2000; Bergan & Kratochwill, 1990; Gresham & Davis, 1988). Furthermore, interventions implemented within behavioral consultation have been found useful for remediating a variety of academic and social behavior problems (Bergan & Tombari, 1976; Elliott & Busse, 1993; Kratochwill et al., 1995; Kratochwill, Sheridan, Carrington Rotto, & Salmon, 1991).

The behavioral consultation model is well established as a form of assessment and service delivery in schools. It has been limited in that both research and practice within the model typically center on parallel (i.e., teacher or parent) implementation, with most research focusing on consultation interviewing with teachers. This specific informant-setting method of assessment, however, leaves untapped the ecological nature of a child's behavior. Given that the level of communication between parents and school may be part of a child's difficulties, and the importance of assessing multiple behavior settings, a potentially useful interviewing strategy is to hold a *conjoint* interview with both parents and teachers (Sheridan, Kratochwill, & Bergan, 1996). Conjoint behavioral interviewing follows the same framework as traditional teacher-only or parent-only interviewing and is predicated on behavioral therapy and principles. Consultations including conjoint interviewing have been successful in treating social withdrawal (Sheridan, Kratochwill, & Elliott, 1990), social behaviors of children with attention-deficit/hyperactivity disorder (ADHD; Colton & Sheridan, 1998), and academic behavior problems (Galloway & Sheridan, 1994).

Conjoint interviewing has several potential advantages in functional as-

sessment and in designing and implementing interventions (Sheridan et al., 1996). First, it may promote greater cooperation and coordination among parents, teachers, and the interviewer/practitioner, thereby enhancing home–school collaboration. Second, conjoint interviewing allows the interviewer to obtain information across settings and sources to aid in the formation of hypotheses regarding the strength, frequency, duration, and function of problem behaviors. Third, this method provides a unique opportunity to examine different perspectives on behavior and to develop more comprehensive and cohesive interventions. Finally, from a practical standpoint, interviewing parents and teachers simultaneously allows efficient use of the practitioner's time.

Although, from our perspective, conjoint interviewing is a potentially useful and preferred method of assessment, there clearly are situations in which simultaneous interviewing of parents and teachers is contraindicated. For example, parents and/or teachers may exhibit dysfunctional behaviors (e.g., mental illness) that obviate a conjoint approach. Relatedly, teachers and parents historically may have negative attitudes toward one another that preclude their ability to work cooperatively (Sheridan & Kratochwill, 1992). (Awareness of these types of parent and teacher behaviors is obviously valuable in understanding a child's behaviors!) In such cases, parallel teacher-only and parent-only interviews can be conducted separately. Regardless of whether the method is conjoint or parallel, a behavioral interviewing method remains most conducive to a functional assessment.

Before considering specific practical aspects of interviewing, it is important to note that our focus is on the interviewing components used in behavioral consultation. For readers who are interested in the applications of parallel and conjoint consultation processes, two useful practical guides are *Behavioral Consultation in Applied Settings: An Individual Guide* (Kratochwill & Bergan, 1990) and *Conjoint Behavioral Consultation: A Procedural Manual* (Sheridan et al., 1996).

INTERVIEWING PROCEDURES AND SKILLS

Although we emphasize the use of behavioral interviewing in functional assessments, there are several procedural aspects and interviewing skills that are basic to any informant interview.

Procedural Aspects

Prior to beginning an informant interview, it is necessary to decide which informants in the child's life are likely to provide the most useful information and who can be part of the intervention process. Typically, informants will

include one or both of the child's parents, guardian(s), or other parent figures. For many children, the appropriate parental source may be a stepparent, grandparent, or other relative. It may also be necessary to consider the involvement of parent figures who do not live with the child, but who may still have significant contact or impact on the child's life. In the school setting the choice of informant varies with the child's grade level. In preschool through elementary grades, the informant typically is the child's lead teacher. In middle and high school settings, the informant may be a teacher with whom the child has the most contact or a teacher in whose class the child is experiencing difficulty. There may also be situations in which two or more teachers participate in the interview. These situations may arise for children in classrooms with team teachers, in settings such as high school where multiple teachers are involved, or for mainstreamed children with disabilities who have a special education teacher. Unfortunately, little is known about which informants are most appropriate or most conducive to productive interviewing. The interviewer must use clinical judgment in considering how many informants to involve without overwhelming the process, which informants are willing and able to provide useful information, and the interpersonal dynamics among the interviewees.

Once the informants are chosen, informed consent must be obtained from the parent informants. Rather than simply being a perfunctory measure, written consent protects the parents, practitioner, and school and sets the stage for the assessment process. A potentially sensitive issue arises when parents are separated or divorced and share legal custody of the child. In these instances, it is prudent to inform both parents and, if necessary, to engage in separate interviews. Ideally, the interviewer will have had prior contact with parent and teacher informants via phone calls, memos, or letters. Contact prior to the interview can be used to establish rapport, state the purpose of the interview, and provide information about the interview process. Practical aspects of the interview also should be described, such as who will be participating, time allotments, and scheduling of the interview.

During these initial contacts, and possibly during the interview, parents and teachers may be anxious about the assessment and concerned that they will be blamed in some way for the child's problems. It is important that the interviewer be careful not to blame either source but to attempt to diffuse any blame parents and teachers assign to each other. It is useful to state at the outset that the child's problems are probably related to a variety of home, community, and school factors, and that the focus of the interview is on helping the child in each of these settings. It is also important to point out that parents and teachers probably know the child better than anyone else, which makes them important sources of information. To maximize the likelihood that they will want to share that information, it is important that they feel comfortable with the interviewer—ideally, as a partner in the inter-

view (and intervention) process. Parents and teachers form an important system in the child's life. It is necessary that the interviewer join this system, rather than expecting the informants to accommodate to the interviewer. Accomplishing this alliance requires the interviewer to be warm and friendly, to avoid jargon, and to suspend judgment of the informants' behavior and beliefs (Orton, 1997). Obviously, these behaviors should carry over into the interview.

Interviewing Skills

Conducting any informant interview involves several basic interviewing skills, among which are active listening and observing. It is crucial that the interviewer attend to both what the informant says and to how he or she says it. For example, a parent may express concern for the child's problems while nonverbally expressing anger and frustration. Specific features to notice are the volume and pitch of speech, the rate of speaking, and the fluency of speech. The interviewer should be attentive to other nonverbal communication as well, such as posture, gestures and other motor behaviors, facial expressions, and eye contact (Sattler, 1998). A skilled interviewer will also monitor his or her own verbal and nonverbal behaviors to be alert for subtle signs of his or her own interfering values and judgments.

At the opening of the interview, the interviewer should greet the parents and teacher, giving his or her name and professional role. The next step is to give an introductory statement to provide structure for the interview and begin the process. This introduction includes informing interviewees of the goals of the interview (i.e., to identify specific influences on the child's problem; to begin to develop a plan for intervention). Confidentiality and its limitations also should be addressed. The interview itself may begin with an open-ended request for information, such as "Tell me about your child," "Please tell me about your concerns for your child," "I understand that your child has been having difficulties; please tell me more about what's been going on." (Sattler, 1998). These openings give parents and teachers the opportunity to begin with their areas of greatest concern.

As the interview progresses, the skills of the interviewer are of great importance. Drawing from several sources on interviewing skills (e.g., Bergan & Kratochwill, 1990; Cormier & Cormier, 1985; Ivey, 1994; Rogers, 1951; Sattler, 1988, 1998; Sheridan et al., 1996), we offer the acronym PACERS to facilitate recall of the basic components of effective listening and interviewing skills. This acronym stands for Paraphrasing, Attending, Clarifying, Eliciting, Reflecting, and Summarizing. *Paraphrasing* involves restating for the interviewee the essence of what has been said. It does not mean simply repeating whatever the person has said; rather the interviewer integrates and restates key words and phrases from the parent/teacher's comments. Para-

phrasing gives the parent or teacher the opportunity to correct misunderstandings while demonstrating the interviewer's understanding of their concerns.

PARENT: There are just so many things. I just can't get him to sit still. Meals are a circus; he's in and out of his chair constantly, running into the other room, knocking things over. No one in the family can eat peacefully. And it's the same problem when we try to get him to do his homework or sit in church.

INTERVIEWER: So it seems that Bill is always on the go and it's disruptive for the family at home and other places, like church.

The goal of *attending* is to convey to the parents and teachers that the interviewer is listening and interested in what they have to say. Showing them that the interviewer wants to understand their viewpoint is just as important as his or her actual ability to understand their concerns. While listening to the interviewees, the interviewer may want to use "minimal encouragers," which are verbal and nonverbal responses used to prompt the clients to continue. These prompts may include head nods (be careful not to overdo!), gestures, phrases like "uh-huh," and repetition of one or two key words.

PARENT: Yes, he is very disruptive. And I'm getting so frustrated with him.

INTERVIEWER: Uh-hm.

PARENT: I'm afraid my anger is going to get away from me. I've noticed that I've been yelling much more than I used to and I don't like that, but I can't seem to help it. He just makes me so mad that I . . . (*trails off*).

INTERVIEWER: You feel so mad . . .

PARENT: I get so mad I just want to scream and throw things.

Clarifying is used to ensure that the interviewer is accurately understanding the comments of the parents and teachers. Clarification may involve paraphrasing their statements to allow them to correct the interviewer (e.g., "Do you mean to say that Jill *always* refuses to do her homework?"). It is also likely to involve asking informants to provide specific examples of their concerns. Similarly, it may be desirable for the interviewer to clarify his or her own statements with specific and concrete examples, rather than giving a summary statement of the child's problem. For example, it is better to say that "Jill has hit other children on the playground at recess every day this week" rather than noting that "Jill has a problem with aggressive behavior."

When clarifying the statements of interviewees and gathering informa-

tion and data, the interviewer will need to ask questions. *Eliciting* information through the use of questions and soft commands (e.g., "Tell me about John's behaviors") can move the interview along and allow the interviewer to obtain necessary data. The interviewer must take care, however, because elicitors also have the potential to turn an interview into a cross-examination that is unpleasant for the parent or teacher.

Interviews involve a combination of "open questions," which encourage talking and cannot be answered in just a few words, and "closed questions," which may be answered briefly and tend to keep the focus on the interviewer. Closed questions can be useful in trying to focus the interview or to obtain specific information (e.g., "How often does Billy hit his brother?"). Open-ended questions are useful in beginning the interview and encouraging the teachers or parents to elaborate on their comments. The first word of an open-ended question will influence the type of information obtained. For example, "what" questions often lead to facts ("What are you going to do?"), whereas "why" questions are likely to lead to a discussion of reasons or causes ("Why do you think that happened?"). One must be careful, however, because "why" questions may lead to negative feelings or put teachers/parents on the defensive (Ivey, 1994). It is often more useful to ask parents "how" they came to a particular decision or "what" leads them to think a particular way about their child rather, than ask "why" something occurred.

Although obviously useful, questioning can pose several potential problems if not phrased appropriately. When questioning, the interviewer must be careful not to disguise statements or judgments as questions (e.g., "Don't you think Kira would do better if you supervised her homework more directly?") or to lead the informant with the question. Useful questions keep the interview on topic and are well connected to the comments and concerns of the informants. The interviewer should also monitor the number and frequency of questions. Too many questions, particularly if several are asked at once, are likely to increase defensiveness and discomfort in the parents/teachers and may result in negative treatment outcomes (Busse, Kratochwill, & Elliott, 1999). Cultural factors must also be considered. Members of non-Western cultural groups are likely to react negatively to the rapid questioning style that is fairly typical of North American interviewers, which may result in the informants' discomfort and distrust of the interview process (Ivey, 1994).

Another interviewing skill, *reflecting*, involves rephrasing the affect of interviewees' statements. Reflecting is similar to paraphrasing, but rather than focusing on content or the cognitive component of a statement, it emphasizes the affective component to validate or clarify emotional responses or messages. For example, in response to a teacher's statement, "It takes so much time to work with Jill, and I have 25 other children to teach," the interviewer

may reflect, "It's frustrating for you when you have limited time and assistance." Reflecting the interviewee's affect, when used judiciously, shows empathy and concern for the difficulties faced by teachers and parents. Reflecting has the added effect of maintaining rapport and allowing the parents and teachers to "vent" feelings that may otherwise interfere with the interview process. As with paraphrasing, reflection should not be a simple parroting of the informant's statements or comments about emotion. To reflect well, the interviewer must be aware of the informant's nonverbal behaviors as well as verbal indications of emotion. Facial expression, gestures, and such vocal qualities as tone of voice and rate of speech can give important clues to underlying emotions, including emotions that are in conflict with the informant's words.

The final effective interviewing skill, *summarizing,* can be useful throughout the interview. Summarizing alerts parents/teachers to the key issues and themes of concern and provides opportunities to check understanding. Summarizing is similar to paraphrasing, but it covers more information and a longer time span. When parents/teachers are providing long statements without pause or are getting off track, summarizing can help the interviewer to maintain the focus and pace of the interview and to organize the statements for both parent/teacher and interviewer. Summarizations also are useful for beginning and ending interviews and for transitions to new topic areas.

COMPONENTS OF A CONJOINT FUNCTIONAL ASSESSMENT INTERVIEW (CFAI)

This section includes an example of a conjoint functional assessment interview, with accompanying structure and guidelines for engaging in effective interviewing. Table 9.1 presents a standardized functional assessment interview with objectives and examples of statements for each objective. The semistructured format and objectives are drawn from the conjoint behavioral consultation model of Sheridan et al. (1996) and a functional assessment interview format adapted by Larson and Busse (1998). The overall goals of this interview, based on the consultation model of the Problem Identification Interview (PII), are to (1) establish a positive working relationship among the parent, teacher, and interviewer, (2) define the problem behavior in operational terms, (3) identify behavioral antecedent, situation, and consequent conditions across settings, (4) provide a tentative identification of the frequency and duration of the behavior across settings, (5) set goals for behavior change across settings, and (6) establish a procedure for data collection (Sheridan et al., 1996). To expand these goals for a specific functional assessment interview (see Table 9.1), we included ascertaining informant

TABLE 9.1. Conjoint Functional Assessment Interview–Problem Identification (CFAI-PI) Objectives, Definitions/Rationales, and Examples

Objective	Definition/rationale	Examples
Opening salutation	General opening statement. Expand as needed depending on familiarity of participants.	"Hello! Thanks for coming in today."
General overview of the interview	General summary statement to introduce the interview process and provide a brief rationale for the interview.	"What I'd like to accomplish today is to get an idea about the behavior of concern and to get very specific about the behavior and where it occurs."
General statement to open the interview	General statement to begin discussion related to referral concerns.	"What seems to be the problem?" "What is it that you are concerned about?"
Behavior specification	Behavioral descriptions of client functioning are elicited and prioritized, with a focus on specific behaviors. Several examples of the general problem should be requested. Whenever possible, a problem that occurs across settings should be targeted.	
	◆ Describe behaviors	"What does Jamie do when he's 'angry?'" "Tell me what you mean when you say he gets upset with himself easily." "Give me some examples of what you mean by 'self-abusive' behaviors."
	◆ Elicit examples	"What are some more examples of Jamie's 'self-abuse' at home/at school?"
	◆ Prioritize behavior	"We've discussed several behaviors, such as hitting himself, kicking objects, ripping up papers, and screaming. Which of these is most problematic at home? School?" "Do you both agree?"
Target behavior definition	Specific operational definition of target behavior. An operational definition is one that is objective, concrete, and observable.	"Let's define exactly what we mean by Jamie hitting himself—he raises his arm, clenches his fist, and slaps the side of his head with force . . . is that right?"

TABLE 9.1. *Continued*

Objective	Definition/rationale	Examples
History of problem	An estimate of the duration of the problem behavior, including how long it has been occurring, any changes in its topography or frequency, and other unique characteristics.	"How long has this behavior been a problem?" "Has the behavior always presented itself this way, or has it changed over time?"
Behavior setting	A precise description of the settings in which the target problem behavior occurs. Ask for as many examples of settings at home and at school as possible. Prioritize the settings from the most to the least severe.	
◆ Describe general setting		"Where is Jamie usually when he hits himself?" "Give me some examples of where Jamie does this at school." "Where does the head slapping occur at home?"
◆ Elicit examples		"What are some more examples of where this occurs?"
◆ Prioritize settings		"Which of the settings at school is most problematic?" "Which of the settings at home is most problematic?"
Functional/ conditional analysis		
◆ Antecedent conditions and setting events	Events or variables that precede the child's behavior. These events can immediately precede the behavior, or they may be removed in time (e.g., events at home in the morning that affect the child's behaviors at school).	"What typically happens at home/at school before Jamie starts to hit himself?" "What things do you notice before he starts that might be contributing to its occurrence?" "What is a typical morning like before Jamie goes to school?"
◆ Consequent conditions	Events that occur immediately following the behavior. These can be environmental in nature or reactions/responses of parents, teacher, or peers. They can occur immediately following the behavior or at a later point in time (e.g., at home after school).	"What typically happens after Jamie hits himself at home/at school?" "How do others react when Jamie slaps his head?" "What types of things do you notice at home/at school after Jamie hits himself that may be affecting its occurrence?" "How are school-related problems handled at home?"

(*continued*)

TABLE 9.1. *Continued*

Objective	Definition/rationale	Examples
◆ Environmental/ sequential conditions	Situational events or environmental conditions occurring when the behavior occurs. A pattern or trend of antecedent/consequent conditions across a series of occasions (e.g., time of day, day of week). This may include activities, persons, situations, or other variables that appear to be related to the target behavior.	"What else is typically happening when Jamie hits himself?" "What patterns do you notice in Jamie's head-slapping behavior?" "What time of day or day of week seems to be most problematic at home/at school?" "Who else is usually present?" "Is the head slapping more frequent in some situations than in others?"
Existing procedures	Procedures or programs/rules in force that are external to the child and to the behavior. Elicit information on the effectiveness (i.e., child's reaction) of the procedures.	"What are some programs or procedures that are currently operating in the classroom/at home?" "How is the problem currently dealt with at home/school?" "How does Jamie react to the praise?"
Behavior strength	The level or incidence of the behavior. The most common features concern how often (frequent) or how long (duration) the behavior occurs. The question format (i.e., whether to ask about frequency, duration, latency, intensity) will depend on the specific behavior and the focus of the consultation.	"How often does Jamie hit himself at home/at school?" "How long does the hitting last?"
Behavioral goal	Appropriate or acceptable level of the behavior. Both long- and short-term goals should be discussed.	"What would be an acceptable level of head slapping at home/ at school?" "Is any hitting okay?" "What would you like to see for Jamie?" "Is there general agreement on our goal for Jamie at both home and school?"
Informant attribution for the behavior function	Parent/teacher perceptions of the function of the target behavior. Important for assessing function and beginning a link to intervention.	"Why do you think Jamie is slapping himself?" "What function do you think the head slapping serves?"
Child's strengths/ assets	Strengths, abilities, or other positive features of the child.	"What are some of the things Jamie is good at?" "What are some of Jamie's strengths?"

TABLE 9.1. *Continued*

Objective	Definition/rationale	Examples
Potential reinforcers/ resources	Social, concrete, or activity-based reinforcers that may be used in a behavioral program. Resources (e.g., aide, computer) available for intervention.	"What are some things (e.g. events, activities) that Jamie finds rewarding?" "What are some things Jamie likes to do?" "What kinds of resources are available that we might use to help with the behavior?"
Skill deficits/ replacement behaviors	Parent/teacher perceptions of skills the child may be lacking and potential behaviors to replace the deficits.	"What skill deficits might be causing the occurrence of this behavior?" "What might replace Jamie's head slapping?"
Rationale and procedures for data collection	A purpose or rationale for data collection.	"It would be very helpful to watch Jamie for a week or so and monitor how often he hits himself on the head. This will help us key in on some important facts that we may have missed, and also help us document the progress Jamie makes."
◆ Cross-setting data collection procedures	Procedural details regarding data recording, including the kind of measure, what is to be recorded, and how to record. Specific details of data recording should be provided. Consistent data collection procedures across settings should be encouraged. A written plan that incorporates the target behavior operationalization for parents and teacher is helpful.	"What would be a simple way for you to keep track of the number of times Jamie hits his head at home/at school?" "We've decided that at home, you will keep a count of the number of times Jamie hits his head each evening, including the time and preceding events. At school, you will chart the number of times Jamie hits himself, as well as what happens before and after, and who is present and how they respond."
◆ Date to begin data collection	Procedural details regarding when to begin collecting data.	"When can you begin to collect data at home/at school?" "Can you both start the recording procedures tomorrow?"
Next appointment/ closing the interview	Meeting time and summary of the next interview.	"When can we all get together again to discuss the data and determine where to go from here?"
◆ Closing salutation	General statement closing the interview.	"Thanks for your time and hard work! See you soon!"

Note. Adapted from Sheridan, Kratochwill, and Bergan (1996). Copyright 1996 by Plenum Publishing Corporation. Adapted by permission.

attributions for the problem behavior, functions of the behavior, and establishing hypotheses about skill deficits and replacement behaviors (Larson & Busse,1998). Within these goals, one of the interviewer's roles is to guide the direction of the interview by maintaining the focus of the interview, ensuring that all parties provide input, and creating a collaborative atmosphere.

At the start of the interview it is important to provide a summary of the objectives of the interview and to set the stage by stating that a major purpose of the interview is to be as specific as possible regarding the behavior, because specificity will help in understanding the behavior and facilitating an intervention. We suggest that this summary include an overview of the general components of the interview: identifying the problem, identifying when and where the behavior occurs, what function the behavior serves, and whether more information must be gathered. It is also useful to remind parents and teachers that their input and questions are important and that all parties are working together toward the common goal of helping the child. Throughout the interview, it is useful to provide transition statements and rationales for the interview segments to keep the interview flowing naturally and to create a "mind-set" for the participants. For the interview to be successful, it is imperative that the interviewer engage in several summarizations and clarifications to ensure understanding and to keep the interview focused. The interviewer should frequently use elicitors to adequately specify behavior and behavior setting variables (Bergan & Tombari, 1975).

On the basis of this general overview, we present a case example of a CFAI that follows the format outlined in Table 9.1, with accompanying analyses of the components of the interview. For illustrative purposes, we have created a composite of actual and simulated interview data drawn from Sheridan et al. (1996), Larson and Busse (1998), and our own practical experiences.

In this case example of a relatively common problem, the referral centers on the behavior of an 8-year-old, third-grade boy named "Scott Smith." Scott lives with his biological mother and father, and a sister (age 6) and brother (age 10). Scott's teacher, "Mr. Jones," initiated a referral to the school's building consultation team, who assigned a team member to the case. Mr. Jones identified the problem as "oppositional and hyperactive behaviors." Records indicate that Scott achieved satisfactory academic marks through second grade, with comments that he tended to "rush" through schoolwork and had poor organizational skills. Scott also has a history of disruptive (e.g., "tends to blurt out answers," "bothers other students") and overactive behaviors. Currently, Scott is in the second month of third grade; he is falling behind in his schoolwork and fails to turn in assignments, and his disruptive behaviors have recently become more problematic at home and school.

CASE EXAMPLE

Opening Salutation

INTERVIEWER: Hello! Thanks for coming today. I think we all know one another, so let's get started.

This general opening statement may have to be expanded, depending on the level of communication prior to the interview. Introductions may be necessary, and the opening may include a brief period of small talk (e.g., about the weather) to establish comfort and beginning rapport. The interviewer should be certain that the seating arrangement is as comfortable as possible, and that the participants are sitting near and facing one another.

General Overview of the Interview

INTERVIEWER: The purpose of our meeting is to better understand Scott's difficulties at home and school, and to figure out how to help. So it's important that everyone feels free to provide input and ask questions. What we'll be doing is talking about Scott's behavior and trying to get pretty specific about when and where it occurs, what seems to be happening before and after the behavior, agreeing on goals for Scott, and whether we need to collect more information.

This overview provides a good summary of the interview and prepares the participants for what will follow. It is typically a good idea for the interviewer to inform the participants that he or she is taking notes and to place the response paper or clipboard in a comfortable, open manner. If using a structured protocol, it may be useful for the interviewer to inform the participants that a format is being followed so that the interviewer does not forget anything.

General Statement to Open the Interview

INTERVIEWER: From the referral, it appears that the main issues are Scott's oppositional and hyperactive behaviors and his lack of progress in school. Does that sound right? Or are there other concerns?

The interviewer opens with a general summary based on the referral and perhaps previously gathered data, but should be careful about using terms such as "oppositional," which may not be readily understood. The

TEACHER: That sounds about right to me.

PARENT: I think that covers it pretty well.

question appropriately asks for general clarification, although the question may need to be expanded if the behavior is misidentified or new concerns have arisen, and the interviewer should wait for a response to each question. If this is an initial contact interview, the statement will be more general—for example, "Let's start with Mrs. Smith. Tell me about your concerns with Scott."

Behavior Specification

INTERVIEWER: Let's try to get a general idea of these behaviors. Mrs. Smith, please describe Scott's behavior problems at home.

PARENT: Well, at home he's just so impulsive and always on the go. He doesn't stop for a minute and doesn't think about what he's doing. Like this morning, he rushed out of the house with his shirt on backwards and forgot his backpack, again!

The interviewer uses a good elicitor to gather a general behavior description. It is often useful to begin with the parent to put him or her more at ease in the school setting.

INTERVIEWER: It sounds as if that can be pretty frustrating. What are some other examples?

PARENT: More examples? You mean like what he does in the morning?

A good use of a reflective statement, followed by an eliciting question.

INTERVIEWER: Well, anytime, really. I'm just trying to get a general sense of his overall behavior.

PARENT: Okay, well, um, I have a difficult time with him at night too. He's always late for dinner and doesn't come in when I call him, and he constantly pesters his brother and sister and a big fight takes place. And he's the devil to get into bed. Is that what you mean?

At this point, the interviewer keeps the topic open to gather general examples and provides a brief rationale. The interviewer may need to give more specific direction if the parent has difficulty proceeding—for example, "Tell me about his behaviors during the rest of the day."

INTERVIEWER: Yes, that's fine. Mr. Jones, tell me about his hyperactive behaviors at school.

TEACHER: Well, I see similar kinds of things. Scott's one of the most hyperactive kids I've seen in 5 years teaching third grade. I mean, he's like a human tornado who comes flying into the classroom at the start of school and doesn't stop until he flies out at the end of the day.

Here the interviewer decides that the general examples are sufficient for the moment, briefly validates the parent's responses, and transitions with an elicitor to gather general examples of the child's behavior at school. A brief summary of the parent's responses may be useful—"Yes, that's fine" may seem dismissive.

INTERVIEWER: Mm hmmm.

Good use of a minimal encourager to convey attending.

TEACHER: He's got almost no attention span for seat work and only slightly more during group projects. I've tried seating him near my desk, calling Mrs. Smith—we've talked a lot recently, haven't we?

PARENT: We sure have!

The interviewer may want to nod and/or smile to convey attending and reinforce cooperative behaviors.

TEACHER: But nothing has worked. They could heat the building on the energy Scott lets loose!

INTERVIEWER: He sounds like a real handful. Tell me more about what he does when he's hyperactive.

Good use of reflecting, followed by a general behavior elicitor.

TEACHER: Okay. In the morning we have reading from 8:25 to 9:00. I get him and his group seated at the table, and he immediately begins to poke and jab the other children. He can't keep his feet to himself. I spend most of the time telling him to stop and to pay attention while other children are reading. Later, he'll blurt out a silly question or something during a test, or start playing with a toy, or tapping his pencil. Yesterday he stood on a table in the library and yelled, "I'm king of the

The interviewer should judiciously intersperse attending behaviors such as nods and verbal encouragers.

world!" The librarian won't even let him in anymore.

INTERVIEWER: He *does* seem to be a handful. It sounds as if you both are seeing similar kinds of behavior at home and at school. What about his academic progress? Mrs. Smith?

PARENT: Well, I have a hard time getting him to do his homework. He's either playing video games or watching some cartoon channel, and he refuses to get to work. When I do get him down, he'll work for a few minutes and then start fiddling with his pencil or paper, humming to himself. And his work is so sloppy. I tell him Mr. Jones won't be able to read it. After a while, I just kinda give up.

Another reflective statement, followed by a good, brief summary that also serves to validate the participants' perceptions of the problem. Good use of a general behavior elicitor and directing the interview.

TEACHER: And Mrs. Smith and I have talked about that, you know, setting a time for schoolwork, turning off the boob tube, and using videos as reinforcement.

INTERVIEWER: And do you see similar work behaviors at school?

The interviewer uses an elicitor to direct the interview to the school setting.

TEACHER: Definitely! He doesn't get any work done, and when he does work it's usually unreadable or he crumples it up in a ball and hands it to me.

INTERVIEWER: Okay. We've discussed several behaviors. At home he has difficulties getting himself ready for school, coming home when called, fighting with his brother and sister, getting to bed, and doing his homework. At school he has problems in reading group, blurts out questions, plays with toys during class, and is disruptive in the library. Does that summarize it pretty well?

Appropriate time for a summarization, followed by a clarification to ascertain agreement about the behaviors of concern.

PARENT: I think so. He also tends to talk back to me, you know, he'll tell me "No!" He doesn't want to come in or whatever.

INTERVIEWER: Do you also see that kind of refusal at school, Mr. Jones?

TEACHER: He doesn't usually say he won't do something, he just doesn't do it or goofs around and kinda avoids it, like during math.

Again, the interviewer uses an elicitor to direct the interview and ascertain similarities in behavior across settings.

INTERVIEWER: Okay. There obviously are several concerns you both have, and it sounds as if you've been communicating well about them. Now, we can't address all the problems at once, so what I'd like to do is prioritize the behaviors. Considering all the problems you have mentioned, which is of the greatest concern?

The interviewer validates cooperative behaviors and elicits prioritization of behavioral concerns. Given the number of concerns, the interviewer should list the behaviors and ask for priorities for each setting— for example, "Mrs. Smith, considering all the problems you mentioned, on a scale of 1 to 10, with 10 being the greatest concern, how would you rate getting himself ready for school? Getting ready for bed? . . ."

PARENT: The biggest problems are the fighting and getting him to school in the morning; it's such a battle, and I have to get to work.

INTERVIEWER: Okay. And at school?

TEACHER: I'd say the disruptive behaviors during reading group.

It is usually advantageous to target a behavior that occurs across settings, although this will not always be the case. The interviewer may need to elicit consensus on a target behavior that is of higher priority for one of the parties—for example, "I'd like to see if we can start with a similar behavior . . ."

Target Behavior Definition

INTERVIEWER: Okay. There seem to be similarities in the reading group difficulties and the fighting at home. Let's focus on that behavior first. What I'd like to do is get a pretty specific definition of the behavior

Here the interviewer briefly clarifies the similarities at home and school, directs the interview to focus on the most problematic behavior, and provides a brief rationale for behavior specification. It is useful to ask on

so we all know we are looking at the same thing and so we can monitor it. Mrs. Smith, please describe what Scott does specifically when he fights with his brother and sister.

PARENT: Well, he pokes at them when we're eating and kicks them under the table, and then the squabbling begins. The same thing happens in the car. He pushes and nudges them.

INTERVIEWER: Does he hit them with his fists or hit them hard?

PARENT: Not really. It's more shoving and pushing. You know, normal brother and sister stuff, but more out of hand than normal.

INTERVIEWER: Okay, at home he pushes, shoves, nudges, and kicks at them. So it seems it's physical poking and shoving and not keeping his hands and feet to himself. Is that right?

PARENT: Yes.

TEACHER: It's the same at school. He pokes at the other kids as though he's trying to get a rise out of them. You expect some of that behavior, but with Scott it's disruptive and happens all the time.

INTERVIEWER: Okay. Would you describe the behaviors in the same way as Mrs. Smith? Poking, kicking, shoving—not keeping his hands and feet to himself?

TEACHER: Yes. It's not as if he's necessarily trying to hurt any of the kids, it's more as though he just can't control himself.

which behavior the interviewees want to focus and to work toward consensus, using rationales such as "Let's try to find similarities so we can work on the same behaviors one at a time." The interviewer also needs to use judgment in deciding on targeting behaviors that are topographically related and on which there is a greater likelihood that an impact can be made. For example, with multiple behaviors it may be useful to note, "Sometimes it is best to start with a behavior that is less problematic to gain some success and then work toward the worst behavior."

After eliciting specifics about the behavior, the interviewer operationalizes the behavior and elicits agreement. The interviewer should mentally note the words used by the parent and teacher to describe the behavior, such as "normal" and "expected." Superlatives such as always, never, and so forth, should also be noted.

While taking notes, the interviewer should record the operationalization for the behavior.

History of Problem

INTERVIEWER: And how long has he been doing this?

TEACHER: Ever since the beginning of the year. We started having problems right away the first week. He did some of the same things last year, although it seems to be even more of a problem this year.

INTERVIEWER: And at home?

PARENT: Scott's always been a bit of a handful, but I agree, this last year has been even worse.

The interviewer transitions to ascertain duration of the behavior. It may be useful to further explore changes that may have occurred at the beginning of the year.

Behavior Setting

INTERVIEWER: Okay. So, we're going to focus on keeping his hands and feet to himself, and that involves not hitting, kicking, poking, jabbing, or shoving others. What I'd like to do now is to get an idea of the settings or places where this occurs. For instance, does it occur at other people's homes, on the playground, or at other places?

Summarization, followed by an eliciting statement to focus on where the behavior occurs.

PARENT: It happens just about everywhere! It's usually okay until he gets comfortable, then blam! He'll start poking away.

The interviewer could have pursued or should at least note that the behavior can come under control of a setting before the child becomes "comfortable."

INTERVIEWER: So you don't really see differences in, say, the grocery store, restaurants, relatives' homes, movies?

PARENT: No, not really.

Good use of an elicitor to clarify "everywhere."

INTERVIEWER: Okay. And at school?

TEACHER: It's pretty pervasive at school too. As I said, it happens at

The interviewer may want to summarize the parent's and teacher's earlier comments about settings, to convey attending and understanding—for

reading group, and at lunch and recess, or if we go to the library.

INTERVIEWER: So the poking
and shoving occurs in every setting.
What I'd like to do is get a sense of
priorities to help us stay focused and
provide us a place to start. Which of
the settings is most problematic?
Mrs. Smith?

PARENT: I'd say the dinner
table. It always turns into such a big
fight, and his father and I get upset
because we'd like a nice family meal.

INTERVIEWER: That's certainly
understandable. And at school?

TEACHER: Reading group is
probably the most problematic for
me.

Functional/Conditional Analysis

INTERVIEWER: Okay. Let's focus,
then, on dinnertime at home and
reading group at school. There are
usually things that happen before a
behavior that might trigger the behavior or set it off. So what typically
happens at home before Scott starts
poking at his siblings?

PARENT: Let me see if I can get
a picture. We always try to have the
kids sit down with us during dinner.
It's kind of a family time that we
think is important. The kids are usually playing or doing homework, and
I call them to dinner. Robert and
Molly usually come right away. Scott
I have to call a few times and then

example, "You said earlier it happens
in the lunchroom . . . is that right?
Where else do you see it occurring?"

As with prioritizing the behavior, a
less problematic target setting,
wherein more control can be exerted
for purposes of an intervention,
should be explored. The interviewer
also should elicit more specific information on setting variables such as
where people sit, room layouts, and
so on.

At this point, the interviewer should
ask the parent and teacher whether
the behavior and setting are adequately targeted and defined, and
are agreed upon. Good use of a
brief rationale for exploring antecedent conditions. The interviewer
should also consider exploring tem-
porally removed setting events that
may serve as stimuli for the behavior,
such as whether Scott is usually doing something enjoyable prior to
dinner, whether his siblings or other
children seem to pick on him, and so
forth.

send his brother to get him. Once I get him to the table, we say grace and pass dishes around . . .

INTERVIEWER: And do you notice anything else that happens before the poking?

PARENT: Not really. Sometimes he'll walk past his brother and ruffle his hair or something. Then we'll start eating, and he will kick under the table or something and the squabbling begins.

INTERVIEWER: Okay. And at school? What is happening just before Scott starts poking other kids during reading?

TEACHER: Well, there are six children, and we all sit around a large table at the back of the room. It usually happens when I'm helping another child to sound out a word or read a sentence. I'd say it's usually when my attention is on another child.

INTERVIEWER: Does that seem similar to what happens at home? I mean, when you are paying attention to someone other than Scott, is that when he pokes?

PARENT: I'm not sure. It could be, but I've never really looked for that specifically.

INTERVIEWER: Okay. Now what typically happens after the poking starts at the dinner table?

PARENT: As I said, the kids start squabbling, you know, "Mom, Scott's kicking me under the table" and, "Cut it out," and Scott denies it and

Although the interviewer is attempting to concentrate on antecedent variables, it often helps to allow the interviewee to describe the situation in his or her own words. In addition, sequential conditions may be important to ascertain, such as how the situation appears during the first moments of dinner/reading group, how soon after dinner begins does Scott start kicking, and so forth.

Good use of elicitors to explore a hypothesis about diverted attention as an antecedent event.

The interviewer elicits information about consequent events. It would have been useful to provide a rationale such as "I'd like to get a sense of what happens after the behavior that may be maintaining it or keeping it going." It is also important to ascer-

we get into the "did too, did not" argument.

INTERVIEWER: And what do you and your spouse do?

PARENT: Fred yells at Scott and tells him to keep his hands to himself and let his brother alone. I do the same thing. Sometimes I try to ignore it, and other times I just try to talk to them all, you know, explain that we're trying to have a family dinner.

INTERVIEWER: So the kids squabble, Fred yells, and you try different things. How about what happens after the poking in school?

TEACHER: The child who was poked reacts in pretty much the same way as your kids, and I'll have to stop what I'm doing and tell Scott to keep his hands to himself.

tain how the target child reacts to the consequent events—for example, "And how does Scott react when you tell him to stop?"

Again, the interviewer may want to ascertain how the child reacts to the consequences.

Existing Procedures

INTERVIEWER: How else have you dealt with the problem? Have you tried other procedures at home or school?

PARENT: We tried putting him at another table in the kitchen or sending him to his room, but I don't like that because I want the family to eat together. Besides, he just gets into mischief and I end up having to deal with him in the same way. Other than talking to him and trying to keep a lid on things, we haven't tried anything else.

INTERVIEWER: And at school?

TEACHER: We've tried sending notes home, but not necessarily for this behavior. You know, overall be-

The interviewer should consider a transition rationale such as, "I'd like to turn now and talk about some of the other things you've tried, to get a sense of what works and what doesn't." Eliciting information on existing procedures can provide information on the acceptability of potential interventions and on interventions that could be used but implemented differently.

havior during the day. I've called Mrs. Smith and I've tried moving him away from the other children and sitting him next to me, but the moment my back is turned he's right back at it.

INTERVIEWER: Have you tried different seating arrangements at home?

PARENT: We do that, and sometimes it works. But if I'm not watching, he'll poke on the way to the table or squirm around—we've got a pretty small table and dining area, so it's easy to get to his brother and sister.

The interviewer may want to validate and paraphrase the attempts the parent and teacher have made: "Sounds as if you've tried several things but nothing has worked consistently."

Behavior Strength

INTERVIEWER: And how many times during dinner, would you say, this behavior occurs?

PARENT: Probably a couple times or so.

INTERVIEWER: And how often during reading group?

TEACHER: Maybe three or four times. By the fourth time, I send him back to his desk.

A natural transition to ascertain the strength of the behavior. To get a better description of the behavior, the interviewer may want to ask about the intensity, duration, and/or whether each event typically is a single occurrence or a series of poking.

Behavioral Goal

INTERVIEWER: What do you think is an acceptable level of poking, if any?

PARENT: I know that kids poke one another once in awhile, but at the dinner table no poking is acceptable to me.

TEACHER: I agree. A little shoving and poking at recess and lunch is

The interviewer elicits perceptions of acceptable levels of behavior. It is useful to distinguish potential long- and short-term goals—for example, "I understand poking is unacceptable and we want to get rid of the behavior. In the short term, what do you think would be an interim goal that might show progress?"

normal. This behavior interrupts instruction.

Informant Attribution for the Behavior Function

INTERVIEWER: Okay. We've been talking for quite a while about Scott's poking. I'd like to get a sense of what the payoff is for this behavior. What function do you think the behavior serves for Scott? What need do you think he is expressing by poking his brother and sister?

The interviewer may want to rephrase this statement to provide a stronger rationale to help the informants understand: "Kids often do things for a purpose, such as trying to get something like attention or avoiding something they dislike. Why do you think Scott acts this way?"

PARENT: I'm not sure. He gets yelled at, but he sometimes gets his brother and sister in trouble because it escalates. I think he likes to get a rise out of people.

TEACHER: I think so, too. Hyper kids always fidget and fool around, but Scott! I think he wants to get a rise out of the other kids. I also think he wants my attention, if you want to know the truth.

The interviewer should make judicious use of verbal (uh-huh) and nonverbal attenders.

PARENT: Yeah, he does get a lot of attention, even though it's negative. I think the attention getting we talked about before is what he's after. You know, negative attention from just about everyone. Maybe we don't pay enough attention to him.

INTERVIEWER: It sounds as though you pay a lot of attention to him, but it's often to his negative behaviors.

TEACHER: I really think it's attention-getting behavior also. Getting attention from me and maybe to make friends, in an awkward way.

Good use of a paraphrase statement to diffuse the potential blame the parent perceives. To get a complete picture of the function of the behavior, the interviewer should ask whether the behavior serves an avoidance function, such as avoiding work (because of skill deficits), food the child dislikes, or talk about him at the dinner table.

INTERVIEWER: We've covered a lot of information here! Let me just recap a bit so I'm sure we're all working with the same information. Scott's poking behavior happens about three or four times during reading group and a couple times at dinner. Kids react by telling you, and telling him to stop. At home, you tell him to stop or try talking to him, and at school you end up removing him from the reading group. You'd like to see the poking stop, and it seems he does it to get a reaction from other kids and attention from you. Does that sound right?

PARENT: Yes.

TEACHER: Um-hmm.

Whenever a series of questions have been asked and information has been gatherered, it is appropriate to provide a summary such as this to be certain the information is correct and agreed upon.

Child's Strengths/Assets

INTERVIEWER: So far we've been talking about Scott's problems. What are his good points?

PARENT: Oh, he can be a real joy. He can be very loving and fun. . . .

TEACHER: And he has a great smile!

The interviewer should use encouragers such as smiles and nods.

PARENT: . . . and he loves to draw and figure out how things work, like clocks and motors.

TEACHER: That's true. He's very creative, and he really can be sweet when he wants to be.

Potential Reinforcers/Resources

INTERVIEWER: Sounds as though Scott has some endearing qualities. Now, what other kinds of

The interviewer will need to listen and watch carefully the reactions to the possible use of reinforcers in case

things does he like to do? I'm trying to get a sense of some things we might use to reinforce positive behavior in him. Mrs. Smith?

PARENT: He loves to play video games and watch cartoons, probably like any other boy his age. He also collects superhero cards. He likes to listen to music, but I won't let him have CDs because I just don't know what's on them. He also loves to eat, and he likes to stay at friends' houses, although he's not invited very often.

INTERVIEWER: And what does he like to eat?

PARENT: Pizza most of all. But he likes candy and soda—I try to keep his sugar and caffeine intake down, though!

INTERVIEWER: And at school?

TEACHER: At school, he likes recess and going to gym. I guess he gets to run out his energy. He also likes computer time and likes to show me what he can do.

INTERVIEWER: Staying with that a minute, are there other kinds of programs or resources at school that we could access?

TEACHER: You or the counselor could put him in one of your groups!

INTERVIEWER: Any other resources that might help?

TEACHER: Not that I can think of.

INTERVIEWER: How about at home? Do you have a computer or other kinds of support?

the parent or teacher objects to their use. The interviewer may need to discuss the appropriate use of reinforcers and fading procedures. Rephrasing the rationale to "things that might help to increase positive behavior or keeping his hands to himself" may offset potential misunderstanding.

It may be useful to ask whether the parent or teacher has used any of the potential reinforcers: "Have you tried having him earn any of these to help with his behaviors?" Although the question may open negative perceptions of reinforcers as "bribes," it is useful to know such acceptability issues.

The interviewer should acknowledge this statement; "That's certainly a possibility. I think it's also important for us to come up with some things that can help us figure out what to do at home and in the classroom."

PARENT: No, we don't have a computer. All the kids want one, but we just can't afford it.

INTERVIEWER: I understand, computers are expensive. Okay. I think we have a pretty good list. If anything else occurs to you, we can talk about it at the next meeting.

A summarization of the reinforcers and resources would be useful at this point.

Skill Deficits/Replacement Behaviors

INTERVIEWER: What skills does he seem to be lacking that cause him to resort to poking to get your attention or to make friends?

This elicitor could be worded more positively: "What skills do you think Scott needs to learn so he can seek attention appropriately or make friends?"

TEACHER: Well, if he could learn to wait for a more appropriate time, or learn a better way of getting my attention—or maybe he just doesn't know how to interact with the other kids.

INTERVIEWER: Mrs Smith?

PARENT: It seems to me he just doesn't know what else to do or that it's just an automatic reaction. I agree he doesn't seem to understand that his behaviors cause other kids to dislike him and us to get mad at him, even though it seems obvious. And it's too bad, because he really is a likeable little guy. I think if he could learn to get the attention without bothering other people. . . . I try to give him as much as I can, but I end up getting frustrated and upset.

Minimal encouragers and/or a reflective statement would be appropriate.

TEACHER: I'm in the same boat! He needs to learn to get attention at a better time and to keep his hands and feet to himself.

INTERVIEWER: So we're think-
ing he does this to get attention, and
what we will need to focus on is helping him to learn more appropriate
ways to get attention and to keep his
feet to himself. Does that sound
about right?

PARENT/TEACHER: Um-hmm.

Here the interviewer summarizes
the perceived function of the behavior, sets the stage for the intervention
phase, and asks for agreement.

Rationale and Procedures for Data Collection

INTERVIEWER: It will be helpful
to watch Scott for a week or so to
get a better idea of how often he
does the poking and to help us
key in on some important things
we may have missed, such as what's
happening to set the behavior off
or what may be keeping it going.
We also can use that information to
monitor improvement once we get
a plan in place. I know this is extra
work and we'd like to get a plan
in place right away, but it's important that we have a very clear picture so we can come up with a
plan that has a better chance of
working, one that we can design
specifically for you and Scott. So a
simple way for you to keep track
of the number of times he pokes is
to keep a count of the number of
times he does it. It is also helpful if
you watch carefully what happens
before and after. Does that sound
doable?

This is a very good use of a summary and rationale for data collection.
The interviewer may, however, want
to ask the parent and teacher for
more input on the procedure—for
example "What might be a good
way to keep track of the poking?"
The level of directiveness will depend on the interviewer's judgment
of the informants' skills.

PARENT: That's sounds easy
enough. Should I do this every
night?

INTERVIEWER: That would be

The interviewer should provide a
written data collection plan that includes the operationalized target behavior, the method of data collec-

best. And each day at school during reading time.

TEACHER: Okay.

INTERVIEWER: Can you both start right away tomorrow? Good. I'd also like to get into the classroom for an observation or two if that's okay. Then next week we'll have a good idea of what's going on.

tion, the time(s) for collection, and a space for recording antecedent and consequent events: "I'm going to write all this down so we don't have to try to remember it."

Next Appointment/Closing the Interview

INTERVIEWER: So let's set a time for next week when we can get together—thanks for coming.

The interviewer should provide a brief summary of the plan for the following interview: "In our next meeting we'll take a look at what we've seen during the week and decide where to go from there."

CASE ANALYSIS AND SUMMARY

For an analysis of this functional assessment interview, we refer to the interview goals introduced before the case example. As we analyze the components of the interview, we consider whether the interviewer has effectively met each of the goals.

◆ *Establish a positive working relationship among the participants.* As noted in the accompanying case comments, the interviewer appropriately incorporated several effective interviewing tactics, or PACERS (paraphrasing, attending, etc.). These tactics, along with the use of transition statements, kept the interview moving within the semistructured format and interview goals and appeared to bring both the parent and teacher comfortably into the problem-solving process.

◆ *Define the problem behavior in operational terms.* For this goal, it is fruitful to ask oneself whether the information is sufficient for identifying the behavior and its functional components. That is, are the target behavior and setting agreed upon and identified so that the behavior can be observed? The answer here is yes; the target behavior of poking and where it occurs were observable.

◆ *Identify behavioral antecedent, situation, and consequent conditions across settings.*

The interviewer ascertained some potential antecedent and consequent conditions, but failed to fully explore setting events and the child's reactions to the consequences—that is, the behavioral effects of the consequences. The conditional analysis of the behavior is the crux of functional assessment; therefore, the question to ask is whether there is a solid picture on which the interviewer can build hypotheses regarding manipulable variables. The answer here is that the level of information *may* have been adequate, but several pieces of the "behavior puzzle" were missing.

◆ *Provide a tentative identification of the frequency and duration of the behavior across settings.* Behavior strength across settings was tentatively identified, although more information on the duration of the behavior would have been helpful.

◆ *Set goals for behavior change across settings.* The interviewer set behavioral goals; however, the goals were set at zero occurrence without consideration of short-term goals.

◆ *Ascertain informant attributions for the behavior and its function.* Informant attributions were ascertained and led to the viable hypothesis that the poking behavior functioned to gain attention for the child. Although this goal was met, it could have been more fully explored by including avoidant functions of the behavior.

◆ *Establish hypotheses about skill deficits and replacement behaviors.* The interviewer adequately met this goal by discussing appropriate behaviors for receiving attention.

◆ *Establish a procedure for data collection.* This goal was met by incorporating an event-recording procedure across settings. It would have been helpful, however, to have the parent and teacher observe and record antecedent and consequent conditions to strengthen the information gathered during the interview.

◆ *Summary.* No problem-solving interview is perfect, as is the case with our example. This interview was adequate in that it met the major goals for a CFAI, but it lacked some specificity for more fully exploring the behaviors of concern and generating hypotheses regarding maintaining variables. With the semistructured format one may miss some information; however, it is important to remember that this is not a static process. The interviewer can always contact the parent and/or teacher to gather more information or to redefine the behavior and hypotheses once additional data are gathered.

CONCLUSION

In this chapter we have presented an overview of interview methods and a model for engaging in functional assessment interviews in school settings. We presented an example of a problem identification interview to provide an il-

lustration of interviewing skills and considerations for engaging in a functional assessment interview. We focused on problem identification because it is clearly the first important aspect of a functional assessment; if the behavior is not adequately identified, the likelihood is lessened that an effective intervention can be constructed (Witt & Elliott, 1983). Furthermore, the skills and procedures presented are used throughout the assessment process. Thus, these skills remain important whether one concludes after problem identification or continues in the problem-solving model and conducts a problem analysis and treatment evaluation interview (see Sheridan, et al., 1996).

It is important to note that the components (i.e., functional attribution, skills deficits, resources) we added have not been specifically evaluated in conjunction with the standardized consultation interviewing objectives, although these components are obviously similar in content to components in the established model. Furthermore, there are limited studies on whether the addition of functional components enhance treatment outcomes. Indeed, Schill, Kratochwill, and Elliott (1998) found that consultation treatment outcomes were the same whether a functional assessment occurred or a self-help treatment package was used without identifying functional aspects of behavior. Interestingly, the interviewers (consultants) in the study perceived greater improvement in child outcomes when using functional assessment methods and believed their relationships with the consultees were improved. Thus, although functional assessment interviewing appears to increase treatment validity, researchers have yet to provide compelling evidence to support its use over potentially less time-consuming methods or other interview formats.

As noted in this chapter and throughout this volume, assessment should be an ongoing, multidimensional process with data-based treatment decisions grounded on hypotheses drawn from converging assessment evidence. Interview data obtained from multiple informants provide integral information to be used in conjunction with other direct and indirect assessment procedures. Therefore, from a functional assessment standpoint, informant interviews are necessary but not sufficient for understanding functional variables and/or designing interventions. Regardless of whether the purpose is diagnosis, placement, or intervention, informant interviews have withstood the tests of time and research and will continue to be useful assessment tools.

REFERENCES

American Psychiatric Association (1980). *Diagnostic and statistical manual of mental disorders* (3rd ed.). Washington, DC: Author.

Angold, A., Cox, A., Rutter, M., & Siminoff, E. (1996). *Child and Adolescent Psychiatric Assessment* (CAPA): Version 4.2—Child Version. Durham, NC: Duke Medical Center.

Beaver, B. R., & Busse, R. T. (2000). Informant reports: Conceptual and research bases of interviews with parents and teachers. In E. S. Shapiro & T. R. Kratochwill (Eds), *Behavioral assessment in schools* (2nd ed): *Theory, research, and clinical foundations* (pp. 257–287). New York: Guilford Press.

Bergan, J. R (1977). *Behavioral consultation.* Columbus, OH: Merrill.

Bergan, J. R., & Kratochwill, T. R. (1990). *Behavioral consultation and therapy.* New York: Plenum Press.

Bergan, J. R., & Tombari, M. L. (1975). The analysis of verbal interactions occurring during consultation. *Journal of School Psychology, 13,* 209–225.

Bergan, J. R., & Tombari, M. L. (1976). Consultant skill and efficiency and the implementation and outcomes of consultation. *Journal of School Psychology, 14,* 3–14.

Busse, R. T., Kratochwill, T. R., & Elliott, S. N. (1999). Influences of verbal interactions during behavioral consultations on treatment outcomes. *Journal of School Psychology, 37,* 117–143.

Colton, D. L., & Sheridan, S. M. (1998). Conjoint behavioral consultation and social skills training: Enhancing the play behaviors of boys with attention deficit hyperactivity disorder. *Journal of Educational and Psychological Consultation, 9,* 3–28.

Cormier, W. H., & Cormier, L. S. (1985). *Interviewing stategies for helpers* (2nd ed.). Monterey, CA: Brooks/Cole.

Edelbrock, G., & Costello, A. J. (1990). Structured interviews for children and adolescents. In G. Goldstein & M. Hersen (Eds.), *Handbook of psychological assessment* (2nd ed., pp. 308–323). New York: Pergamon Press.

Elliott, S. N., & Busse, R. T. (1993). Effective treatments with behavioral consultation. In J. E. Zins, T. R. Kratochwill, & S. N. Elliott (Eds.), *Handbook of consultation services for children* (pp. 179–203). San Francisco: Jossey-Bass.

Galloway, J., & Sheridan, S. M. (1994). Implementing scientific practices through case studies: Examples of home–school interventions and consultation. *Journal of School Psychology, 32,* 385–413.

Gresham, F. M., & Davis, C. J. (1988). Behavioral interviews with teachers and parents. In E. S. Shapiro & T. R. Kratochwill (Eds.), *Behavior assessment in schools: Conceptual foundations and practical applications* (pp. 455–493). New York: Guilford Press.

Groth-Marnat, G. (1997). *Handbook of psychological assessment* (3rd ed.). New York: Wiley.

Hodges, K. (1997). *Child Assessment Schedule* (CAS). Ypsilanti, MI: Eastern Michigan University.

Ivey, A. E. (1994). *Intentional interviewing and counseling: Facilitating client development in a multicultural society.* Pacific Grove, CA: Brooks/Cole.

Kratochwill, T. R., & Bergan, J. R. (1990). *Behavioral consultation in applied settings: An individual guide.* New York: Plenum Press.

Kratochwill, T. R., Elliott, S. N., & Busse, R. T. (1995). Behavioral consultation training: A five-year evaluation of consultant and client outcomes. *School Psychology Quarterly, 10,* 87–117.

Kratochwill, T. R., Sheridan, S. M., Carrington Rotto, P., & Salmon, D. (1991). Preparation of school psychologists to serve as consultants for teachers of emotionally disturbed children. *School Psychology Review, 20,* 530–550.

Lapouse, R., & Monk, M. A. (1964). Behavior deviations in a representative sample of children: Variations by sex, age, race, social class, and family size. *American Journal of Orthopsychiatry, 34,* 436–446.

Larson, J., & Busse, R. T. (1998). *Outcomes-focused school consultation: Practical training on how to make the pre-referral building consultation team process work.* Workshop presented at the fall convention of the Wisconsin School Psychologist Association, Eau Claire, WI.

Lentz, F. E., & Wehmann, B. A. (1995). Best practices in interviewing. In A. Thomas & J. Grimes (Eds.), *Best practices in school psychology* (3rd ed., pp. 637–649). Washington, DC: National Association of School Psychologists.

Lewis, T. J., & Sugai, G. S. (1996). Functional assessment of problem behavior: A Pilot investigation of the comparative and interactive effects of teacher and peer social attention on students in general education settings. *School Psychology Quarterly, 11,* 1–19.

Orton, G. L. (1997). *Strategies for counseling with children and their parents.* Pacific Grove, CA: Brooks/Cole.

Orvaschel, H. (1995). *Schedule for Affective Disorders and Schizophrenia for School-Age Children—Epidemiological Version 5 (K-SADS-E5).* Ft. Lauderdale, FL: NOVA Southeastern University.

Reich, W. (Ed.). (1996). *Diagnostic Interview for Children and Adolescents—Revised* (DICA-R) 8.0. St. Louis: Washington University.

Reynolds, C. R., & Kamphaus, R. W. (1992). *Behavior assessment system for children.* Circle Pines, MN: American Guidance Service.

Rogers, C. R. (1951). *Client-centered therapy.* Boston: Houghton-Mifflin.

Sattler, J. M. (1988). *Assessment of children* (3rd ed.). San Diego, CA: Author.

Sattler, J. M. (1998). *Clinical and forensic interviewing of children and families: Guidelines for the mental health, education, pediatric, and child maltreatment fields.* San Diego, CA: Author.

Schill, M. T., Kratochwill, T. R., & Elliott, S. N. (1998). Functional assessment in behavioral consultation: A treatment utility study. *School Psychology Quarterly, 13,* 116–140.

Shaffer, D. (1996). *Diagnostic Interview Schedule for Children* (DISC-IV). New York: New York State Psychiatric Institute.

Shapiro, E. S. (1996). *Academic skills problems: Direct assessment and intervention* (2nd ed.). New York: Guilford Press.

Sheridan, S. M., & Kratochwill, T. R. (1992). Behavioral parent–teacher consultation: Conceptual and research considerations. *Journal of School Psychology, 30,* 117–139.

Sheridan, S. M., Kratochwill, T. R., & Bergan, J. R. (1996). *Conjoint behavioral consultation: A procedural manual.* New York: Plenum Press.

Sheridan, S. M., Kratochwill, T. R., & Elliot, S. N. (1990). Behavioral consultation with parents and teachers: Delivering treatment for socially withdrawn children at home and school. *School Psychology Review, 19,* 33–52.

Witt, J. C., & Elliott, S. N. (1983). Assessment in behavioral consultation: The initial interview. *School Psychology Review, 12,* 42–49.

CHAPTER 10

◆◆◆

Cultural and Linguistic Issues

◆

ELISA M. CASTILLO
STEPHEN M. QUINTANA
MANUEL X. ZAMARRIPA

Ethnic and linguistic minority (ELM) children constitute the most rapidly growing segment of the youth population in the United States. In fact, ethnic minority youth now constitute 35% of the U.S. public school population and more than 50% of the student population in many large urban school districts and several large states (e.g., Texas). Currently, 16% of students are African American, 12% are Hispanic, 3% are Asian or Pacific Islander, and 1% are American Indian or Alaskan Native. About 14% of students in grades K–12 speak languages other than English at home, and it is estimated that another 8% or more may speak a nonmainstream dialect (e.g., Black English).

Some have suggested, however, that psychology is at risk for "cultural malpractice" in its failure to respond effectively to the cultural diversification of the U.S. population (e.g., Hall, 1997). Relatively little information is available to aid psychologists and educators in their assessment of the problems, needs, and strengths of ELM children. The need for appropriate instrumentation and practices in the assessment of children from ELM backgrounds has been considered a pervasive problem in education and psychology (Padilla & Medina, 1996). Inappropriate assessment practices with ELM children and adolescents can lead to misdiagnosis, misguided interventions, or failure to intervene when necessary. Students who are inadequately assessed may be placed at increased risk for poor treatment in the educational system and inappropriate services.

Problems in assessment stem from many sources, including (1) historical bias in the development of psychological assessment procedures that have

been applied to ELM children, (2) disproportionate representation of ELM populations as research participants and as researchers, and (3) ecological or contextual issues that may contribute to a degree of mistrust of the psychological profession by some ELM communities. Traditional models within psychology have tended to view ethnic and linguistic minority groups as deficient and have failed to incorporate two important considerations: (1) the strengths, resources, and resilience of ethnic minority communities and (2) the role of outside forces (e.g. racism, discrimination, and bias) in the creation and maintenance of many of the problems faced by ELM children (García-Coll et al., 1996). Finally, assessment of ELM children may be significantly more complicated than it is for monolingual, English-speaking white children. For example, an examiner attempting to understand the process by which bilingual children process educational material in their nondominant language requires awareness of bilingual issues in addition to the educational issues associated with monolingual children. The American Psychological Association has drawn attention to the importance of providing culturally appropriate treatment, yet problems remain in the training and implementation of culturally appropriate practices (Hall, 1997; Quintana & Bernal, 1995).

The purpose of this chapter is to describe cultural competence for the practice of behavioral assessment of ELM children and adolescents. We focus on the cultural and linguistic aspects of four domains in such assessment: (1) characteristics of the examiner, (2) characteristics of the child, (3) characteristics of the assessment context, and (4) characteristics of the assessment procedures. Figure 10.1 pictorially represents the four domains. Each of these domains is influenced by and reflective of various cultural and linguis-

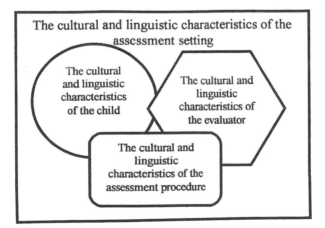

FIGURE 10.1. Four domains in the assessment of ethnic and linguistic minority children.

tic orientations. In each section of this chapter we briefly summarize important information related to cultural competence and make suggestions as to where more information may be obtained. We conclude with recommendations on continued training and development of skills in this area.

CULTURAL COMPETENCY OF THE EXAMINER

Cultural competency is a key concept in the counseling profession (Arredondo et. al., 1996; S. Lopez, 1997; D. W. Sue, Arredondo & McDavis, 1992; S. Sue, 1998). Some have suggested that the cultural competencies of an examiner maybe more important than the purported unbiased nature of an assessment instrument (Ponterotto & Alexander, 1996). In this section we describe the cultural competencies that have been broadly defined within the counseling profession and identify implications for assessment of ELM children using several models (S. Sue, 1998; D. W. Sue, et al., 1992).

S. Sue (1998) defined cultural competence as the practitioner's appreciation, recognition, and ability to work with the cultural characteristics of ELM groups. S. Sue identified three principles that are critical in cultural competency: (1) being scientifically minded, (2) having skills in dynamic sizing, and (3) being proficient with particular cultural groups.

Scientific mindedness refers to the ability of the practitioner to form tentative hypotheses, to develop creative ways of testing these hypotheses, and to act on the basis of collected data (S. Sue, 1998). In cross-cultural relationships between examiners and ELM children, errors are often made because the examiners have failed to test their assumptions about the children. Practitioners must test their clinical inferences by investigating possible cultural and adaptive reasons underlying children's behavioral problems. They can test their clinical inferences by observing an ELM child's behavior in different environments, consulting with other professionals that have expertise in working with the child's cultural group, and discussing the hypothesis with family members and, when appropriate, with the child.

Dynamic sizing refers to the ability to avoid stereotyping individuals, while not ignoring the critical cultural or linguistic features of an individual's psychological functioning (S. Sue, 1998). The examiner finds an appropriate "size" or way to generalize cultural characteristics to a child, but also appreciates the child's individuality, independent of the child's cultural group. Too often examiners stereotype an ELM child by attributing the cause of the child's problem to the child's cultural or linguistic characteristics, but at other times examiners ignore cultural characteristics that may be important factors in the ELM child's adjustment. Examiners must be accurate in assessing the role culture plays in the manifestation of children's behavioral disorders. This concept of dynamic sizing is similar to S. Lopez's (1997) *cultural lenses.* Ac-

cording to Lopez, cultural lenses allow examiners to be able to use both the mainstream cultural lens and a culture-specific lens when assessing an ELM child. To illustrate, consider a Southeast Asian adolescent who attributes her nightmares to a "weak spirit." If viewed clinically within a Western medical model, the nightmares might be understood as symptoms of an underlying disorder and the attributions to a weak spirit might be classified as delusional manifestations. Alternatively, if the nightmares are viewed within a culturally specific reference, the examiner may refer the child to an indigenous healer (e.g., shaman) or spiritual leader. Finally, if viewed interactively among cultural orientations, the nightmares may be conceptualized as a posttraumatic stress reaction attributable to the child's refugee status and expressed in a manner congruent with the way problems are expressed in her culture.

The third characteristic of cultural competence proposed by S. Sue (1998) is *culture-specific expertise*. Culturally skilled examiners have thorough knowledge and understanding of their own worldview, have specific knowledge of the cultural groups with whom they work, and understand the sociopolitical forces that affect such populations. These professionals are also able to use culturally based interventions and to translate interventions into strategies that are consistent with the client's cultural orientation. This characteristic, which appears to be complex, is similar to the model of cultural competency we consider next.

D. W. Sue et al. (1992) identified features of cultural competency for the counseling profession in three categories (knowledge, beliefs/attitudes, and skills) and across three areas (the practitioner's cultural background, the client's cultural background, and the cultural nature of the psychological intervention). This chapter elaborates and discusses the most relevant of these principles for assessment with children and adolescents. Table 10.1 is a summary of cultural competence for examiners based on the model developed by D. W. Sue et al. (1992).

Three areas of competence (attitudes, knowledge, and skills) in three areas (examiner's own culture, children's culture, and intervention strategies) have been identified within the counseling profession. We elaborate on these areas and draw implications for the assessment of children and adolescents in the following sections.

CULTURAL CHARACTERISTICS OF THE CHILD

As mentioned earlier, one of the most important features of cultural competency in the assessment process is the examiner's ability to integrate his or her awareness of the cultural characteristics of the child into the assessment process. Gibbs and Huang (1998) indicated four specific ways in which the child's culture can influence the assessment process (see Table 10.2).

TABLE 10.1. Cultural Competencies of Examiners

I. Examiner awareness of own cultural values and biases
   A. Attitudes and beliefs
      1. Culturally skilled examiners have moved from being culturally unaware to being aware and sensitive to their own cultural heritage and to valuing and respecting differences.
      2. Culturally skilled examiners are aware of how their own cultural backgrounds and experiences and attitudes, values, and biases influence psychological processes.
      3. Culturally skilled examiners are able to recognize the limits of their competencies and expertise.
      4. Culturally skilled examiners are comfortable with differences that exist between themselves and clients in terms of race, ethnicity, culture, and beliefs.

   B. Knowledge
      1. Culturally skilled examiners have specific knowledge about their own racial and cultural heritage and how it personally and professionally affects their definitions of normality–abnormality and the process of assessment.
      2. Culturally skilled examiners possess knowledge and understanding about how oppression, racism, discrimination, and stereotyping affect them personally and in their work. This understanding allows them to acknowledge their own racist attitudes, beliefs, and feelings. Although this standard applies to all groups, for white examiners it may mean that they understand how they may have directly or indirectly benefited from individual, institutional, and cultural racism (white identity development models).
      3. Culturally skilled examiners possess knowledge about their social impact on others. They are knowledgeable about communication style differences, how their style may clash with or foster the assessment process with minority clients, and how to anticipate the impact it may have on others.

   C. Skills
      1. Culturally skilled examiners seek out educational, consultative, and training experience to improve their understanding and effectiveness in working with culturally different populations. Being able to recognize the limits of their competencies, they (a) seek consultation, (b) seek further training or education, (c) refer clients to more qualified individuals or resources, or (d) engage in a combination of these actions.
      2. Culturally skilled examiners are constantly seeking to understand themselves as racial and cultural beings and are actively seeking a nonracist identity.

II. Examiner awareness of client's worldview
   A. Attitudes and beliefs
      1. Culturally skilled examiners are aware of their negative emotional reactions toward other racial and ethnic groups that may prove detrimental to their clients in assessment. They are willing to contrast their own beliefs and attitudes with those of their culturally different clients in a nonjudgmental fashion.
      2. Culturally skilled examiners are aware of the stereotypes and preconceived notions that they may hold toward other racial and ethnic minority groups.

TABLE 10.1. *Continued*

B. Knowledge
  1. Culturally skilled examiners possess specific knowledge and information about the particular group with which they are working. They are aware of the life experiences, cultural heritage, and historical background of their culturally different clients. This particular competency is strongly linked to the "minority identity development models" available in the literature.
  2. Culturally skilled examiners understand how race, culture, ethnicity, and so forth may affect personality formation, vocational choices, manifestation of psychological disorders, help-seeking behavior, and the appropriateness of psychological interventions.
  3. Culturally skilled examiners understand and have knowledge about sociopolitical influences that impinge on the life of racial and ethnic minorities. Immigration issues, poverty, racism, stereotyping, and powerlessness all leave major scars that may influence the assessment process.

C. Skills
  1. Culturally skilled examiners familiarize themselves with relevant research and the latest findings regarding mental health and mental disorders of various ethnic and racial groups. They actively seek out educational experiences that foster their knowledge, understanding, and cross-cultural skills.
  2. Culturally skilled examiners become actively involved with minority individuals outside the assessment setting (community events, social and political functions, celebrations, friendships, neighborhood groups, and so forth) so that their perspective of minorities is more than an academic or helping exercise.

III. Culturally appropriate intervention strategies
  A. Attitudes and beliefs
    1. Culturally skilled examiners respect clients' religious and/or spiritual beliefs and values, including attributions and taboos, because they affect worldview, psychosocial functioning, and expressions of distress.
    2. Culturally skilled examiners respect indigenous helping practices and minority communities' intrinsic help-giving networks.
    3. Culturally skilled examiners value bilingualism and do not view another language as an impediment to assessment (monolingualism may be the culprit).

  B. Knowledge
    1. Culturally skilled examiners have a clear and explicit knowledge and understanding of the generic characteristics of assessment and therapy (culture bound, class bound, and monolingual) and how they may clash with the cultural values of various minority groups.
    2. Culturally skilled examiners are aware of institutional barriers that prevent minorities from using mental health services.
    3. Culturally skilled examiners have knowledge of the potential bias in assessment instruments and use procedures and interpret findings keeping in mind the cultural and linguistic characteristics of the clients.
    4. Culturally skilled examiners have knowledge of minority family structures, hierarchies, values, and beliefs. They are knowledgeable about the community characteristics and the resources in the community as well as in the family.
    5. Culturally skilled examiners are aware of relevant discriminatory practices at the social and community level that may be affecting the psychological welfare of the population being served. (*continued*)

TABLE 10.1. *Continued*

C. Skills

1. Culturally skilled examiners are able to engage in a variety of verbal and nonverbal helping responses. They are able to *send* and *receive* both *verbal* and *nonverbal* messages *accurately* and *appropriately.* They are not tied to only one method or approach to helping but recognize that helping styles and approaches may be culture-bound. When they sense that their helping style is limited and potentially inappropriate, they can anticipate and ameliorate its negative impact.

2. Culturally skilled examiners are able to exercise institutional intervention skills on behalf of their clients. They can help clients determine whether a "problem" stems from racism or bias in others (the concept of health paranoia) so that clients do not inappropriately personalize problems.

3. Culturally skilled examiners are not averse to seeking consultation with traditional healers and religious and spiritual leaders and practitioners in the treatment of culturally different clients when appropriate.

4. Culturally skilled examiners take responsibility for interacting in the language requested by the client or, if not feasible, make appropriate referrals. A serious problem arises when the linguistic skills of an examiner do not match the language of the client. If this is the case, examiners should (a) seek a translator with cultural knowledge and appropriate professional background or (b) refer to a knowledgeable and competent bilingual examiner.

5. Culturally skilled examiners have training and expertise in the use of traditional assessment and testing instruments. They not only understand the technical aspects of the instruments, but are also aware of the cultural limitations. This knowledge allows them to use test instruments for the welfare of diverse clients.

6. Culturally skilled examiners attend to, as well as work to eliminate, biases, prejudices, and discriminatory practices. They should be cognizant of sociopolitical contexts in conducting evaluations and providing interventions and should develop sensitivity to issues of oppression, sexism, elitism, and racism.

7. Culturally skilled examiners take responsibility in educating their clients in the processes of psychological intervention, such as goals expectations, legal rights, and the examiner's orientation.

Note. From Sue, Arredondo, and McDavis (1992). Copyright 1992 by the American Counseling Association. Adapted by permission.

TABLE 10.2. Four Ways Culture Influences the Assessment Process

1. Culture influences a child's belief system about behaviors and characteristics associated with adjustment.

2. Culture influences how disorders (e. g., fear, depression, guilt, and anger) are expressed and manifested.

3. Culture influences help-seeking behaviors.

4. Culture influences treatment acceptability and responsiveness to treatment.

Note. Material abstracted from Gibbs and Huang (1998).

First, a child's cultural worldview plays a role in that child's mental health and school adjustment. Culture and ethnicity provide a framework for children in perceiving and responding to their environments. Culture influences children's worldviews, including their values, beliefs, and attitudes, which serve to organize and shape their perceptions, expectations, and behavior. Cultural heritage also affects children's group identity and self-concept. The worldviews of ELM children in the United States are also, to some extent, shaped by variables related to adapting to the majority culture, which can include coping with racism and discrimination.

Second, ethnicity shapes the child's belief system about what constitutes mental health or appropriate behavior. Ethnic culture also influences a child's manifestation of symptoms, defensive styles, and patterns of coping with a variety of emotions and conditions. Cultures vary in their tolerance and/or encouragement of a variety of behavioral, affective, social, and somatic expressions. Thus, children are socialized into a pattern of behavior that is culturally reinforced. Research has documented important differences across cultural groups in the determination of which behaviors are considered problematic, as well as the bandwidth for behavioral norms (Crijnen, Achenbach, & Verhulst, 1997). For example, Lambert et al. (1992) found cultural differences in the threshold for behavioral problems as judged by Jamaican and U.S. parents, teachers, and clinicians. Jamaican raters were more tolerant of a wider range of behavior in children before considering a behavior problematic, as compared with U.S. raters. Similarly, research has found that whereas white children prefer academic environments that are quiet and subdued over those that are vibrant and active, the reverse pattern was characteristic of African American children (Bell, 1994; Boykin & Allen, 1988).

Third, ethnicity determines the help-seeking behaviors in which children and families engage. ELM families tend to underutilize mental health services in favor of more indigenous methods of healing (Aponte, Rivers, & Wohl, 1995). Fourth, ethnicity is also a factor in the way the child uses and responds to treatment. The attitude toward self-disclosure, the motivation to participate in an assessment or a treatment, the perception of a problem, and the acceptability of a treatment plan are all filtered through the screen of ethnicity. Aponte et al. (1995) have suggested that because Western psychology tends to focus on the individual, it encourages (1) verbal, emotional, and behavioral assertiveness, (2) a linear approach to problems, and (3) a clear distinction between physical and mental functioning. Disparities between this Western model and the worldviews of ELM populations can be found in all of these dimensions (Aponte, et al., 1995).

Clearly, the child's culture has a significant impact on the assessment process. There are several frameworks for conceptualizing characteristics that may have important implications for working with ethnic and linguistic minority children. In this section we discuss primary cultural characteristics,

cultural adaptation, and other factors that influence ELM children, such as migration history, socioeconomic status, social support, and language. We end this section with a summary of information that examiners should know or collect about ELM children with whom they work.

Primary Cultural Characteristics

Primary cultural characteristics are those characteristics in a cultural group that occur prior to contact with another cultural group, whereas secondary cultural characteristics occur because of, or in response to, contact between cultural groups. Examples of primary cultural characteristics of Mexican Americans are the Spanish language and cultural values that can be traced to Mexico. Several theorists (e.g., Trandis, Bontempo, Villareal, Asai, & Lucca, 1988; Greenfield & Cocking, 1994) have established frameworks for understanding primary cultural characteristics. They have identified the individualism/collectivism continuum as a critical dimension that characterizes differences in primary cultural characteristics in cultures throughout the world. Collectivism is characterized by the tendency to give priority to the goals of a collective unit, such as the family, village, or group, and is associated with cooperation, in-group cohesion, deference to authority, emotional attachment to the group, and a sense of self defined as a representative of the group (Triandis et al., 1988). Conversely, individualism is defined as the tendency to give priority to the goals of individuals and is associated with competition (between individuals), self-reliance, hedonism, and assertiveness (Triandis et al., 1988). The ELM cultural groups within the United States vary in adherence to collectivist goals, although many are more collectivist, in a general manner, than English-speaking white children in the United States. For example, some Asian (e.g., Japanese, Chinese, and Korean) cultures in particular tend to emphasize group harmony, personal modesty, obedience to authority, and filial piety (see Greenfield & Cocking, 1994). Children who are descendants from Latin America tend to value respect, preservation of dignity, and cooperation (Triandis et. al., 1988). Research has found, for example, that Latino children in the United States were willing to share lunch money even with peers whom they did not like (Rotheram-Borus & Phinney, 1990). Some African-descent children may be socialized toward individual expressiveness (e.g., demonstrate individual talents), but be collectivist in many other characteristics (Boykin, 1986). Some American Indian tribes (e.g., Navajos) tend to emphasize holistic cognitive processing (Tharp, 1994).

Clearly, there are many more cultural differences between and within ELM groups in the United States than we can describe here. Interested readers may wish to find other sources detailing these cultural differences (e.g., Greenfield & Cocking, 1994). See Table 10.3 for ideas on basic information on cultural characteristics that can be collected in an assessment.

TABLE 10.3. Basic Information Examiners Should Know about Primary Cultural Characteristics

---

◆ What are the predominant religious and spiritual beliefs?

◆ How do members of this culture communicate (verbal/nonverbal, high context/low context)?

◆ What are social norms governing social interactions (e.g., respect, dignity, formality, cooperation, etc.).

◆ What are the socialization norms within families (e.g., parental authority)?

◆ What are the age- and gender-related expectations for children?

◆ Where do members seek medical, psychological, behavioral, and spiritual guidance?

Cultural Adaptation

Besides acquiring knowledge on a child's primary cultural characteristics, it is important to understand how the child has adjusted to the mainstream culture and is able to negotiate living within more than one cultural context. Three factors influence cultural adaptation: acculturation, second culture acquisition, and other sociocultural influences.

Acculturation

Acculturation is the process of adjustment and adaptation that occurs when two cultural groups have contact (Berry, 1993). Contact between two cultural groups often results from immigration, migration, or other sociological trends. Through this contact, each cultural group responds to, adapts to, and, in many cases, adopts some of the characteristics of the other. Although we usually think of minority cultural or immigrant groups adjusting or adapting to the more dominant cultural groups, Berry (1993) stressed that acculturation processes affect both minority and dominant groups.

The degree of acculturation in a cultural minority child is a rough guide to the extent to which this child has adopted cultural characteristics of the more dominant group, as well as the extent to which the child (or child's family) can access resources that are controlled by the dominant cultural groups. Originally, the process of acculturation for minority groups was thought to proceed toward the gradual replacement of the characteristics of the minority group's native culture with the adoption of cultural characteristics of the dominant group. However, research has suggested that adoption of some dominant cultural characteristics does not necessarily imply the loss of native cultural characteristics (e.g., Berry, 1993). In the same way that children can become bilingual, they can also become bicultural, becoming conversant and comfortable in two cultures. This bicultural orientation has been associated

with positive adjustment (Berry, 1993). Nonetheless, for the purposes of assessment, it may be useful to assess the child's level of acculturation to dominant cultural norms, as these characteristics have been found to be critically important in assessment (Velasquez, Ayala, & Mendoza, 1998).

The strongest markers of a child's degree of acculturation to dominant cultural norms are (1) the child's language ability and usage, (2) the length of stay in the dominant culture of the child or the child's family, and (3) the extent of exposure to members of the dominant culture. Children whose first language is that of the dominant culture tend to be more acculturated than children whose first language is not. Similarly, those children who are fluent in the language of the dominant culture tend to be more acculturated than are children who are not fluent. The generational status of the child or the child's family is often associated with the level of acculturation to dominant culture, with recent immigrants being less acculturated than second- or third-generation families. Finally, the degree of the child's extended and intimate exposure to members of the dominant culture also tends to be associated with acculturation status. Children who live in integrated neighborhoods tend to be more acculturated than those who live in segregated ethnic enclaves. For any individual child, these sociological markers must be supplemented with a more individualized exploration of the child's behavioral, social, attitudinal, and ideological dimensions of acculturation. Information regarding the child's culture is useful, but examiners should be careful not to stereotype any child because of acculturation status.

Second Culture Acquisition

Biculturalism involves the capacity to function in more than one culture and to integrate various cultural influences. LaFromboise, Coleman, and Gerton (1993) have suggested that attention be given to one particular dimension of acculturation: the process of second culture acquisition. They identified several strategies for coping with cultural diversity, which range from cultural segregation, to assimilation, to bicultural integration (see Table 10.4). Examiners can use this framework to conceptualize the way in which an ELM child or family is coping with cultural diversity. Children who cope by separating or segregating themselves from other cultural groups may do so in response to racism and discrimination (Quintana, Vera, & Cooper, 1999). For these children, it seems important for the examiner to consider the role of racism, the children's perception of it, and the children's response to it, in the assessment process. Children who segregate themselves from other cultural groups may have difficulty in trusting members of other cultural groups. If the children's teachers are ethnically or racially different, the children who use separation may resist their power and influence.

In other ELM children, there may be an attempt to assimilate or accul-

TABLE 10.4. Styles for Coping with Cultural Diversity

Coping style	Description of style
Fusion/integration	Child attempts to integrate or fuse two or more cultural orientations simultaneously.
Alternation	Child attempts to integrate two or more cultural orientations sequentially.
Separation	Child becomes immersed in own cultural group and avoids interaction with other cultural group.
Acculturation/assimilation	Child immerses self in other cultural group—and may minimize contact with own cultural group.

Note. Based on LaFromboise, Coleman, and Gerton (1993).

turate into the dominant culture by adopting the characteristics of the dominant group while abandoning or losing the cultural characteristics of their own group. However, the push to assimilate and abandon their home culture may be associated with negative feelings about their native culture (i.e., internalized racism). This potential negativity can be reinforced by the school culture, which often encourages an assimilation orientation (Davidson, 1996). Thus, a child may begin to look upon his or her culture as a source of shame or anger. Children who follow an assimilation strategy may encounter conflict with other children of their own cultural group; that is, children who choose to assimilate may be viewed as "traitors" or "sellouts" by those of their culture.

Between these two extreme orientations to coping with diversity, there is a range of strategies for integrating two cultures. Some may choose to try to fuse the two cultures by including simultaneous components of each culture in their social relationships and activities. This kind of fusion or integration of two cultures may be most easy to implement if the child's environment has a multicultural orientation in which cultural differences are appreciated and accepted. The extent to which children's environments encourage or reward one culture over another will determine the level of stress created for children who are coping with an integrative cultural style.

A particularly important means of coping with cultural diversity for children of immigrant or refugee parents is the alternation strategy. Children of parents who have recently arrived in the United States are often exposed to two very different cultures: a dominant school culture and their parent's culture. For these children, an attempt to fuse the two cultures may appear difficult, and they find themselves alternating between the two. The alternation strategy involves, for example, the child's conforming to the school culture when at school and following the parent's cultural patterns while at home. Although this strategy may be particularly viable for children of immi-

grants, children of groups experiencing tensions with other cultural groups may also benefit from using this strategy. In a recent study, Quintana et al. (1999) found that African American children following the alternation strategy evidenced positive signs of adjustment in their cultural coping.

Other Sociocultural Influences

Further information about a child's cultural context can be useful in understanding the environmental factors that affect the child: migration history, socioeconomic status, educational attainment, and social support. Such variables should be considered separately from the role of the family's culture in the child's behavior.

The family's reason for moving to this country can provide insight into the child's behavior and the dynamics of the child's family. Although cultural groups tend to share similar migration trends, each family's story is unique and is a rich source of information for the examiner. Ogbu (1994) classified three types of minority status in terms of how and why people came to this country. Voluntary or immigrant minorities are those who enter a new country by choice. For Ogbu, voluntary minority status means that the immigrants perceive that they were not forced, but chose to become a minority in another country. Consequently, voluntary minorities are receptive to acquiring and adjusting to the dominant cultural patterns, much like a tourist to a new country is willing to learn about the new country and is likely to attribute cultural conflicts that may arise to his or her own lack of knowledge about the host country's culture.

Conversely, Ogbu classified involuntary minorities as those groups who were initially incorporated into the host country against their will through conquest, slavery, or colonization. Native Americans and African Americans are examples of involuntary minorities. Ogbu described secondary cultural characteristics that may emerge in involuntary minority groups. Secondary cultural characteristics are those cultural characteristics that emerge in a cultural group in response to cultural conflict and tension with the majority cultural groups. As a result of the legacy of slavery, discrimination, and racism experienced by involuntary minority groups, coping mechanisms (i.e., secondary cultural characteristics) develop, which include distrust of the dominant cultural group and the development of oppositional identity. That is, for involuntary minorities, acquisition of the cultural characteristics of the dominant culture may be viewed as a threat to their identity, and, consequently, they may resist assimilation influences. Social psychologists (e.g., Crocker and Major, 1989; Osborne, 1997) have examined some of these secondary cultural characteristics, such as the coping with stigmatization and academic disidentification that may occur with some involuntary minority groups.

Refugees cannot be included within this involuntary/voluntary minority

group classification, because, unlike voluntary minority groups, they were forced to migrate, and, unlike involuntary groups, they do not have a history of discrimination with their host country.

The process of migration and acculturation is difficult for each member of an ELM family, and these varying responses to the process often create problems within the family. Research has found that family members were often unaware that some of their difficulties resulted from their migration and acculturation experiences. Thus, parents tended to attribute the cause of conflict to their children's having been negatively influenced by American culture (Aponte et al., 1995).

Socioeconomic status (SES) variables are important mediators in students' adjustment in schools. Although the majority of poor children are white, a disproportionate number of poor children are African American, Native American, and Latino (McLoyd, 1998). Families of lower SES, as compared with their peers, are disadvantaged by reduced accessibility to jobs, high-quality private and public services (schools, day care, parks, community centers), and informal social supports (Mash & Barkley, 1996). They are also more likely to be exposed to environmental stressors such as street violence, illegal drugs, and negative role models. Research has found that income and SES have been linked to differences in cognitive development, school achievement, and socioemotional functioning (McLoyd, 1998).

A particularly important component of social class is the educational background of a family. The parent's familiarity with the school system, and success within that system, will have a great impact on the child's academic achievement. Some families may value their child's education but may be unfamiliar with the expectations and demands placed on the child in the school setting, may be unable to assist the child with schoolwork, may have difficulty communicating with the school personnel regarding the child's educational needs, and may give mixed messages to the child about their expectations. A study by Okagaki and Sternberg (1993) found that parents from different cultural backgrounds differed in beliefs about child rearing, intelligence, and education. For example, parents from ELM groups differed from white parents in that the former suggested that noncognitive characteristics (e.g., motivation) were as or more important than cognitive characteristics of academic performance (Okagagi & Sternberg, 1993). Hence, information about the family's economic and educational backgrounds and their expectations and hopes for the children's education may be critical to consider in an assessment.

Considerations Specific to Children's Language Characteristics

Linguistic ability varies considerably among children in the United States who are raised in homes in which standard English may not be the dominant

language (limited English proficiency, or LEP). Children from these homes may not develop fluency in English prior to their entry into public schools. Fortunately, there has been substantial research into second language acquisition, which has identified several trends in the development of verbal and academic skills. Unfortunately, there has been relatively little research into the implications of second language acquisition specific to assessment purposes.

Research into second language acquisition has made an important distinction between the development of a second language (e.g., English) and the development of verbal reasoning abilities, including the understanding of academic concepts. This distinction is, of course, unnecessary in developing curriculum for children whose native language is the dominant language. However, for bilingual children the comprehension of advanced verbal and academic concepts may be in either their first or second language. In the United States, educators attempting to promote the English language skills of LEP children have often recommended to parents—who often have only limited proficiency in English—that they speak more English to their children (Ortiz, 1997). This recommendation can have unintended consequences. For example, parents who have limited English proficiency may be unable to provide the critical language stimulation for advanced verbal concepts in English that they could provide in their native language. In these cases, children may be robbed of an important source of stimulation, which may stunt their language development. Hence, parents should be advised to speak more, not less, of the children's native language to provide complex and stimulating language models for their children and thereby promote children's cognitive and intellectual development (Ortiz, 1997).

Similarly, research investigating bilingual education suggests that children who are integrated into English classrooms later, as compared with children who have early entry into English immersion classrooms, have high scores on achievement skills (e.g., reading, math) even though these skills are assessed in English (Padilla et al., 1991). This pattern of findings indicates that proficiency in LEP children's native language is a critical basis for learning English proficiency (Cummins, 1984). Research also suggests that ELM children need strong educational experience in their own language and traditions before they can cope and succeed in mainstream society.

Language is associated with cultural, social, and cognitive variables. Bilingualism has been linked to positive cognitive characteristics. Bilingual youth score significantly higher on verbal and nonverbal measures of intelligence and achievement, are more flexible in their cognition, are more creative, and have increased problem-solving ability (Lambert, 1981). These positive characteristics of bilingual children only occur if the two languages are accorded similar social value and respect. Language minority children in the United States are often pressured to develop English language skills at the

expense of the home language. Such a case is referred to as the *subtractive* bilingual, wherein the individual is forced to put aside or subtract out his or her ethnic language for the more prestigious national language (Hamers & Blanc, 1989). This form of bilingualism can be devastating, because it can place the youth in a psycholinguistic limbo where neither language is a useful tool of thought and expression (Lambert, 1981). The subtractive bilingual person can also experience identity conflict and acculturative stress when the person's culture is stigmatized by the society (Hamers & Blanc, 1989).

Language assessment should address emotional, as well as cognitive and academic, concerns. If children cannot identify cultural norms for expression and cannot regulate emotional displays, they are likely to experience difficulties. Vano and Pennenbaker (1997) examined the relationship between emotion vocabulary and school adjustment. They found that problems associated with acting out were most common among students with a wide disparity in emotional vocabulary between English and their native language (Spanish).

Bilingual children show a range of linguistic competencies, and their expertise in either language is dependent on their age, ability level, language(s) of instruction, and amount of exposure to specific languages (Rogers, 1998). The ability to converse socially in a language is different from the ability to engage in an academically demanding task. It is important that a child's speaking, writing, and reading skills be evaluated in both English and the child's native language to determine the child's language proficiency as well as the language in which an assessment should be conducted. Language assessment is discussed further in a following section.

In addition, it is important to note that language not only influences the performance of ELM children but also influences other people's perceptions of such children. Many studies have shown that individuals and groups may be positively or negatively evaluated according to the language they speak. Children who speak with a French accent (a valorized language) are perceived in a more positive light than students speaking with an accent of a less valorized language (Hamers & Blanc, 1989).

Ortiz (1997) and Stockman (1986) generalized the principles of second language acquisition to those situations in which children are exposed to Black English rather than Standard English as the main basis for oral and written communication prior to beginning formal schooling. Clearly, it is critical for those conducting assessments and making recommendations for language minority children to become familiar with research on second language acquisition.

All of the considerations mentioned in this section regarding primary cultural characteristics, sociocultural adjustment, social mediating variables, and language are important in understanding the cultural context of ELM children. Table 10.5 includes questions for practitioners to use as a guide in

TABLE 10.5. Questions for an Evaluator to Consider in the Assessment of an ELM Child

What is the child's ethnic or cultural background?

What is his or her degree of English proficiency? What is the client's preferred language?

Is the client first or second generation? What is his or her acculturation level?

How does the child cope with different cultural contexts?

When did the family migrate? What were the reasons for migration?

Is the family living in the United States legally?

Has the child lost relatives because of separation or violence?

Who lives with the family? Has the family been separated during or because of immigration?

How long has the family been in the current residence?

What is the family's socioeconomic status? What are the parents' occupations?

Is the child living in an environment of multiple stressors?

What are the parents' attitudes toward education?

What are the parents' educational background and experience?

In what ways can parents help the child with his or her adjustment to school (e. g., homework)?

What are the consequences to the child for school success or failure?

What are the child's responsibilities to the family?

In what ways is the child encouraged to be independent?

Are there differences in expectations between males and females because of gender role socialization?

How is the child expected to interact with adults? How is the child disciplined?

In what ways does the child demonstrate collectivisitic and individualistic goals?

How involved is the family in the community?

What is the child's support system?

Does the child interact comfortably with other cultural groups?

What are the child's past experiences with mental health professionals, psychologists, academic settings, and other professionals?

What are the cultural explanations for the child's condition or problem?

What forms of treatment are indigenous to the culture?

How do language and cultural differences affect the examiner's ability to communicate with and understand the client's concern?

In what ways can the clinician modify the interview or the assessment to establish rapport and perform an adequate assessment?

Does the clinician share the majority culture's stereotype of the client's culture? Does the client hold a culturally biased view of the clinician?

Note. Material abstracted from Rogers (1998) and Mendez-Villarubia and Labruzza (1994).

gathering information about ELM children with whom they are working. In answering these questions, the evaluator should develop a good understanding of a child's cultural context.

CULTURAL CONTEXT OF THE ASSESSMENT ENVIRONMENT

Many have stressed the value of ecologically or contextually based assessment approaches (Armour-Thomas & Gopaul-McNichol, 1997). Ecological assessment approaches emphasize the impact of children's behavior on the culture of the various environments in which the children are engaged, and vice versa. Rogers (1998) has viewed environmental assessment as an essential component of the process to help the examiner understand the social context of the child. An environmental assessment includes a systematic analysis of the characteristics of the classroom, school, home, and community environments in which the child functions. Assesors should also examine the norms, culture, climate, and power relationships that exist within the schools. They should be aware of the factors within the school that promote achievement and health in ELM children, and of the barriers to success.

García Coll et al. (1996) described an ecological, integrative model conceptualizing the developmental context of ELM children. They identified the ecological factors that inhibit or promote children's adjustment and development. These factors include environmental stress resulting from segregation (residential, economic, social, and psychological) and discrimination (racism, oppression, and prejudice), local communities (neighborhoods and schools), and social services (medical and psychological services). These ecological factors may be important to the assessment process (1) as possible contributing factors to a behavioral problem, (2) by influencing the process for the referral, and (3) by affecting recommendations and interventions.

Evaluators conducting behavioral assessments in schools should be aware of the cultural context of the school setting. Culture influences a school environment as much as it does children. Schools, like other institutions, are places where bias occurs, and examiners must evaluate the degree to which bias is affecting a child's experience in the school environment. Examiners must be skilled in developing, implementing, and evaluating techniques designed to eliminate the bias, prejudice, and oppression that exists on both an individual and an institutional level (Rogers, 1998).

It is important that examiners consider how the assessment process is influenced by differences between the school culture and cultural norms of ELM children. Weisz and Weiss (1991) found significant cultural differences for "referability" of child problems. Referability refers to the ratio of the fre-

quency of a behavior pattern being referred for professional attention, divided by the incidence of the behavior pattern in the population. Uncontrolled behavioral problems (e.g., swearing, lying, cheating, arguing) were referred for treatment or assessment in the United States more often than in Thailand; there were no cultural differences for overcontrolled behavioral problems (e.g., depression). Hence, the U.S. culture in general, and school cultures within the United States in particular, may be less tolerant of undercontrolled behavioral problems as compared with other cultures. In some situations it may be appropriate for examiners to work with school personnel to revise their cultural expectations for children's behavior or help them revise their pedagogy in order to be compatible with the cultures of ELM children. Some referrals may possibly reflect ethnic bias or stereotyping by the person making the referral. In these situations, it may be important for the examiner first to work with the person making the referral to address this bias. It may be helpful to have an examiner observe the child's behavior, using behavioral norms reflective of the child's ELM group, to detect the presence or absence of a behavioral problem independent of the referral source. It is also possible that prejudice or bias within the school environment is responsible for or contributes to the manifestation of behavioral problems. In these situations, the assessment of behavioral problems would be incomplete without addressing the prejudice or bias to which the children are exposed. Similarly, in situations in which children's resistance to assimilation pressures contribute to the manifestation of behaviors, it is important that examiners supplement their assessment of the child with consideration of such pressures within the school culture.

Clearly, it is important that examiners consider the historical context of relations between ELM communities and the educational system. Indeed, Baker and O'Neil have reported on their experiences in attempting to enact educational reform (i.e., performance assessment) that they believed would increase the cultural fairness of the educational system for ELM children. They were surprised by the response from the ELM community, which considered the reform to be the "creation of the majority community intended to hold back the progress of disadvantaged children" (Baker & O'Neil, 1996, p. 185). Obviously, the response of the ELM community was not based solely on the nature of the proposed reform, but rather reflected a long history of the ELM community's responses to previous educational initiatives, which were viewed as undermining the interests of the community. Moreover, because psychological examiners are likely to be perceived as the latest representatives of the educational system, this mistrust may undermine the educational goals being addressed in a behavioral assessment.

We recommend that the evaluator consider the impact of the relationship between the ELM community and the school or the conceptualization of the behavior problem of the child, the assessment process, and the will-

ingness to seek treatment. The examiner should consider the child's having to cope with racism, stigmatization, and other ecological factors affecting adjustment. Examiners should be prepared for the ELM children, parents, and community to respond to them as members of the educational system with which there has been a long history of interactions potentially marked by misunderstanding and mistrust. Examiners may need to make particular efforts to establish credibility before receiving ELM members' trust and cooperation. Ideally, examiners should have a history of visible involvement and participation in support of the community. They may need to take additional time and care to understand the community's relationship with the educational system. Obviously, it may be unwise to assume that the efforts of the examiner will be viewed as serving the interest and benefit of ELM children. Credibility with ELM communities is not established simply by being careful not to be discriminatory. Rather, credibility is based on demonstrating that the efforts of the educational establishment give priority to the welfare of the child. Finally, examiners may have to establish collaborative working relationships with children, parents, and other members of the ELM community, in which the interests and welfare of the ELM child are central.

CULTURAL AND LINGUISTIC CHARACTERISTICS OF ASSESSMENT PROCEDURES

The fourth major area of cultural competency is the examiner's awareness of the cultural implications of psychological assessments and his or her ability to implement culturally and linguistically appropriate assessment procedures. This kind of competency requires the examiner to be aware of the underlying cultural assumptions of the assessment procedures. That is, an assessment procedure may have been implicitly developed for one particular cultural population. In addition, there may be critical modifications needed for tailoring assessments for a cross-cultural context. For example, additional time or procedures may be required to develop the necessary rapport in a cross-cultural context that may not be required in a monocultural situation. There may also be some procedures indigenous to a child's culture that can be implemented to obtain the most relevant information about the psychological functioning of the child. For example, in extended kinship contexts, the examiner may need to include more than the "nuclear" family in the procedures and instead include, for example, *padrinos* (godparents), religious leaders, or other influential persons in the child's culture. There may also be necessary adjustments related to language to ensure cultural equivalence in generalizing cross-culturally. Finally, multicultural assessment models are recommended to help practitioners arrive at sound assessment decisions.

Behavioral Assessment Procedures

For a practitioner conducting a behavioral assessment, it is vital to examine the cultural assumptions underlying this form of assessment. Behavioral assessment, like most psychological interventions, is derived from Western European/North American worldviews. Examining such assumptions is crucial in conducting culturally competent assessments. There are various reasons that behavioral assessment has been found, in some ways, to be culturally appropriate for ethnic and linguistic minority (ELM) children. Behavioral assessment traditionally gathers information on the role of the environment in the child's identified problem and integrates information about the child's strengths. These two areas are often lacking in traditional assessments of ELM children. Moreover, behavioral assessment has been described as an effective strategy in the assessment and treatment of culturally diverse populations because of certain inherent characteristics that tend to be culturally congruent with such populations. For example, behavioral strategies tend to be concrete, action oriented, and focused on the immediate and on learning (Paniagua, 1994). The integration of these factors into an assessment procedure is a positive step toward cultural competence.

Tailoring the Assessment Procedure To Be More Culturally Congruent

It is important to be aware that the format for an assessment may be alien and potentially threatening to children of ELM cultures. The examiner can inform children of expectations and strategies related to test-taking procedures, provide freedom of movement for children who are particularly active, and establish a comfortable and cooperative environment to facilitate accuracy in the assessment process (Thomas-Presswood, Sasso & Gin, 1997). Culturally biased attitudes weigh heavily on a client's expectations regarding assessments. Rosenberg-Ostereld and Haber (1997) found that ELM parents were suspicious about the purpose and the effects of assessment of their children. One family may be relieved that a child is being assessed, because they believe that the assessment will provide a greater understanding of the child's needs and connect him or her with beneficial services. Such parents will encourage the child to be truthful and express him- or herself freely. Another family, however, may feel ashamed that the child is being singled out for an assessment, may fear loss of face (respect) in their community because of the child's failure to comply with school expectations, and may encourage the child to behave properly in the assessment and minimize the problem. It is crucial that examiners attempt to clarify and reconcile their expectations of an assessment with those of the child and family.

In order to obtain important information about an ELM child, the ex-

aminer may have to collect data from a variety of sources and settings. Information regarding the child should be gathered from various teachers, professionals, relatives, and members of the child's cultural groups. Some researchers recommend a multisource, multilevel, and multimethod approach to assess the capacities, potentials, and limitations of the client (Ridley, Li, & Hill, 1998). This method of collecting data can access the various cultural contexts that influence the child's experience.

It is important for the examiner to establish rapport with the family. It may be helpful to speak with the family to explain the reason for the assessment and the role of the examiner and to enlist the family's participation. The competencies in establishing this relationship have been divided into three levels (Paniagua, 1994). The first is the *conceptual level,* which includes the client's and the practitioner's perceptions of sincerity, openness, honesty, motivation, empathy, and credibility. The *behavioral level* includes the client's perception of the practitioner as competent in the particular assessment and intervention procedure. This level also includes the practitioner's perception of the client's ability to participate effectively in the intervention. The final level is the *cultural level,* which includes two approaches. The cultural compatibility approach minimizes ethnic and cultural barriers between the practitioner and the client. (i.e., the examiner and the client share similar cultural backgrounds). The other approach is the universalistic, which involves the examiner's ability to display cultural sensitivity and cultural competence. Because the first approach may not be feasible in many situations, the second approach has been more widely adopted in the field (see D. W. Sue et al. 1992).

Examiners are encouraged to establish credibility and competence on each of these three levels. Another important consideration in the cultural context of the testing situation is how the results are going to be used. Assessment should yield necessary and sufficient evidence regarding the nature and quality of the problem, as well as the ecological or environmental factors that facilitate or impede its expression (Armour-Thomas & Gopaul-McNicol, 1997). When a child is initially referred by the school, close attention must be paid to the reasons for the referral. Examiners are advised to consider (1) bias as the reason for the referral, (2) the context of the child's current experience, and (3) the severity and chronicity of a problem before proceeding with the assessment. Many presenting issues may be situational issues associated with adjusting to new surroundings (Rogers, 1998).

The results of all assessments and the implications should be simply and clearly communicated to the parents and other professionals who work with the child. Parents should be given an opportunity to ask questions and give feedback. Parents' input regarding decisions should be sought, noted, and incorporated into the treatment plan. The family should be able to be involved as much as they choose to. The examiner should also monitor the child's progress by consulting with teachers and family members on an ongoing ba-

sis. The examiner can also communicate with the family regarding the child's progress. These guidelines represent the hallmark of a collaborative and co-operative relationship between the examiner and the child.

Considerations Specific to Language in Assessment Procedures

Several practical guidelines have been recommended for psychologists in conducting assessments of bilingual children and those with limited English proficiency. First, it is critical that the child's language dominance be determined, as well as the child's level of English proficiency. It is important not to assume that the child's native language is his or her dominant language. As previously mentioned, as children are exposed to a second language, their linguistic skills in the first language may regress (E. C. Lopez, 1997). Consequently, the level of proficiency in each of the child's languages has to be assessed prior to the formal assessment. The assessment of language proficiency should be conducted in different contexts, as language usage may vary depending on context (with family at home, with peers in recreation, in formal classrooms, etc.). In addition to being evaluated as to the general level of proficiency in each language, the child can be assessed for the dynamic integration of linguistic skills. For example, children may prefer their first language for social contexts, but rely on the second language skills for academic tasks, especially if they learned these academic skills in their second language. Results obtained from assessments conducted in one language may not be replicated when the child is assessed in another language. For example, some examiners have noted that bilingual children performed at a higher level in a nondominant language than they did when assessed in their apparent dominant language. Hence, the current state of science may not allow examiners to assess bilingual children with the same level of consistency or reliability as achieved with monolingual children.

It is ideal, yet unrealistic to expect, that the examiner be able to speak all of the languages spoken by the children they assess. If an examiner is not fluent in the same language as the child, there are other ways to effect clear communication. Ridley et al. (1998) encourage practitioners to develop other skills: assessing language dominance and preference, mastering key idioms and phrases specific to the client's language, becoming knowledgeable regarding different communication styles and dialect variants. Examiners may also need to develop the ability to use alternative communication modes such as drawing, music, or other media. Perhaps the most common way examiners manage linguistic differences is to rely on interpreters.

Use of Interpreters

Trained interpreters can be helpful in the assessment practice when the examiner is not fluent in the child's dominant or preferred language. However,

TABLE 10.6. Guidelines for Using Interpreters

1. Use interpreters who share the client's racial and ethnic background.
2. Use interpreters trained in mental health and culture-related syndromes.
3. Ensure that the translator and the client become acquainted and comfortable with each other.
4. Interpret sentence by sentence to avoid the loss of detail.
5. Avoid technical language, and encourage clients to use their own words.
6. Allow for twice as much time for an interview.
7. Consider the potential effects of interpreter bias in the interpretation of the information.
8. Consider the level of acculturation of the translator as well as the client.
9. Do not use relatives or friends as translators, if possible.
10. Determine the client's dialect before recruiting interpreters.

problems can and do occur if the translator is untrained or examiners are inexperienced in the use of translators. Lopez and Rooney (1997) found that most interpreters used in schools had no formal training as interpreters. Common problems with untrained interpreters are that they may misinterpret information and add their own opinions. E. C. Lopez (1997) and Ortiz (1997) have discussed guidelines in the use of translators to minimize miscommunication, as summarized in Table 10.6.

Multicultural Assessment Model

To properly integrate cultural and linguistic issues into any assessment procedure, Ridley et al. (1998) have proposed a framework for cultural sensitivity in assessment. Their model consists of four phases: identifying cultural data, interpreting cultural data, incorporating cultural data, and making sound decisions informed by the data. For an assessment to be effective, it must incorporate cultural data in a way that leads to an accurate, comprehensive assessment decision. These phases are listed in Table 10.7.

TABLE 10.7. Multicultural Assessment System

Phase 1: Identify cultural data.
Collect salient clinical information.

Phase 2: Interpret cultural data.
Formulate working hypotheses.

Phase 3: Incorporate cultural data.
Test working hypotheses.

Phase 4: Arrive at sound assessment decision.

Note. Based on Ridley, Li, and Hill (1998).

During the first phase cultural data are collected and identified. The cultural data can be obtained from children, parents, teachers, or others who are familiar with the child and his or her cultural environment. It is important that multiple data collection methods be used so as to avoid neglecting important kinds of information. For example, consider an assessment conducted with a child, using an alternation strategy to cope with cultural diversity: If data were obtained only from school, the child's other cultural frame of reference could not be incorporated into the assessment. Similarly, if a bilingual child was observed only while engaged in academic tasks, the child's linguistic preferences and abilities in social contexts may not be reflected in the assessment. Consequently, involving multiple sources in collecting cultural information can provide a more complete cultural context for the child.

The second phase involves interpreting the cultural data. Several features of the cultural data must be considered and distinguished. The examiner must differentiate characteristics that are idiosyncratic to the child from characteristics that are specific to the child's cultural group (Ridley et al., 1998). This kind of differentiation may require the examiner to be intimately familiar with the child's cultural group. The examiner may also have to differentiate characteristics of the child's cultural group that have developed in response to acculturation experiences from those characteristics that were present prior to contact with nonminority cultural groups. For example, children of refugee parents may manifest many of the characteristics associated with the acculturation process, whereas parents may manifest more strongly the primary cultural characteristics that were present prior to their becoming refugees. While cultural data are being interpreted, the examiner may wish to consult with the child, the child's parents, and other members of the child's cultural group to add their perspectives to that of the examiner. Finally, during the interpretation phase, examiners formulate working hypotheses about the role of culture and language in the child's overall adjustment.

The third phase of the multicultural assessment model involves integrating the working hypotheses concerning the child's cultural context with the working hypotheses formulated from the findings of traditional sources of assessment. For example, when a child is referred for assessment by a teacher, the examiner may have to integrate formulations about the role of culture in the child's life with the information provided by the referral source—this is particularly important when the referral source has failed to adequately consider the cultural context of the child. In some cases, the cultural information may be more crucial than that provided by the traditional assessment sources. In other cases, the cultural information may have little relevance for the assessment (Ridley et al., 1998). Nonetheless, the process of identifying, formulating, and incorporating cultural information into the assessment

process allows for the fourth phase in the multicultural assessment model, arriving at a sound assessment decision. This final phase represents the culmination of considering and integrating cultural information along with other personal and individual information about the child. Ridley et al. (1998) emphasized that in this phase, as well as in each of the previous phases, it is critical that examiners invoke debiasing strategies. Debiasing strategies attempt to correct for potential biases in the assessment process. Research into assessment decision making has suggested pernicious problems (Spengler & Strohmer, 1994). Examiners may be particularly susceptible to a confirmatory bias in which their preliminary hypotheses are confirmed prior to searching for or reviewing disconfirming information. Consequently, it is important for examiners to refrain from drawing conclusions or making decisions about interventions until all of the information has been considered. To this end, it is critical that examiners devote substantial effort to proceed through the phases of the multicultural assessment model prior to reaching conclusions about the children they are assessing.

INTEGRATING CULTURAL CONTEXTS TO ACHIEVE A CULTURALLY COMPETENT ASSESSMENT: A CASE EXAMPLE

Ramon was an 11-year-old Dominican child who was attending a primarily white school. He was referred for assessment because of frequent absences, failure to complete homework assignments, and some recent behavioral outbursts involving fistfights.

Cultural Competence of the Evaluator

Before meeting with the child, the evaluator assessed her cultural competency in regard to her skills, behaviors, and attitudes, her understanding of her own worldview and the cultural worldview of the client, and her understanding of culturally sensitive interventions with respect to this particular assessment context. The examiner, a bilingual white psychologist, had experience with other Latino populations, children of Puerto Rican and Mexican descent, but this would be her first experience with a Dominican child. Many of the skills and attitudes and much of the knowledge that she found helpful with other Latino children and families could be helpful with this child. She had engaged in consciousness-raising about her own cultural background and was aware of the cultural influences shaping her life. Equally important, she had gained perspective on many of the customs, behaviors, expressions, and values with which she was socialized and was able to respect the fact that others may have life-style and cultural differences. She had become sensitive

to the impact of discrimination and prejudice on the lives of many of the children with whom she worked. In addition, she became aware of how other cultural groups may view her and that she may need to work to gain their trust, to let them know that she truly cares about their welfare. Although many of her cultural competencies related to her awareness of her worldview would likely transfer to this case, she realized that she may need to increase her awareness of this Dominican child's worldview. She anticipated that Dominican families would share some of the worldviews of other Latino families. Some cultural values, such as familism, respect for authority, importance of dignity, and spirituality are common across Latino cultural groups. Nonetheless, she sought consultation with others who had experience in working with Dominican populations to gain their advice. Through this consultation and further reading she learned about some migration experiences particular to Dominicans and the sequelae of these differences in the psychological adjustment of Dominican families. Finally, she inquired about possible referral sources specifically addressing Dominican populations, which she added to her list of agencies that she has found helpful in providing services to her other Latino clients.

Cultural Characteristics of the Child

Through school records and interviews with Ramon it was determined that he was born in the Dominican Republic and migrated to the United States when he was 7 years old. His family had moved from Santo Dominigo to Puerto Rico and then to the United States. He currently lives with his grandmother, while his mother is staying with relatives in another state and his father remains in the Dominican Republic. According to Ramon, his mother will send for him and his father as soon as she secures stable employment and residence. Ramon seems more comfortable using Spanish, but knows enough English to maintain a conversation. According to achievement tests conducted in English, Ramon's academic skills cluster between the second- and third-grade level, but he was placed in fourth grade as a compromise between his academic abilities and chronological age. He misses his home, family, and neighborhood in the Dominican Republic. He has expressed his hope that his mother will abandon the family's plan of living in the United States and return home.

Through a meeting with his grandmother at her apartment, it was found that many of his absences were due to his having to act as translator for her visits to social service agencies. It was also discovered that she felt uncomfortable meeting with his teacher because she was embarrassed that his behavior was the source of special attention and because of her limited English verbal skills. She admitted that she did not understand much of what the teacher had communicated to her in regard to the concerns about Ramon.

Cultural Context of the Setting

The cultural context of the school setting was predominately white and English oriented. There were few resources within Ramon's school for children from different backgrounds. Ramon had been placed in an early English-immersion classroom upon his arrival in the United States, and he has been in predominately English-oriented classrooms ever since. His teachers do not speak Spanish to him, and there are few Spanish-speaking resources available to him in his school. In other words, there is pervasive encouragement of assimilation to a white, English-language culture. Outside the school, but within the school district, there is a parent–teacher liaison service that could be utilized to facilitate communication and adjustment between Ramon's grandmother and his teacher.

To evaluate the cultural context of Ramon's classroom setting, the examiner observed Ramon in his classroom. Through some behavioral observations made by the examiner subsequent to her initial meeting with Ramon and the grandmother, she detected Ramon's social isolation and difficulty in interacting with his English-speaking peers. Their verbal fluency was confusing to Ramon, and his cultural differences were the subject of taunting and derision by his peers. Peers also teased him because of his low socioeconomic status (e.g., participation in the free lunch program). Ramon appeared to attempt to assimilate, but his familiarity with U.S. culture and limited verbal fluency made these efforts impractical. In an interview, Ramon's teacher indicated that she had attempted to meet with Ramon's grandmother to discuss his problems and potential solutions, but believed that the grandmother was not interested in meeting. The teacher was aware of Ramon's cultural isolation, but was not aware of potential resources to ameliorate it.

Assessment Procedures and Integrating the Information

The assessment process involved a series of interviews with Ramon, his grandmother, and his teacher and observations made in the classroom. The teacher had had difficulty arranging a meeting at school, and it was judged important to meet with Ramon's grandmother at her home to increase her comfort in the interview. Conducting the interview in Spanish was seen as critical because of the grandmother's limited English and because it could facilitate the access of critical information. The interview with Ramon was conducted in a combination of English and Spanish, partly to accommodate his own preference but also to assess his fluency in each language. The observations made in the classroom provided particularly important information about how cultural differences were critical components in his behavior. His teacher and grandmother were asked to complete the Child Behavior Checklist (CBCL), with the grandmother completing the Spanish version.

The examiner used the results from the CBCL to help explain to Ramon and to his grandmother some of the teacher's observations of Ramon. The examiner worked with Ramon and his grandmother to focus on several goals: to increase homework completion and to reduce physical conflict between Ramon and his peers. A procedure was established whereby a report of the teacher's monitoring of Ramon's progress was sent home to the grandmother so that she could be involved and assist in the attainment of these two goals. In addition, to address his cultural isolation, Ramon was offered services at the local Latino community center, where tutoring by Latino individuals was available. Family counseling services, also available, were recommended to the grandmother to help Ramon cope with the acculturative stress he was experiencing. Finally, Ramon's grandmother was introduced to a Spanish-speaking parent–teacher liaison to assist in communications with the school. A follow-up meeting was scheduled for Ramon, his grandmother, and his teacher for 3 months later to monitor progress and determine whether further evaluation would be required.

CONCLUSION

Authors on cultural competency (Rogers, 1998; Ridley et al., 1998; Arredondo et. al., 1996) have made various suggestions on how to continue developing and expanding cultural competencies. Recommendations are made for readings, conferences, and other activities that can enhance professional development. These suggestions are not limited to the field of psychology, but are intended to provide information from a variety of resources. Thus, feature films, documentaries, novels, and Internet resources are included. Table 10.8 provides an overview of information regarding ELM populations. This table lists information from the psychological literature as well as from popular literature and film.

Assessment of ELM children is a complex task that, if done competently, includes the awareness and incorporation of the various cultural contexts at play. The long-range solution frequently recommended for appropriate assessment of language minority children is the training of bilingual examiners (Lopez & Rooney, 1997) and development of instruments indigenous to the child's linguistic group. Perhaps more challenging is to apply our current knowledge of assessment and cultural competence to make each assessment intervention culturally appropriate. Examiners need to be very strategic in the collection of information about the child and must rely on multiple sources, make observations in different contexts, scrutinize the appropriateness of norms and standardized procedures, and work with multidisciplinarian assessment and treatment teams that include language and cultural experts (E. C. Lopez, 1997; Ortiz, 1997).

TABLE 10.8. Additional Information on ELM Populations

Recommended readings in the psychological literature	
Racial identity	Carter (1995); Helms (1995); Pedersen (1987); Pope-Davis & Ottavi (1992)
Working with diverse populations	Aponte, Rivers, & Wohl (1995); Collins (1990); Dana (1993); D. Sue (1989); Sue & Sue (1990); Ramirez (1991, 1999); Walsh (1993)
Culturally appropriate interventions	Atkinson & Gim (1989); Atkinson, Morten, & Sue (1993); Katz (1976); LaFromboise, Trimble, & Mohatt (1990)
Working with ethnic minority children and adolescents	Gibbs & Huang (1998); Canino & Spurlock (1994); Lynch & Hanson (1998)

Recommended popular literature and films	
Feature films	*El Norte / The North; Stand and Deliver; Mi Familia / My Family; The Joy Luck Club; A Raisin in the Sun; The Milagro Beanfield War; Double Happiness; The Wedding Banquet*
Documentary films	*The Color of Fear* by Lee Mun Wah; The Frontline specials *A Class Divided* and *True Colors; Mountains, Mist and Mexico, Made in China,* and *The Trial Model* by Paul Pederson
Novels	*Bless Me, Ultima* by Rodulfo Anya; novels by Amy Tan; *Occupied America by* Rodulfo Acuna; *Face of an Angel* by Denise Chavez; novels by Terry McMillan; novels by Native American authors Sherman Alexie and Leslie Marmon Silko; *Lakota Woman* by Mary Crow Dog and Richard Erdoes; *I Know Why the Caged Bird Sings* by Maya Angelou; *The Spirit Catches You and You Fall Down* by Anne Fadiman; *When I was Puerto Rican* by Esmeralda Santiago

Several models have been recommended to assist examiners in incorporating the cultural context of each aspect or component of the assessment process. These models emphasize the integration of attitudes, skills, and knowledge, which when applied in a systematic and scientific manner will assist in obtaining valuable information about the cultural variables affecting the problem at each step. The integration of these cultural variables in the assessment procedure, as well as in its results and the impact it may have on the child, constitutes what we consider to be a culturally competent assessment with ELM children.

For behavioral assessment (or any form of assessment) to be adminis-

tered in a culturally competent manner, the examiner must possess cultural competency skills and the procedure must be able to take into account the cultural context of the child in the evaluation and treatment recommendation. Although behavioral assessment procedures have been considered non-biased, in large part, because some sources of cultural bias have been removed from the procedures, it seems impossible and undesirable to render assessment procedures void of any cultural characteristics. The inclusion of cultural features in assessment procedures is problematic only when they are incompatible with the culture of the child. Consequently, we recommend that behavioral assessment not be stripped of culture, but reflect the culture of the target population. Some aspects in which culture may be reflected in the assessment process include the cultural background of the examiner, the language or linguistic style used by the examiner, the context in which the behavioral assessment is made, the goal of the assessment, and the cultural framework used to interpret behavior. If performed appropriately, behavioral assessment can provide a method for changing an ELM child's behavioral, academic, or social problems, but it can do so more effectively by taking into consideration all of the cultural variables and implementing a culturally sound plan of behavior modification. Psychologists need certain skills to be able to use the cultural context of the child in every step of the assessment procedure. A culturally competent examiner can understand and identify the cultural nature of the child's problems, interpret the cultural forces that affect the child, identify the child's cultural strengths, increase cultural understanding and communication between the family and the professionals, implement appropriate treatment that is congruent with the child's and family's culture, and enable positive outcomes. Many of these goals may be accomplished by increasing examiners' cultural competency, fostering examiners' awareness of the impact of culture on the child, the assessment context, and the assessment procedures.

REFERENCES

Aponte, J., Rivers, R. Y., & Wohl, J. (1995). *Psychological interventions and cultural diversity.* Boston: Allyn & Bacon.

Armour-Thomas, E., & Gopaul-McNichol, S. (1997). In search of correlates of learning underlying "learning disability" using a bio-ecological assessment system. *Journal of Social Distress and the Homeless, 6,* 143–159.

Arredondo, P., Toporek, R., Brown, S. P., Jones, J., Locke, D. C., Sanchez, J., & Stadler, H. (1996). Operationalizing of the multicultural counseling competencies. *Journal of Multicultural Counseling and Development, 24,* 42–78.

Atkinson, D. R., & Gim, R. H. (1989). Asian-American cultural identity and attitudes toward mental health services. *Journal of Counseling Psychology, 36(2),* 209–212.

Atkinson, D. R., Morten, G., & Sue, D. W. (1993). *Counseling American minorities.* Madison, WI: WCB Brown and Benchmark.

Baker, E. L., & O'Neil, H. F., Jr. (1996). Performance assessment and equity. In M. B. Kane & R. Mitchell (Eds.), *Implementing performance assessment: Promises, problems, and challenges.* Mahwah, NJ: Erlbaum.

Bell, Y. R. (1994). A culturally sensitive analysis of black learning style. *Journal of Black Psychology, 20,* 47–61.

Berry, J. (1993). Ethinc identity in plural societies. In M. E. Bernal & G. P. Knight (Eds.), *Ethnic identity: Formation and transmission among Hispanics and other minorities* (pp. 271–296). Albany, NY: SUNY Press.

Boykin, A. W. (1986). The triple quandary and the schooling of Afro-American children. In V. Neisser (Ed.), *The school achievement of minority children.* Hillsdale, NJ: Erlbaum.

Boykin, A. W., & Allen, B. A. (1988). Rhythmic-movement facilitation of learning in working class Afro-American children. *Journal of Genetic Psychology, 149,* 335–347.

Canino, I. A., & Spurlock, J. (1994). *Culturally diverse children and adolescents: Assessment, diagnosis, and treatment.* New York: Guilford Press.

Carter, R. T. (1995). *The influence of race and racial identity in psychotherapy.* New York: Wiley Interscience.

Collins, A. O. (1990). A conceptual model for culturally appropriate health education programs in developing countries. *International Quarterly of Community Health Education, 11*(1), 53–62.

Crijnen, A. A. M., Achenbach, T. M., & Verhulst, F. C. (1997). Comparisons of problems reported by parents of children in 12 cultures: Total problems, externalizing, and internalizing. *Journal of the American Academy of Child and Adolescent Psychiatry, 9,* 1269–1277.

Crocker, J., & Major, B. (1989). Social stigma and self-esteem: The self-protective properties of stigma. *Psychological Review, 96,* 608–630.

Cummins, J. (1984). *Bilingualism and special education: Issues in assessment and pedagogy.* Clevedon, Avon, England: Multilingual Matters.

Dana, R. H. (1993). *Multicultural assessment perspectives for professional psychology.* Boston: Allyn & Bacon.

Davidson, A. L. (1996). *Making and molding identity in schools.* Albany, NY: SUNY Press.

García Coll, C., Crnic, K., Lamberty, G., Wasik, B. H., Jenkins, R., García, H. V., & McAdoo, H. P. (1996). An integrative model for the study of developmental competencies in minority children. *Child Development, 67,* 1891–1914.

Gibbs, J. T., & Huang. L. N. (Eds.). (1998). *Children of color: Psychological interventions with culturally diverse youth.* San Francisco: Jossey-Bass.

Greenfield, P. M., & Cocking, R. R. (1994). *Cross-cultural roots of minority child development.* Hillsdale, NJ: Erlbaum.

Hall, C. C. I. (1997). Cultural malpractice: The growing obsolescence of psychology with the changing U. S. population. *American Psychologist, 52,* 642–651.

Hamers, J., & Blanc, M. H. (1989). *Bilinguality and bilingualism.* Cambridge, UK: Cambridge University Press.

Helms, J. (1995). An update of Helms's white and people of color racial identity

models. In J. G. Ponterotto, J. M. Casas, L. A. Suzuki, & C. M. Alexander (Eds.), *Handbook of multicultural counseling.* Thousand Oaks, CA: Sage.

Katz, P. A. (1976). The acquisition of racial attitudes in children. In P. A. Katz (Ed.), *Towards the elimination of racism* (pp. 125–147). New York: Pergamon Press.

LaFromboise, T., Coleman, H. L., & Gerton, J. (1993). Psychological impact of biculturalism: Evidence and theory. *Psychological Bulletin, 114,* 395–412.

LaFromboise, T. D., Trimble, J. E., & Mohatt, G. V. (1990). Counseling intervention and American Indian tradition: An integrative approach. *Counseling Psychologist, 18,* 628–654.

Lambert, M. C., Weisz, J. R., Knight, F., Desrosiers, M., Overly, K., & Thesiger, C. (1992). Jamaican and American adult perspectives on child psychopathology: Further exploration of the threshold model. *Journal of Consulting and Clinical Psychogy, 60,* 146–149.

Lambert, W. E. (1981). Bilingualism and language acquisition. *Annals of the New York Academy of Science, 379,* 9–22.

Lopez, E. C. (1997). The cognitive assessment of limited English proficient and bilingual children. In D. P. Flanagan, J. L. Genshaft, & P. L. Harrison (Eds.), *Contemporary intellectual assessment: Theories, tests, and issues* (pp. 503–516). New York: Guilford Press.

Lopez, E. C., & Rooney, M. E. (1997). A preliminary investigation of the roles and background of school interpreters: Implications for training and recruiting. *Journal of Social Distress and the Homeless, 6,* 161–175.

Lopez, S. (1997). Cultural competence in psychotherapy: A guide for clinicians and their supervisors. In C. E. Watkins, Jr. (Ed.), *Handbook of psychotherapy supervision.* New York: Wiley.

Lynch, E. W., & Hanson, M. J. (1998). *Developing cross-cultural competence: A guide for working with children and families* (2nd ed.). Baltimore: Brookes.

Mash, E. J., & Barkley, R. A. (Eds.). (1996). *Child psychopathology.* New York: Guilford Press.

McLoyd, V. C. (1998). Socioeconomic disadvantage and child development. *American Psychologist, 53,* 185–204.

Mendez-Villarubia, J., & Labruzza, A. (1994). Issues in the assessment of Puerto Rican and other Hispanic clients, including attaques de nervios. In A. Labruzza & J. Mendez-Villarubia (Eds.), *Using the DSM IV: A clinician's guide to psychiatric diagnosis.* Northvale, NJ: Jason Aronson.

Ogbu, J. U. (1994). From cultural difference to differences in cultural frame of reference. In P. M. Greenfield & R. R. Cocking (Eds.), *Cross-cultural roots of minority child development* (pp. 365–392). Hillsdale, NJ: Erlbaum.

Okagaki, L., & Sternberg, R. J. (1993). Parental beliefs and children's school performance. *Child Development, 64,* 36–56.

Ortiz, A. A. (1997). Learning disabilities occurring concomitantly with linguistic differences. *Journal of Learning Disabilities, 30,* 321–332.

Osborne, J. W. (1997). Race and academic disidentification. *Journal of Educational Psychology, 89,* 728–735.

Padilla, A. M., Lindholm, K. J., Chen, A., Durán, R., Hakuta, K., Lambert, W., & Tucker, G. R. (1991). The English-only movement: Myths, reality, and implications for psychology. *American Psychologist, 46,* 120–130.

Padilla, A. M., & Medina, A. (1996). Cross-cultural sensitivity in assessment: Using tests in culturally appropriate ways. In L. A. Suzuki, P. J. Meller, & J. G. Ponterotto (Eds.), *Handbook of multicultural assessment* (pp. 3–28). San Francisco: Jossey Bass.

Paniagua, F. A. (1994). *Assessing and treating culturally diverse clients.* Thousand Oaks, CA: Sage.

Pedersen, P. B. (Ed.). (1987). *Handbook of cross-cultural counseling and therapy.* Westport, CT: Greenwood Press.

Ponterotto, J. G., & Alexander, C. M. (1996). Assessing the multicultural competence of counselors and clinicians. In L. A. Suzuki, P. J. Meller, & J. G. Ponterotto (Eds.), *Handbook of multicultural assessment.* San Francisco: Jossey Bass.

Pope-Davis, D. B., & Ottavi, T. M. (1992). The influence of white racial identity attitudes on racism among faculty members: A preliminary examination. *Journal of College Student Development, 33*(5), 389–394.

Quintana, S. M., & Bernal, M. E. (1995). Ethnic minority training in counseling psychology: Comparisons with clinical psychology and proposed standards. *The Counseling Psychologist, 23,* 102–121.

Quintana, S. M., Vera, E., & Cooper, C. (1999, August). *African-American children's racial identity and inter-racial coping strategies.* Poster session presented at the American Psychological Association, Boston.

Ramirez, M. (1991). *Psychotherapy and counseling with minorities; A cognitive approach to individual and cultural differences.* New York: Pergamon Press.

Ramirez, M., III. (1999). *Multicultural psychotherapy: An approach to individual and cultural differences* (2nd ed.). Boston, MA: Allyn & Bacon.

Ridley, C. R., Li, L. C., & Hill, C. L. (1998). Multicultural assessment: Reexamination, reconceptualization and practical application. *Counseling Psychologist, 26,* 827–910.

Rogers, M. (1998). Psychoeducational assessment of culturally and lingustically diverse children and youth. In H. Vance (Ed.), *Best practices in assessment for school and clinical settings* (2nd ed.). New York: Wiley.

Rosenberg-Oesterheld, J., & Haber, J. (1997). Acceptability of the Conners Parent Rating Scale and Child Behavior Checklist to Dakotan/Lakotan parents. *American Academy of Child and Adolescent Psychiatry, 36,* 55–66.

Rotheram-Borus, M. J., & Phinney, J. S. (1990). Patterns of social expectations among black and Mexican American children. *Child Development, 61,* 542–556.

Spengler, P. M., & Strohmer, D. C. (1994). Clinical judgment biases: The moderation roles of clinical complexity and clinician client preferences. *Journal of Counseling Psychology, 41,* 1–10.

Stockman, I. J. (1986). Language acquisition in culturally diverse populations: The black child as a case study. In O. L. Taylor (Ed.), *Nature of communication disorders in culturally and linguistically diverse populations* (pp. 117–155). San Diego: College-Hill.

Sue, D. W. (1989). Racial/cultural identity development among Asian-Americans: Counseling/therapy implications. *AAPA-Journal, 13*(1), 80–86.

Sue, D. W., Arredondo, P., & McDavis, R. J. (1992). Multicultural counseling competencies and standards: A call to the profession. *Journal of Counseling and Development, 70,* 477–486.

Sue, D. W., & Sue, D. (1990). *Counseling the culturally different.* New York: Wiley Interscience.

Sue, S. (1998). In search of cultural competence in psychotherapy and counseling. *American Psychologist, 53,* 440–448.

Tharp, R. G. (1994). Intergroup differences among Native Americans in socialization and child cognition: An ethnogenetic analysis. In P. M. Greenfield & R. R. Cocking (Eds.), *Cross-cultural roots of minority child development* (pp. 87–106). Hillsdale, NJ: Erlbaum.

Thomas-Presswood, T., Sasso, J., & Gin, G. (1997). Cultural issues in the intellectual assessment of children from diverse cultural backgrounds. *Journal of Social Distress and the Homeless, 6,* 113–127.

Triandis, H. C., Bontempo, R., Villareal, M. J., Asai, M., & Lucca, N. (1988). Individualism and collectivism: Cross-cultural perspectives on self-ingroup relationships. *Journal of Personality and Social Psychology, 54,* 323–338.

Vano, A. M., & Pennenbaker, J. W. (1997). Emotion vocabulary in bilingual Hispanic children: Adjustment and behavioral effects. *Journal of Language and Social Psychology, 16,* 191–200.

Velasquez, R., Ayala, G. X, & Mendoza, S. A. (1998). *Psychodiagnostic assessment of U. S. Latinos with MMPI, MMPI-2, and MMPI-A: A comprehensive resource manual.* East Lansing, MI: Julian Samora Research Institute.

Walsh, F. (1993). (Ed.). *Normal family processes* (2nd ed.). New York: Guilford Press.

Weisz, J. R., & Weiss, B. (1991). Studying the "referability" of child clinical problems. *Journal of Consulting and Clinical Psychology, 59,* 266–273.

Index

♦